HERBAL

Healing for

WOMEN

Simple Home Remedies for Women of All Ages

ROSEMARY GLADSTAR

ILLUSTRATIONS by ANNA VOJTECH

A Fireside Book   Published by Simon & Schuster
New York London Toronto Sydney Tokyo Singapore

FIRESIDE

Rockefeller Center
1230 Avenue of the Americas
New York, New York 10020

Designed by Bonni Leon
Artwork by Anna Vojtech
Manufactured in the United States of America
8   10   9
Library of Congress Cataloging-in-Publication Data is available.
ISBN: 0-671-76767-4

This book is lovingly dedicated to four wise elders
who brought me the magical gifts of wisdom and laughter:

Jasmine Karr, my mother, whose joy and laughter always helped me live
in the lightness of being
Juliette de Bairacli Levy, my mentor and friend, who taught me the wisdom
of the simplers
Tasha Tudor, my inspiration for magic and delight in all life
and Adele Dawson, my neighbor and marvelous friend, who passed on to
the other side as this book was written

And to three open-hearted young women whom I've been blessed to know
and who have allowed me to share the wisdom that was passed on to me:
Jennifer Slick, Melanie Slick, and Celeste Pinney

Acknowledgments

Many people contribute to the birth of a book. To these people I offer special thanks and appreciation:

My husband, Karl Slick, without whose encouragement and help this book would forever have remained a dream in sleep. As well as inspiring me deep in my soul, he helped me through endless hours of computer frustration.

My fellow herbalists and dear friends, Jane Bothwell and Cascade Anderson Geller, who, amidst babies, families, and herbal work found time to proofread *Herbal Healing for Women* and who helped tremendously with their support and feedback to make this a better book.

Wabun Wind for making it possible. And Sheila Curry for her support and fine editing advice.

And the women of Sonoma County, whose faith and trust in me in my early days as "the river herbalist" helped me to flower into the herbalist I am today. I am forever thankful for the friendships, support, and teachings from my Sonoma County family.

Contents

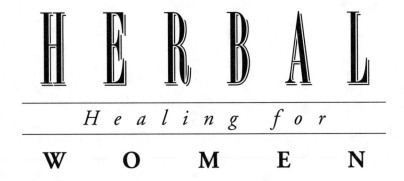

HERBAL

Healing for

WOMEN

Part One

HERBALISM

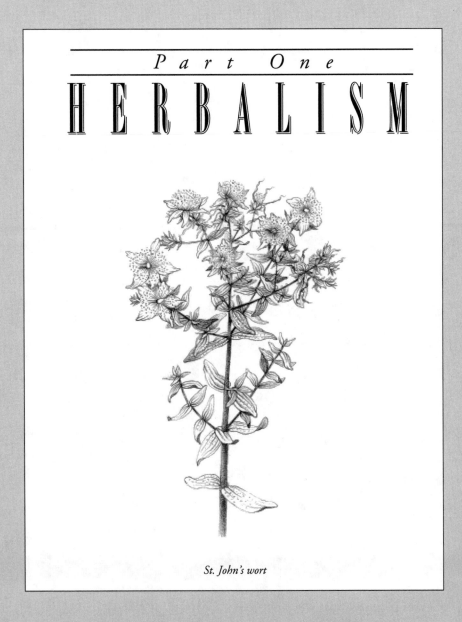

St. John's wort

An Introduction to Herbalism

If it is the greatest and highest that you seek, the plant can direct you. Strive to become through your will what, without will, it is.
—Goethe

Honoring the Wisdom of Our Ancestors

In every culture throughout the world you will find a great body of folklore concerning the indigenous plants of that region and the wise women who used them. For thousands of years women collected plants from meadows and woodlands and used them to create healing medicines. They gathered herbs by the waning and waxing of the moon, artfully created preparations, and developed herbal formulas. Through an intuitive communication with the plants, women learned the healing powers of these green allies. Their wisdom developed over countless years as remedies were tried, proven, and passed on. The best of these remedies were added to the lore, and the wisdom was transferred from mother to daughter, from wise woman to apprentice for countless generations. This is the legacy we have inherited. Healers, wise women, simplers—these women were the center and source of medicine and healing for their communities. They understood the cycles of the seasons, the ebb and flow of the universe, the sun, the moon, the stars, and the natural rhythms of their bodies.

Herbalism, rooted in the earth and honored as a woman's healing art, survived the natural catastrophes of time. It wasn't until the fourteenth century, when a wave of witch-hunts began in Europe, that herbalism encountered its first great obstacle. The quiet influence of the wise women—their inner power and their healing skills—began to be feared by the largely patriarchal Roman Catholic Church, and for the next three hundred years women were burned at the stake and tortured to death simply for being healers. Just being a woman during these times was dangerous; using herbs was a sure invitation to be persecuted. Thousands of women were killed in Europe during the height of the witch-hunts.

In spite of recurrent waves of repression, herbalism flourished right up until the dawning of the twentieth century, when it encountered its second great challenge. With the onslaught of the Industrial Revolution and the introduction of technology, a new tradition of medicine emerged, and herbalism's popularity began to wane. Through the influence of Newton and Descartes, Western culture entered a period wherein people believed they could understand and control nature by dissecting and quantifying it. The science of medicine was going to replace the art of healing. In the space of a century, allopathic or modern, Western technological medicine established itself as the number-one medical system in the Western world. Though it offered a remarkable technological and "heroic," or emergency-oriented, medicine, its monopoly on health care posed a serious problem: no one system of medicine could answer the needs of all people or every health situation. As a result, in spite of the technology and resources offered by allopathic medicine, we gradually became less healthy and—not unrelatedly—more disconnected from our feminine sources of healing.

For almost a century, the practice of herbalism, viewed as antiquated and outdated by the scientific community, became illegal in the United States. Women forgot the art of gathering plants and making their own medicines. Saddest of all, women lost both the knowledge and the initiative to heal themselves. We became totally dependent on doctors and doctors' "orders." No longer in touch with our own healing power, we came to rely on external sources for answers to our deeply personal health problems. A particularly insidious aspect of this situation was the way we began to downgrade and disregard our own intuitive powers. My grandmother used to tell me "tools not used are tools abused"—all too often, they also became "tools we lose." Out of neglect, we began to forget the inherent gifts of the Wise Woman, a tradition of healing that relies on the remarkable feminine powers of intuition, ancient wisdom, and herbal knowledge.

But the wheels of change are turning again. Dissatisfaction with Western medicine, coupled with a herbal renaissance in America, is reawakening the healing instincts that have lain dormant for so long. Women are rediscovering their relationship with medicinal plants and the satisfactions of healing.

Many women begin their herbal studies unsuspectingly in the safety of their gardens. They plant their herb gardens simply because gardens are enchanting and beautiful, full of life and spirit. Then something inexplicable begins to happen. As the women quietly weed, water, and work within the garden, the plants seem to instruct, teach, and guide them. Often, in spite of themselves, women develop a strong curiosity about the healing energies of the plants they're growing and, before they know it, they are reading medicinal herb books, signing up for classes, and treating their families with simple remedies when all they thought they wanted to do was grow some tasty culinaries.

For other women the path to discovering herbs is through their own illnesses. Though allopathic medicine offers an exceptional crisis- and emergency-oriented medicine, it does not offer women with recurring feminine health problems long-term solutions or remedies. Nor does Western medicine address the cause of these imbalances. Frequently problems treated with allopathic chemical drugs recur soon after the effects of the drugs wear off. Women are discovering that herbs offer a sane, safe, and effective alternative and/or complement to allopathic medication.

Some women simply seem to "remember" something deep within them—their age-old herbal legacy. They first remembered it as children, playing in the fields. For long periods, perhaps, they forgot what they knew, but it was there nonetheless, ready to be rekindled by a special memory or circumstance. Because the knowledge of plants is an old knowledge and easily accessible, some women simply "remember" how to find it buried in the fertile soil of their hearts.

Herbalism is definitely flourishing today. Women are once more growing, gathering, and making their medicines. They are again cultivating their ancient healing traditions. Going back into the closets of our grandmothers to see what jewels of wisdom rest there, we are unearthing our heritage. Working with herbs, digging in the earth, making herbal preparations, and using them for health and healing is the best way possible to reestablish our connection to our Wise Woman tradition.

I had the good fortune to grow up with a woman who never forgot that tradition. My grandmother Mary was born in Armenia and came to this country during the Turkish invasion of her country. She and my grandfather escaped the death march and the almost complete annihilation of the Armenian people. She always credited the plants and her belief in God with saving her, and she passed her beliefs on to her children and grandchildren. We were instructed at an early age which plants were good for food and which for illnesses. Her teachings were without fuss, strong and powerful like herself. The lore she taught me in the garden of my childhood has stayed with me throughout my life.

A magical, intangible process, healing is an art, not a science. The same treatment regimen used on different patients for the same illness can sometimes cure, sometimes have no effect, and sometimes exacerbate a problem. If we are to heal the many levels of imbalance in the female world today we must make some overall changes in our attitudes and beliefs. We must first and foremost remember and accept that for countless generations we carried the wisdom and the magic of healing within ourselves. And we must find a way to reconnect with that ancient place of wisdom and power.

Working with herbs is one of the steps toward discovering that place of wisdom and reclaiming our tradition as wise women and healers. The plants do teach us. They take us to the heart and soul of Mother Earth. They offer a system of healing that is gentle, imbued with "soft power," and attuned to the feminine spirit. To relearn this tradition takes a certain commitment, but it is a wonderful, joyful process that often leads one into the fields and gardens of our gentlest memories. As herbalism resurges in the hearts of women, it is my hope that this book may serve as a guide to the healing way of herbs, providing not only remedies and recipes for women's health, but also opening the door that leads women to the ancient art and legacy of herbalism.

Herbalism and Western Medicine

Having been a practicing herbalist for over twenty years in an extremely diverse and colorful community, I've had an excellent opportunity to witness both alternative and orthodox systems of healing and their effects on our health. Though herbal medicine is the system closest to my heart, I do not ignore or exclude other systems of medicine. Diet, exercise, shamanic healing, visualizations, allopathic medicine, acupuncture; all of these practices and many others have an intrinsic place in the organic wholeness of medicine. This book focuses primarily on herbs and dietary suggestions, not because I do not believe in the validity of other systems of medicine but because herbalism is the system of healing I know best. I believe in it, I know it deep in my heart, and I love to share it with others.

Allopathic medicine and herbalism are frequently seen as the antithesis of one another, and people assume that they are incompatible. On the contrary, the two systems of medicine can work very effectively together and do, in fact, complement one another. Representative of the female and male energies, both are needed for harmonious balance. And both have much to learn from one another. Unfortunately, there is a schism between these two systems of medicine. Herbalism is viewed as antiquated, old-fashioned, and ineffective. Allopathic medicine is viewed as mechanical and impersonal, treating symptoms rather than causes. One is right brain; the other left brain.

Working in concert, allopathic medicine and herbalism can enhance our possibilities for well-being. Though some of the most powerful herbs (these are indicated in herb books) should not be used with allopathic drugs, most herbs do not interfere with the action of chemical drugs and can be used to augment allopathic treatments. While chemical drugs are actively killing bacteria and viruses, herbal medicines build and restore the system. Chemical drugs generally have a specific agenda, while herbs, through a complex biochemical process, take the whole person into consideration and replenish the body on a cellular level. Herbs, when taken correctly, do not upset the body's innate sense of harmony, so there are little or no side effects. Using herbal therapy with chemical drugs often helps eliminate or lessen the side effects of drug therapies.

About 3000 years ago Asclepius of Thessaly, one of the great minds of ancient medicine, gave the following sequence for the use of therapeutic agents: "First the word. Then the plant. Lastly the knife." Several hundred years later, Dr. Rudolf Weiss, a highly respected medical herbalist from Germany and author of *Herbal Medicine,* expanded on Asclepius's theme by adding radiation and chemotherapy to the armamentarium of healing techniques: "First the word. Then the plant. Next the major synthetic chemotherapeutic agents. And finally the knife." What both of these wise physicians advised was a sequence of medical intervention beginning with least invasive substance and progressing only if necessary to the most invasive. Counseling first, then herbs. If neither of these work, then hospitals, doctors, and surgery should be considered.

Applying the sage words of these two physicians as guidelines, it becomes easier to determine when herbs may be most appropriate as a first-choice medicine.

❦ As preventive medicine, herbs are inimitable. They build and strengthen the body's natural immunity and defense mechanisms. They nourish the deep inner ecology of our systems on a cellular level. Our bodies are comfortable with herbs, recognize them, and efficiently utilize them.

❦ Herbs support our life force. They are effective when used over an extended period of time to strengthen the immune system. They may also be used to quickly perk up the immune system when it is under attack by cold and flu viruses. Herbs are also powerful "adaptogens," increasing the body's ability to adapt to the ever-changing environment and increasing stresses of life.

❦ Most nonemergency medical situations also respond well to herbalism. Simple everyday problems such as bruises, swellings, sprains, cuts, wounds, colds, fevers, burns, and so forth are easily treated with herbs. If your grandma would have treated it at home, chances are that you can too. Herbs can also be an effective first-aid treatment for emergency situations when medical help is unavailable or is on its way.

❦ For treating serious illnesses such as AIDS, cancer, and autoimmune disorders, herbs serve as excellent secondary therapeutic agents. They provide necessary fundamental support for the body while it is undergoing more radical forms of treatment that may sap its life energy. Herbs and allopathic medicine can and do work compatibly in these critical situations, complementing and enhancing each other's effects.

❦ Herbs are a first-choice medicine for many women's health problems. For years I have talked to women who, tired of rounds of antibiotics and orthodox treatments, have tried alternative health remedies. They would use simple herbal remedies, often unaware that women had been using these remedies for centuries, and were amazed by the results. I think herbs act in a particularly impressive way on women's health because there's a natural affinity between women and the plant world. Plants spring from the heart of the earth; they are nourished by the seasons and whims of Mother Nature. Beautiful, strong, and powerful, herbs are in sympathy with women's spirit. They provide a deep source of nourishment and vitality to the female organs and have an innate ability to heal imbalances that have lodged in those deep, moist places of our female being. Herbs can also be used to support and nourish the female system when a woman chooses to use allopathic medicine. While allopathic medicine provides symptomatic relief, herbs often provide the impetus for lasting change. They seem to heal on a cellular level.

Herbs in the Test Tube

As herbs regain a place of recognition and honor in the healing community, they are also encountering skepticism and attack in the scientific community. Western science attempts to analyze herbs in the same deductive way it evaluates synthetic drugs. Technicians extract the chemicals in herbs and analyze them as single, separate components. These chemicals are frequently used in the horribly inhumane animal experimentation that still wracks our medical world in the name of "healing."

Much misinformation has been collected about herbs in this manner. Two classic examples of this laboratory technique, which time and again produces results at odds with centuries of empirical proof, are the recent tests conducted on sassafras and comfrey.

Sassafras, long valued as a "blood purifier" and "liver herb," is an important ingredient of many old-fashioned root-beer drinks. It contains safrole, a very potent plant chemical that is largely insoluble in water (in other words, you can't extract it when making tea). When safrole was isolated from the herb and injected in extremely high doses into laboratory animals, it produced carcinogenic cells. Based on this information, sassafras was banned from use in all soft drinks. (Synthetic chemicals are now used instead.) It is interesting that the southern United States, where sassafras grows naturally and has been enjoyed as a beverage tea and a blood cleanser for generations, has the lowest rate of cancer in our country. It is even more interesting to note that there is not one recorded case of sassafras poisoning or of sassafras-related cancer.

The comfrey controversy is another case in point. For centuries comfrey has been valued throughout the world as a food and medicine. Rich in mucilage, allantoin (a cell proliferant), and vitamins and minerals, it's been recommended for treating stomach disorders, mending bones, and healing the lungs. Never in history has there been any question of comfrey's safety and efficacy as a healing plant.

Recently, pyrrolizidine alkaloids have been identified and isolated in the young leaves and roots of comfrey. When injected into laboratory rats in ridiculously high doses, these alkaloids have produced carcinogenic cells and liver toxicity (hepatic veno-occlusive disease). But Richard De Sylva states, in the *Canadian Journal of Herbalism,* "The original research [on the presence of pyrrolizidine alkaloids in comfrey] was seriously flawed. The laboratory rats that developed tumors on the liver were only six weeks old. At this age, quite a number of substances would be inappropriate for them to ingest. As well, the total amount of comfrey ingested formed 30–50 percent of their basic diet. This could be compared to human consumption of several platefuls of comfrey daily. This daily regimen did eventually cause tumors to grow on their livers and proved only one of the standing laws of science: that every substance or chemical is a poison if we consume enough of it." Or as Paracelsus said several years ago, "All things are poison and nothing is without poison. It is the dosage that makes a thing poisonous or not." Because of these laboratory findings, an attempt was made to locate cases of individuals who used comfrey and later developed liver toxicity. Of the thousands of people who use comfrey worldwide, only three somewhat questionable cases have been identified, none of which conclusively point to comfrey as the culprit.

The small amounts of pyrrolizide alkaloids found in comfrey are balanced by the abundance of allantoin, a cell proliferant, calcium salts, and mucilage it contains. All these components are very nutritious to the cells and serve to counteract the cell inhibiting action of the pyrrolizidine alkaloids. Though there is no concrete evidence of its toxicity after centuries of recorded use, comfrey has been banned in Canada and is awaiting its verdict in the United States. (For further information on comfrey, see its listing in the Materia Medica in Part VII of this book.)

It would be naive to believe all plants are safe to use. They absolutely are not. Some are incredibly potent and are not recommended for use by the unskilled or inexperienced healer. Some are so toxic they shouldn't be used at all. But these plants have been identified as such for centuries by herbalists. Such information has been handed down to us as part of our herbal tradition. What laboratory science has primarily proven is how accurate the intuitive wisdom of the ages has been. Scientists are now able to isolate certain chemicals from the herbs and turn them into "wonder drugs," using them for the same illnesses as have herbalists for countless generations.

Alchemy and magic are integral parts of herbalism and healing. It is essential to recall when reading these test results that the whole is *always* greater than the sum of the parts. As more and more tests are conducted on herbs and their chemicals are isolated, it is important to be open-minded about the results—open-minded to the fact that science can be just as fallible as it can be infallible. If a plant has been found safe and effective for a thousand years of human use, it may be wise to question the validity and applicability of the scientific tests now being used. There is generally some unidentified magic in the plant in the form of another chemical or an innate natural wisdom that allows the medicine, when taken as a whole, to function in a safe and beneficial manner.

T W O
Beginning Your Herbal Studies

Come forth into the light of things, let nature be your teacher.
—William Wordsworth

Where to Begin?

How does one approach the vast study of herbs? Where does one begin? At first it may seem like an overwhelming project to learn about this subject from which we've become so culturally isolated. In previous decades, older women taught herbalism as naturally as they taught their daughters and granddaughters how to sew and cook. But without the teachings of the grandmothers, we must find new ways to learn this ancient tradition. Thankfully, it is a remarkably easy and joyful skill to learn. Rooted in common sense and natural laws, much of what there is to learn about herbalism comes simply and naturally. In fact, I've never met anyone who did not thoroughly enjoy the study of herbs. Herbalism seems to capture the heart and spirit of its students and guides them along. Primarily an intuitive art, much of the learning involves working directly with plants, gardening, making tea, using herbal remedies for health and healing, and allowing the herbs to teach us. In the process, we learn to awaken and trust our intuition.

The method I've found that works best when teaching herbalism is a mixture of the basic art of herbalism as taught by the old-time "simplers," peppered with a touch of science. Long ago herbalists were called "simplers" because they understood the basic laws of life and learned through common sense and life experience. Simplers used noncomplex remedies. They utilized the herbs that grew around them that were effective and nontoxic. Meanwhile, over the centuries, science was developing weights and measures and clinical studies to comprehend, measure, and explain the art of life. A tablespoon or two of this scientific knowledge is appropriate to the study of herbs and adds a touch of proficiency to the art. Combining the simpler's approach with research and study is the best way I know to blend the worlds of herbal wisdom and knowledge.

Though there are many marvelous herbal instructors, I think the best teachers of herbalism are the plants themselves. They may not be able to teach us about how much vitamins and minerals they contain, or what their chemical constituents are (though you can often tell this by tasting them), or what they are specifically used for, but they teach us about the magic and beauty of life, the life force inherent in the green world. When you sit with a plant, observing its color and scent, aware of the community of different plants it grows with, sensing its relationship to the world, you begin to develop a deep sense of peace, joy, and wisdom. Believe me, this happens for almost everybody who enters humbly into the world of "the green nations"—the plant world. Often this communication with plants develops into a keen relationship that helps one to awaken and trust one's own intuition.

Studying about herbs from some of the great books available and from actual herb teachers, who, more often than not, are lively characters, is a wonderful learning process. But I have watched people accumulate so much information about herbalism, yet know little about herbs. Often herbalists get so busy being herbalists they have almost no time to be with the subject that fills the wellspring of their heart and is the source of their inspiration. The best way to receive the deepest gratification from your herbal studies and to step into the wisdom of the plants is to spend time with them.

Spending time with herbs means stopping to "smell the flowers." When you're gardening, stop once in a while to listen to the plants. When you're on a walk, notice every living green thing around you. The very air we breathe is a gift from the plant world. Pause now and then and give thanks to our green allies for the air we breathe.

For many women, the opportunity to spend time with the plant world is limited, either because of time or location. If you live in the city, a walk often doesn't take you along an herb-bordered pathway. But there are many ways to spend time with plants. This morning when I was mixing my favorite tea (a mixture of rose hips, chamomile, and a pinch of stevia), it struck me how beautiful the herbs looked in their jars, and how joyful I felt standing there with them. When I held the warm cup of tea in my hands, I could feel the fusion of my world with that of the plants. Being with the herbs and learning from them means simply making time for them and using them in so many ways for health and healing. And even if you've no time or space for a garden it's always possible to have a few pots of herbs growing about your house.

There are several exercises I love to do with students to help them develop their intuitive skills with plants. I believe that this kind of information is as valuable, if not more so, than all the book learning and educating we do. One of my favorite exercises is very simple, but so profound. Go for a walk. Find a tree that beckons to you. Put your arms around it and hug tightly. Pull yourself close to the tree and allow yourself to smell it, feel it, hear its heartbeat. Trees have very strong energy and you will feel as if you are well supported, that you can surrender and let go. Often people feel they can tell the tree anything and it will hear them and help them. Trees also have strong voices and it is easy to hear them singing back to you. When you walk into a woods, have you ever thought you heard the trees talking? They probably were!

Creating Your Herbal Pantry

One of the first steps in learning herbalism is selecting a small group of herbs you wish to "be with" and learn about. These herbs will form the basis of your herbal work. There are so many herbs to choose from that the difficulty is limiting your choices. It is wiser to select just a few herbs and know them well than to have a large selection of herbs you know little about. If you will be using your herbs primarily for women's problems, you may wish to select herbs from the Materia Medica in Part VII of this book. If you prefer a more general list, the following are some of my favorite all-purpose herbs. These herbs are all commonly available in natural food and herb stores or you can order them from several of the sources listed in Appendix II. Many are easily grown in the garden.

Cayenne (Capsicum frutescens) Hot and fiery, cayenne is often used to improve poor circulation and sluggish bowels. Rich in vitamin K, a blood coagulant, cayenne will stop bleeding almost instantly. It will sting when applied externally. It is great for constipation, and is a good heart tonic, improving blood circulation to the heart and increasing overall body warmth and energy. It is easily cultivated in hot climates.

Chamomile (Matricaria chamomilla and related species) A gentle herb long valued for its ability to relieve stress and nervous tension. Even Peter Rabbit's mother knew of the value of this gentle stress-relieving plant. Camomile is served in hospitals throughout Europe to calm and relax the patients, a practice I would like to see established in our medical facilities. It is excellent for stomach tension, indigestion, and for inflammation. It is easily cultivated and makes a fragrant and lovely ground cover. (See the Materia Medica in Part VII for more information.)

Comfrey (Symphytum officinale) A rich source of allantoin, calcium, iron, and vitamin A, comfrey is highly prized for its wound-healing properties and is used to help mend broken bones, torn ligaments, and injured tissue. Its high mucilage content makes it an excellent remedy for lung, stomach, and dermal inflammation and it is considered one of the best remedies for stomach ulcers. It is easily cultivated, though beware: comfrey can soon take over a garden. Please note: there is currently a controversy over the safety of comfrey and it is best to avoid using it during pregnancy. (See the Materia Medica in Part VII for more information.)

Dandelion (Taraxacum officinale) One of the most widely used herbs in the world, dandelion is highly respected, both for its preventive and for its remedial qualities. It is a specific remedy for the kidneys and liver. High in natural potassium, dandelion, unlike

comfrey

pharmaceutical diuretics, does not deplete the body of this essential mineral. The root is used for the liver and liver-related problems. Because of its high concentration of vitamins and minerals, both the root and the leaf of dandelion are considered restorative and adaptogen aids to the body in building and restoring energy reserves. It is easily cultivated. (See the Materia Medica in Part VII for more information.)

Echinacea (Echinacea angustifolia, A. purpurea) The herb supreme for strengthening the immune system. Excellent for building resistance to colds, flu, and infections. A widely used herb, it has gained much respect throughout Europe for its immunological properties. Current research indicates that echinacea holds promise as an AIDS treatment. Easily cultivated, it is a beautiful garden perennial.

Garlic (Allium sativum) Called the "poor man's penicillin," garlic has long been valued for its antibiotic, antiviral properties. High concentrations of volatile oil, mucilage, and germanium make this one of the most effective antimicrobial plants available and one of the best remedies for colds, flu, bacterial, and viral infections. It is also used to lower high blood pressure. Easily cultivated.

Ginger (Zingiber officinale) This versatile and tasty herb is as useful to the medicinal herbalist as it is to the cook. Ginger has warming, stimulating, and antispasmodic properties. It is used frequently for stomach cramps, colds, poor circulation, motion and morning sickness, and for menstrual irregularities and discomfort. (See the Materia Medica in Part VII for more information.)

Goldenseal (Hydrastis canadensis) Indigenous to the eastern woodlands of the United States, goldenseal was a favorite remedy of the Native Americans and early colonists. It is still used in large quantities by pharmaceutical companies and is considered one of the most effective natural antibiotics and infection-fighting herbs. Unfortunately, due to its remedial value, goldenseal has been severely overharvested and is quickly approaching endangered-species status. Demand *only* cultivated goldenseal when purchasing it; do not use "wildcrafted" (grown-in-the-wild) plants because of the extinction threat. Goldenseal is difficult to cultivate.

Caution: goldenseal should only be used for short periods of time. Taken over an extended period, it builds up in the mucosa of the body, causing irritation and inflammation. A suggested dose would be two capsules three times daily for three weeks; stop for three weeks, then repeat dosage if necessary.

Goldenseal should be used during pregnancy with caution. Large doses stimulate the involuntary muscles of the uterus and may cause premature contractions. It can, however, be used in small amounts (one capsule three times daily) during pregnancy for morning sickness or to help fight infections and colds.

Nettle (Urtica dioica) One of the highest sources of digestible iron in plant form, rich in calcium and vitamin A, nettle strengthens and supports the whole body. Long valued as a food and medicine, it is used for anemia, fatigue, edema, menstrual difficulties, and allergies and hay fever. Easily cultivated but not recommended as a garden plant unless you have a lot of space and privacy. The fresh leaves produce a painful form of dermatitis on contact. (See the Materia Medica in Part VII for more information.)

Peppermint (Mentha piperita) and *spearmint* (M. spicata) Both refreshing, energizing herbs, peppermint and spearmint are often used to enhance the flavor of other, less tasty medicinals. Excellent digestive aids, they are used frequently for upset stomachs, poor digestion, and for colds and fever. They are both extremely easy to cultivate.

Skullcap (Scutellaria lateriflora) Another of the powerful herbal nervines, skullcap revitalizes the entire central nervous system. It is one of the most widely used remedies for headaches and nervous stress. A member of the mint family, it is easily cultivated.

Valerian (Valeriana officinalis) Valerian has long been considered *the* herb supreme for nervous stress and tension. It is excellent for insomnia, headaches, and reducing pain. Though a powerfully effective herb, it is nonhabit-forming and nonaddictive. A small percentage of people who use it experience a stimulating rather than relaxing effect when they use it. Easily cultivated. (See the Materia Medica in Part VII for more information.)

Selecting the Best-Quality Herbs

The single most important factor when purchasing herbs is to recognize and obtain the best quality available. The results of your herbal remedies will depend on the quality of the herbs you are working with. In the past, women collected, dried, and prepared their own herbs, so were assured of quality. This is not always feasible or possible today. Herbalism is a big industry these days, and high quality cannot always be taken for granted.

In recent years consumer awareness has done more to improve the quality of herbs than anything else. If you had walked into an herb store years ago, you would most likely have found a variety of brown or yellow stalks in jars. Today, a stroll around an herb store reveals many jars with "wildcrafted" and/or "organic" labels on them, jars whose contents usually have greater color, vibrancy, and scent. The words "wildcrafted" or "organic" are synonymous with quality. They tell you that the herb has been grown and harvested with care and concern for both the quality of the herb and the integrity of the environment. They express a certain conscious responsibility to the environment and avoidance of chemical fertilizers and sprays. And they suggest that the herb was generally picked according to the seasons, at the right time of day, and dried in the best drying conditions.

By contrast, almost all commercial quality herbs that are imported into this country are channeled through a few tonnage warehouses. While in storage and awaiting FDA inspection, they are sprayed several times to kill insects. Most of these herbs were grown in third world countries where the use of heavy dosages of toxic sprays is common practice. Many of the sprays used have been banned in the United States because of their toxicity, then sold to these countries for agricultural purposes.

These commercial-grade herbs are harvested en masse, dried in excessive, damaging heat, and then shipped to America via several ports, where they are usually sprayed again. Many of these herbs then sit in warehouses for several months or years awaiting distribution. People wonder why herbs treated this way don't work. I'm amazed that they work as well as they do. Somehow, despite all this stressful treatment, some of the life force of these herbs may manage to survive, but it pales beside the vitality of its wildcrafted and organically grown cousins.

The very best way to obtain your herbs is to grow or wildcraft your own. Herbs are amazingly easy and rewarding to grow, and they flourish even in limited space and poor soil; you don't need to be born with a green thumb to grow herbs! As for the availability of wild plants, you'd be amazed at the number you can find growing wild, even in the heart of a city (though you wouldn't want to wildcraft them in cities because of heavy traffic and pollutants). When I mention this to city dwellers, they often express disbelief. But the next time you're walking past a deserted city block, check out the wild plants growing there—generally a beautiful, vibrant, and tenacious sampling of plants. Or look at the median along the highway. Some of my favorite little weeds grow happily in that wasteland. Herbs are very cosmopolitan, love to travel, and are carefree wanderers. Discovering wild plants is one of the great joys of herbalism. However, it is neither the purpose of this book nor within its scope to expound on the identification of wild plants. So you'll have to look elsewhere for training. Many herbalists offer herb walks and there are several good books on wild plant identification. (See Appendix I.)

Whether you grow your own herbs, collect them in the wild, or order them from an herb supplier, it's important to have on hand those herbs you are drawn to work with. Procure about two to four ounces of each herb in its dried form and store it in an airtight glass container. Buy herbs from local sources whenever possible, but if you don't have a local supplier, you can obtain them from mail-order herb companies. I have included the names of several companies that are respected for the quality of the herbs they supply. (See Appendix II.)

How to Tell Good-Quality Herbs

Whenever possible, use your herbs fresh. It always makes me smile when innocent beginners ask how they should dry their peppermint so they can make tea with it. It's like asking how to dry lettuce to make salad. Herbs are dried for convenience, storage, and commercial purposes. Good quality dried herbs are acceptable if fresh ones are not available. How do you tell if dried herbs are of good quality? They should look, taste, and smell almost exactly as they do when they are fresh. And they should be effective. Here are the four guidelines for determining good quality herbs.

❦ **Color** Dried herbs should remain almost the same color as they are when fresh. If you are buying green leaves, such as peppermint or spearmint, they should be vivid, bright, and alive. If you are buying blossoms, they should be bright and colorful. For instance, calendula (marigold) should be a bright orange or yellow. Roots, though generally subtle in color to begin with, should remain true to their original shades. Goldenseal should be a bright golden green; echinacea, a silver brown; yellow dock root, a yellowish brown. In the beginning, you may not always know what the correct color of a plant should be, but look for aliveness, vibrancy, deep strong colors. You will soon develop a knack for knowing.

❦ **Scent** Herbs have distinctive odors that offer an effective means of determining quality. They should smell strong, not necessarily "good." Not all herbs smell good. The scent of valerian, for instance, has been compared to that of dirty socks. Good-quality valerian should smell like *really* dirty socks. Good-quality peppermint will make your nose tingle and your eyes water. Some herbs, like alfalfa, just smell "green." But in that green odor is a freshness and unmistakable vitality. Beautiful, exotic, fragile, sometimes offensive, the scents of herbs vary widely, but they are all distinctive and pronounced.

❦ **Taste** Herbs should have a distinctive, fresh flavor. Do not judge them on taste by expecting them to taste "good." You will quickly learn that not all medicinal herbs taste good by any stretch of the imagination! So judge taste on potency rather than flavor. Do they taste fresh? Strong? Vital? Distinctive? Do they arouse a distinctive response from your taste buds?

❦ **Effect** The herb must work effectively. Herbal remedies made from fine quality herbs and used properly are remarkably effective. If the herbs you are using are not working as well as you would expect them to, inspect the quality of the herb first. It may, in fact, not be working for several other reasons (such as being the wrong herbal remedy for the problem) but before checking anything else scrutinize the herb for quality first.

How to Store Your Herbs

Light, heat, air, and age are the villains that destroy the essence of herbs. Insects can also be a problem. Store your herbs in glass jars with tight-fitting lids away from direct light and heat. I find it baffling that good cooks still store their fancy herbs and spices directly above the kitchen stove exposed to bright light and excess heat. The flavors of most culinarys deteriorate rapidly in these conditions. A cool dark kitchen closet or pantry is excellent for storing herbs. Herbs stored this way will last for several months or even years. If you suspect an herb is losing its potency, give it the quality-control test outlined above. And if it doesn't meet the requisites, offer it up to the compost goddess.

Your Medicinal Herb Library

Though it's important to balance your herbal studies with actual experience with plants, the information you gain through researching and gathering data on the herbs you use is invaluable. It provides the necessary background information that allows you to work with the plants themselves. You don't want to start using an herb unless you know something about it. For instance, if you see cascara sagrada in a formula, you should know that it is a laxative. If you see ginger in a formula, you should know that it is warming and stimulating to the system. If you wish to become knowledgeable about the uses of herbs, you need to know about them before using them. This information helps you make clear decisions about which herbs to use, and when and how much to use them. The best way to conduct this research is to have a good herbal library.

Though often not as colorful as the characters who write them, herb books are a wonderful way to research and learn about herbs. When I first began my herbal studies there were just a few good books on herbs available. One, *Back to Eden* by Jethro Kloss, was considered the "herbal bible." Though an excellent book and still one of my favorites, it certainly is not the best book for beginners. Today herbals are flooding the market, and the difficulty is no longer in finding one, but in finding those that are authentic and reliable. The main criteria I use when looking for good medicinal herbals are as follows:

❦ Are they written by *practicing* herbalists, people who were or are herbal practitioners, rather than people who simply research herbs? Though books written by researchers are often full of wonderful information, stories, and scientific facts, they are not written from the priceless experience of someone who actually practices herbalism. As David Hoffman writes, "All too often the plethora of new herbals assailing the public are written by journalists commissioned by publishers to fill their subject catalogues. Whilst they usually write better than herbalists, what they write about will usually come from other books." When seeking medicinal herb books, look for those books written by practicing herbalists past or present.

❦ Do they provide a clear explanation of how herbology as a medical system works? There are many different systems of herbology such as the Chinese, Western, Ayruvedic, Indian, and Wise Woman. A good herb book will take the time to explain the system(s) of herbalism and how the herbs work so that the inquisitive reader begins to grasp the fine art of medicinal herbology.

When you are learning about new herbs, it is important to read about them in more than one herbal. Each herb has so many different facets. To get a comprehensive view of the plant, you need to learn about it from more than just one source. Most of the time the information in different sources is compatible. But sometimes you will find differences, even outright contradictions, that may confuse and fluster you. At these times, remember that herbalism is a living art and, though we attempt to systemize it, it will remain at its core individualistic and unique. Herbs interact with each person who uses them. They are reflections of the environment they grow in. They have their own power, their own life force. How does one standardize the use of such a marvelous healing art, catch its essence, put it in writing? Each herbalist writes about her own personal interaction with the herbs, and in most cases the experiences are similar. But when they are not, compare them with your own experience, and you will begin to discover how and which herbs work best for you.

For an herb library to be effectively used for cross referencing and studying herbs, I recommend having *at least* three good herbals. Three herb books will give you a comprehensive overview of each herb and provide information from enough different sources to give you a fair analysis of the plant. I have included a list of my favorite herb books in Appendix I.

Using Your Herbs

Begin by using your herbs for simple, nonemergency, first-aid situations. Throughout this book there are countless suggestions that have been used successfully by other women. You can try these suggestions and see how they work for you. You can also begin to experiment with herbs for other simple problems. Got an upset stomach? Drink peppermint tea. Head pounding with a stress-induced headache? Try a cup of skullcap/chamomile tea. Not sleeping soundly at night? Take hops/valerian tincture. Through gentle experimentation you will begin to gain invaluable personal experience.

We learn best by doing and by hands-on experience. Continue to expand and discover your knowledge of this ancient healing art by practicing herbalism at every opportunity. Use the herbs daily in your life as preventive teas. Use them for simple illnesses. Make lovely dream pillows filled with herbs and sleep with them. Sharing your bed with herbs is a great way to get to know them intimately! Whenever possible, spend time with the plants. Grow an herb garden. Even if you have only the tiniest yard or a sunny windowsill for space, the growing, living herbs will be your greatest teachers. They will guide you gently into the world of herbs. By providing yourself with the opportunity to learn this powerful women's healing art, you awaken the healer within and reestablish your connection with the oldest system of healing on earth.

red clover

How to Use This Book

Herbal Healing for Women was written from my years of experience in working with women and herbs. Many of my students have shared their experiences and recipes, and through them, have contributed to this book. There are many excellent herbalists practicing in this country today, and a wonderful community has grown up around them. Through the years we've compared cases, notes, and recipes. The best of these have been included to make this as comprehensive a book as I could possibly offer.

I've divided the information into the three major stages of womanhood: adolescence; midlife, which includes pregnancy; and menopause. These three stages of womanhood are often associated with the phases of the moon, and particular goddesses and deities are assigned to each. As the moon journeys through its cycles each month, it mirrors our own cycles.

The first stage of our journey into womanhood reflects the waxing moon, which begins at the birth of the new moon and is completed as the moon grows into her fullness. This cycle represents birth and growth. It is the time of beginnings and emergence. The young woman, the adolescent, is exemplified by the newness of the waxing moon. She is the bride coming into her ripeness. She is Artemis, a woodland nymph, wild and free. She is the daughter. Her dreams are without limits, her possibilities yet undefined.

The second stage of womanhood is represented by the full moon. This is the time in a woman's life when she is at her fullness, her most brilliant. The full moon radiates its magnificent light upon all things. Its very fullness sheds light on all in its presence and symbolized motherhood, nourishment, and manifestation. The full moon is abundant, and through its fiery sensuality creates union with the dark (yin) and the light (yang) forces. This cycle is personified by the goddess Selene, the gracious and all-powerful moon mother.

The final and most powerful cycle of womanhood, the menopause years, is represented by the waning moon, the time when the moon's light returns into itself. This cycle is personified by Hekate, the "crone," the wise old woman who, sadly, is so rebuffed in our society. Yet Hekate is the midwife of the psyche and helps birth all other stages. She is the accomplished shaman, fully trained in her skills. She is the mother of the lost daughter; it is through honoring the spirit of Hekate that we rediscover our inner powers of healing and divination. She contains both male and female energies and balances the light of the moon and the sun between her hands. She knows the secrets of death and rejuvenation and is honored for her powers of healing. When you pause and reflect on these images of the menopause years, you can see this cycle with entirely different eyes.

These three cycles of the moon represent the archetypal stages of a woman's life—those of daughter, mother, and grandmother—and the qualities attributed to each. By coming to understand these cycles of womanhood, we create greater room for understanding our needs and health concerns at each phase.

Many of the suggestions and remedies in one section are applicable to the other stages. For instance, remedies recommended for young women experiencing difficulties with their menstrual cycles may be applicable for older women experiencing the same problems.

I have recommended many different suggestions, recipes, and remedies for each imbalance. Don't get carried away trying to do everything that is suggested. A good health program is one that is comprehensive but simple enough to be carried out by the person following it. If you design a program that is too demanding for you to follow or does not fit your life-style, then you will most likely discontinue it rather quickly. The very best health program in the world won't work unless a person is willing and able to follow it.

When designing a program for yourself for a particular problem, it is wise to plan it on paper. Write out the program completely and thoroughly. Include the foods you are

How to Interpret Measurements Throughout This Book

While many people are converting to the metric system, I've reverted to the simplers' method of measuring. Many herbalists choose to use this system because it is extremely easy and very versatile. Often throughout this book you'll see measurements referred to as "parts": 3 parts dandelion, 1 part nettle, 2 parts raspberry leaf. *The use of the word "part" allows the measurement to be determined in its relation to other ingredients.* For instance, if you decide in this case to define "part" as an ounce, you would use 3 ounces of dandelion, 1 ounce of nettle, and 2 ounces of raspberry leaf. That would give you six ounces of tea. If you wanted to make a smaller amount, you could use a tablespoon as your definition of "part": 3 tablespoons of dandelion, 1 tablespoon of nettle, 2 tablespoons of raspberry leaf. A part is a unit that can be interpreted to mean cups, ounces, pounds, tablespoons, or teaspoons—*so long as you use that definition consistently throughout the recipe.* You simply determine what "part" will stand for before you begin, and then use that unit of measurement all the way through the recipe. (The rule is that you must never change from one unit of measurement to another in any one recipe.)

For example, a formula contains roses, chamomile, and lavender. The following table shows the simplers' method in action, or how the parts blend in relation to each other, first in tablespoons and then blended in ounces. *Remember to keep the measurement quantity consistent throughout a formula.*

SAMPLE FORMULA BLENDED IN THE SIMPLERS' METHOD

Parts	Parts in tablespoons	Parts in ounces
3 parts roses	3 tablespoons roses	3 ounces roses
1 part chamomile	1 tablespoon chamomile	1 ounce chamomile
2 parts lavender	2 tablespoons lavender	2 ounces lavender

to eat, the remedies, vitamins and minerals you are to take, and any other therapies you feel are appropriate. It is, of course, ideal to work out your program under the guidance of a qualified health practitioner. Often we cannot see ourselves clearly or do not have the needed experience to determine the cause of our problems. A qualified, holistically minded practitioner can assist you in identifying the problem and working out a personalized program.

Follow this program diligently. Keep a record of your progress (and any relapses) and make note of any changes. In Appendix V have included a health evaluation questionnaire and a sample form for a treatment program. You may wish to fill them out as you design a program that meets your specific needs. I have also included an example of a successful treatment program for a woman who had fibroids. When in doubt, or if experiencing serious health problems, consult a health care professional.

Choose your primary health care professional carefully. After all, it is your body, your health, and sometimes it's your life that is at stake when you consult a health care person. I recommend, when possible, selecting a doctor who is either holistically minded or, at the very least, sympathetic and responsive toward other systems of healing. It is extremely difficult to work with a health care professional who is from "the doctor is god" school of medicine.

It is also wise, though not many women do it, to choose a health care professional when you are in a state of good health—not vulnerable and emotionally stressed from an illness. When ill, a person is more likely to make decisions or allow medical procedures that would not normally be acceptable to them. It may seem simpler and easier to do so than to question the doctor. After all, these are the "doctor's orders." But often what seems simple may in fact turn out to be quite involved and complex. If you have already developed a relationship of trust and acceptance with a health care person when you are well, she or he will have a better understanding of you and be more willing to work with your needs when you are ill.

In ancient Chinese medical practices, the doctor was hired to keep his patients well. If his clients became ill, he provided medical treatment at no cost. And his primary system of medicine was herbal. Would that we could find medical practitioners like that today!

Herbalism is a marvelous system of healing, but it doesn't work for every situation and it certainly doesn't work for everyone. It would be ludicrous to imagine that any one system of healing would hold the answers to every health concern or that everybody *should* use the same system (which is what the AMA has decided for us). My family is a good example. I have found that herbs answer my almost every need. They *always* help me, so I always choose to use them. My husband has a different relationship with herbs. When ill he finds herbs helpful, but he also relies on allopathic medications to augment the herbs. One of my daughters has found herbalism an excellent system of healing and uses herbs every day for a rather serious condition with which she was born. My other daughter has less patience with herbs, and though she uses them and enjoys them, she's less likely to reach for the tincture bottle at the first sign of a cold or flu. I've come to respect these differences in people over the years and have become less fanatical about thinking that this system—or any system, for that matter—is for everybody. I offer the herbalist system of healing primarily because it has been neglected for so long and because I have found it to be so very effective—especially for women's health problems.

Shopping for Herbs

Luckily, herb stores are springing up around the country and many natural food stores now carry a large selection of herbs. If you have never shopped for herbs before or been in an herb store, it is quite an experience. You may feel a little lost and confused in the beginning. You'll find row upon row of jars filled with herbs of unusual odors, beautiful colors, strange-sounding names. A few of the names will be familiar—basil, oregano, comfrey, thyme. But many will seem peculiar and unusual. There will be herb pills, capsules, syrups, and a variety of tinctures, salves, and ointments. To add to the confusion, there will often be rows of vitamins, minerals, homeopathic remedies, Ayruvedic remedies, and Chinese remedies. You may even feel you've entered a different era! It can be quite a perplexing adventure, to say the least. But don't give up and walk out. Most herb stores employ herbalists or a knowledgeable clerk. Don't hesitate to ask for help. If you don't have a supplier of herbs close by, you can always mail-order them. There are several excellent mail order companies that supply high-quality herbs; some of them are listed in Appendix II. However, though it's simpler and often less confusing to order your herbs through the mail, a visit to the herb store, especially after the initial confusion wears off, is an enchanted delight not to be missed.

How to Determine Dosage

Determining the correct dosage of an herbal remedy can be confusing. It's not as simple as prescribing "two tablets of aspirin three times daily" (though I think prescribing "regular," orthodox medicine is far more of an art than a science and that it requires more intuition and trust than we are led to believe). When using herbs, one needs to take into account the constitution of the person, the strength of the herb(s) being used, and the nature of the imbalance. I have included general recommendations throughout this book, but to make it easier I thought it would be helpful to include the following chart. Remember, it is just for general purposes. Ultimately, you must trust the wisdom of your own body; listen to what it's telling you.

I have generally found that when an herbal formula is not working it is either because the herbs being used are of inferior quality or it is due to insufficient herbal dosages. As long as the herb(s) are considered safe and nontoxic, do not be afraid to increase the dosage. It is always sensible to start with smaller dosages, but perfectly appropriate to increase the dosage as necessary. Research the herbs that you are using to determine if there is any known toxicity from using them. And listen, listen to your sacred sense of knowing; it will guide you.

Amount of tea to take for a chronic problem: 3–4 cups daily for 3–4 months or longer

Amount of tea to take for an acute problem: ¼ cup of tea every ½–1 hour until symptoms subside

Amount of tincture to take for a chronic problem: ½–1 teaspoonful 3 times a day

Amount of tincture to take for an acute problem: ¼–1 teaspoon every ½–1 hour until symptoms subside

Amount of tablets/capsules to take for a chronic problem: 2 "00" capsules or tablets 3 times daily

Amount of tablets/capsules to take for an acute problem: 1–2 capsules every 3–4 hours until symptoms subside

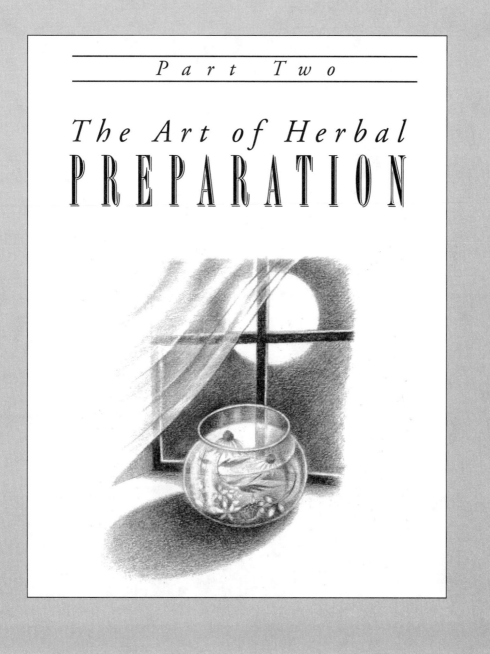

Part Two

The Art of Herbal PREPARATION

The Tools of Herbalism

Just as flowers grow from the Earth, so the remedy grows in the hands of the physician . . . the remedy is nothing but a seed which develops into that which it is destined to be.

—Paracelcus

One of my earliest memories is that of learning to cook. My learning was by doing—an organic process as natural and wholesome as the vegetables my mother brought in from the garden. Our farm kitchen was a warm, friendly place, rich with savory smells of soup simmering, bread baking, and Armenian delicacies steaming in the well-seasoned cast-iron skillet. My mother and grandmother were both large women, not so much in size but in presence, and occupied ample space in that old farm kitchen. But there was always room for us kids, and our presence seldom went unnoticed. We were regularly enlisted for whatever task was under way.

This is the place where I learned to trust the process of creativity and imagination, and to understand the art of preparation. Often sent to the garden, I learned how to dig roots and collect greens, learned to put my hands into the worm-rich earth and to feel the pleasures of life in the soil. I learned to slice onions into silver moons and to peel and chop garlic the quick and easy way. It was here, too, I learned that indispensable skill of life—the fine art of substituting what you do have for what you don't, of making use of what is available.

These early lessons learned informally in the stewpot of my childhood were a great help in learning to work with and prepare herbs. Cooking food and preparing herbs are very similar processes. Both include some basic rules, a generous dash of creativity, and a few simple tools. Both also involve a basic understanding of alchemy, the art of transforming one substance into another.

As natural as cooking and at least as rewarding, herbal preparation is a wonderful art that needn't be lost to contemporary women. Learning this ancient alchemical art of herbal preparation is quite simple. In fact, herbal preparation is really easier to learn than cooking and is every bit as valuable a skill to master and pass on.

Though it is certainly possible to buy almost any good herbal product you need in natural food markets these days, I still maintain that the best-quality products are those that are handmade. And it is so rewarding to know that you can make these herbal products yourself right in your own kitchen. I suggest trying these recipes at least once. Then, if being an herbal medicine maker is not your cup of tea, go to the herb shop or natural food store and stock your shelves with the many prepared herbal products available. (See Appendix II for a list of places that supply high-quality herbal products.)

There are as many methods of preparing herbs for medicinal purposes as there are ways of cooking. Like the basics of cooking, you learn what goes into the recipe, then you close the cookbooks and create. The following methods of preparing herbs are among my favorites. It is a pleasure to pass them on. Having taught them to literally hundreds of people, I know you'll have no problem following the directions and making excellent medicinal preparations yourself. They are simple, easy, and effective and, most of all, they are fun to make. Once you've made an herbal salve or a special medicinal tincture, you'll catch that same fervor that comes when you bake your first loaf of bread or your first batch of cookies. Everything about it just captures your imagination and whets your appetite for more.

The technique I prefer to use in making my herbal products is a mixture of the simpler's approach to herbology, or the *art* as it is often called, blended with a touch of *science*. Over the centuries science has developed weights and measures, detailed techniques, and clinical studies to comprehend, measure, and explain natural phenomena. A tablespoon or two of this clinical knowledge is appropriate to the study of herbs and can add a touch of professionalism, but more than a tablespoon of science hinders the herbal art.

I have developed recipes through trial and error and a dash of scientific seasoning. Use these recipes and directions only as guidelines. The finest student is the one who perceives with the heart and follows the teachings heard from within. I encourage you to create your own unique formulations using these recipes as guidelines. Many years ago, while teaching a class on natural cosmetics, I shared one of my favorite facial cream recipes. It was a formula I had developed and, though I was pleased with it, I knew it wasn't quite perfect. One of the students in that particular class was a talented young artist and an excellent herb student. Using both her creative input and her knowledge of herbs, Dyana improved that basic cream formula so that it became a work of art. Her perfected version has been my favorite cream recipe for many years now.

What I would like most for you to keep in mind as you make these formulas and recipes is to allow your creativity to flow—and to have fun! Making herbal preparations allows us to play with the herbs. The herbs come alive and dance, suggesting new combinations for us to try. We're allowed to tap into the old ways, those ancient roots of the herbalist, to be a little wild and different. Remember to experiment and experience. I've always maintained that the very best and most effective recipes are the ones that flow from the heart of each individual.

Where to Begin

1 The first and foremost place to begin is with the *quality* of the herbs you are using. Try to obtain your herbs and related products from the best sources available. Whenever possible, buy organic and wildcrafted herbs. (See Appendix II.) The quality of these herbs is far superior to that of nonorganic plants, and using them will make you a part of a network of herbalists who are working to upgrade the standard of herbs. You'll be discouraging the widespread use of chemicals and encouraging the growing trend to farm organically, and you'll be helping to support small cottage industries. But most important, the quality of your herbal medicine will be superior because you are using the best quality herbs available.

2 Keep a recipe file of *all* your products. Label each item thoroughly and accurately. Include in your recipe file:

❧ The date made
❧ A list of all the ingredients
❧ The recipe itself
❧ Where you obtained the recipe and
❧ Any special instructions or comments about the recipe

3 When making *any* item for the first time, make it in *small* batches. It is better to lose only a few ingredients in your experimentation than to have to throw away a large batch.

4 Know each of the herbs you are using in your product making. Take a few minutes to research each one in a favorite herb book or two. Not only will this assure you that you are using the correct herbs in your products, but it is one of the best ways to get to know the plants you are using. Reading about them and then working with them will help you develop a relationship with the herbs. (See Appendix I for a list of herb books.)

5 Label your product as soon as it is made. You can do this by using ready-made stick-on labels. But it's much more fun to design your own. Even if you're making products for your own use only, personalized labels are attractive and express a sense of pride in your finished work. If you have children, their help in making labels can be a delightful way to involve them in your herbal work. In this age of computers it's not difficult to find a friend who has a computer. Computers have delightful capabilities for designing labels. In just a few minutes you can design a professional-looking label for your own home products.

INCLUDE THESE "VITAL STATISTICS" ON YOUR LABEL:

❧ Date made
❧ Ingredients, listed in order from the major ingredient down to the least ingredient
❧ Name of product
❧ Instructions for using
❧ Whether for *internal* and/or *external* use (very important)

Proper record keeping and labeling of your products will help you repeat favorite and successful recipes and avoid repeating mistakes.

What You Will Need

Common kitchen tools will supply you with most of the utensils you need for preparing herbal products. Along with a few pots and pans, large spoons, and a measuring cup, you will find the following items useful:

❦ Cheesecloth or fine cotton muslin for finely straining herbs
❦ A large stainless-steel, fine-meshed strainer
❦ A hand grater that you reserve just for grating beeswax
❦ Glass bottles and jars for storing your preparations
❦ A coffee or seed and nut grinder for powdering and grinding small quantities of herbs. Do not use your herb grinder for grinding coffee, or vice versa. Not only will the coffee drinkers in your house be up in arms, but all your herbal products will smell and taste like fine Colombian.
❦ A potato ricer lined with cheesecloth for an excellent, inexpensive hand press

One of the few rules that most herbalists adhere to is to *not* use aluminum or copper pots for preparing herbs. Both metals are injurious to the quality of the herbs. Cooking utensils made with aluminum are especially harmful, as the metal is released in toxic amounts into the preparation during cooking. Copper destroys the vitamin C content of certain herbs. Favored cooking receptacles include glass, stainless steel, ceramic, cast iron, and enamel. I've heard arguments pro and con for each of these also. But rather than get fanatical, do as Carl Jung, the famous Swiss psychologist, did. Talk to your pots and select those that say "good morning" back to you.

FOUR
The Fine Art of Making Medicinal Herb Teas

There is more to that steaming cup of tea than meets the eye. Herbs are as ancient as time itself and capture the magical qualities of fire, air, water, and plant life. Like ancient alchemy, the making of herb tea involves the mixing and brewing of different elemental forces. Though it is a profoundly simple and gracious art, few people really know how to prepare herb teas properly. There are simple guidelines to follow and choices we can make when we brew our herbs that affect the finished quality of the tea. Herb teas, properly prepared, are warming and soothing to the soul. They provide essential medicinal qualities and healing energy. Preparing and drinking herb teas involves us in the personal process of healing and teaches us to be conscious of the role we each play in our well-being.

Today, with so much emphasis placed on speed and efficiency, herb teas—especially medicinal blends—have fallen by the wayside, even amongst herbalists. Yet they are a very important part of herbal medicine, and I am forever encouraging people who are seeking well-being and health to daily brew their pot of herbs. Though useful for short-term health problems, herb teas are most effective for chronic health problems. Used consistently over an extended period of time, herb teas ensure gradual but steady long-term results. Since the menstruum (the substance used to extract the plant constituents) used is water, it is nontoxic and user-friendly.

Proportion of Herb in Water

The standard proportion of herbs to water as stated in most herb books is one teaspoon of dried herb, or two tablespoons of fresh herb, to one cup of water. This amount is arbitrary, however, since the quality and the nature of each herb you use is completely different. In most cases using an exact amount of herb is not crucial since only plants that are safe and nontoxic should be used in your herbal blends. Use your *sense of taste* as well as your *knowledge* of each of the individual herbs you are using as a guide to the amount of herb to use in the formula. When in doubt, use one teaspoon of dried herb or two tablespoons fresh to one cup of water.

I seldom suggest that people make medicinal teas by the cupful. It is impractical and time-consuming. Instead, make a *quart* of tea each morning. Thermoses and quart canning jars are convenient for storing your daily tea. They are handy for carrying your tea with you and making it easy to consume the suggested daily amount. As an added benefit, having the tea on hand will make you less tempted to drink unhealthy beverages like soda and coffee. You can also leave the pot of tea on the stove for easy reheating or for drinking at room temperature. (Warm liquid is much healthier for our systems than the extremes of hot and cold). Again, proportions will vary depending on the herb used, but I generally use about four to six tablespoons of dried herb per quart of water.

Infusions and Tisanes

There are several methods for properly brewing medicinal herb teas. Infusions (also called tisanes) extract the easily rendered vitamins, mucilage, and delicate volatile oils. They are used when preparing the more fragile parts of the plant—the leaves, fruits, seeds, flowers, and those roots with a high concentration of volatile oils. There are *four* methods commonly employed for making infusions. To get an idea of the effectiveness of each method, take one herb, such as nettle or chamomile, and infuse it using each of the different four methods described below. You'll soon choose your favorite method.

❦ *Method 1* Place the herb(s) in a container with a tight-fitting lid and pour boiling water over them. Quickly cover the container. Allow to steep for ten to twenty minutes. The length of steeping time will depend on the herbs being used and the active plant constituents you wish to extract. For instance, tannins are extracted very quickly during preparation, and if allowed to steep longer than three to four minutes, the tea will become bitter and very acidic. This is what happens when you steep your favorite black tea (such as Earl Grey or Jasmine) too long and it becomes bitter.

❦ *Method 2* A stronger, medicinal infusion can be made by placing the herb(s) in a pan with cold water. Place a tight-fitting lid on the pan and *slowly* over a *very low heat,* bring the water to the boiling point. Take the brew off the heat just before it begins to boil. This method makes a stronger and more medicinal infusion but is neither necessary nor appropriate for all herbs.

❦ *Method 3* Sometimes it is most effective to let the tea steep overnight. Follow directions for either Method 1 or Method 2. Remove from the stove and allow to infuse overnight. Quart canning jars are great for steeping herbs because of their tight-fitting lids. This is one of my favorite methods.

❦ *Method 4* Have you ever considered the light sources of the sun and moon as an aid in preparing your herb teas? Both the sun and the moon, though very different in their energy fields, provide a powerful but subtle heat source useful for extracting the healing energy of herbs. Sunlight imparts an inner warmth and vitality to herbs, while moonlight seems to draw on the acute powers of the feminine. Lunar infusions are great for romance, dreaming, and awakening creative endeavors.

To make a solar infusion, place the herb(s) in a glass jar, fill with water, and secure with a tight-fitting lid. Put the jar in a hot, sunny spot in direct contact with the sunlight and let it infuse for several hours.

When preparing lunar teas, you are employing the subtle light of the moon. You are invoking the intuition, the enchanted and mystifying aspects of life. You are calling upon the unknown; unleashing that lunar energy humankind has always feared. Where did the term lunacy derive from? The mystical, wild, enchanted energy of the night!

To prepare a lunar tea, place the herb(s) in an open crystal glass or bowl. It is ideal, if possible, to use fresh herbs and flowers. Cover the mixture with fresh water and place directly in the moonlight. Do not place a cover over the container unless there are a lot of insects around. Allow to infuse in the moonlight all night and drink first thing on rising. The flavor of moon teas is subtle but enchanting.

Decoctions

Decoctions are used to extract more tenacious plant material and are generally used for brewing roots, barks, nuts, and nonaromatic seeds. There are a few exceptions to this rule, however. Some roots are very high in volatile oils that are easily destroyed by high temperatures. Roots such as goldenseal and valerian, both very high in volatile oils, are better infused than decocted.

There are three methods commonly used to decoct herbs.

❦ *Method 1* Bring the water to a boil, add the herb(s), and gently, over a low heat, simmer for fifteen to twenty minutes. Keep a tight-fitting lid on at all times to prevent the escape of steam and important nutrients. Remove from the heat, strain, and drink.

❦ *Method 2* Add the herb(s) to the cold water, place over *low* heat, and slowly bring to a boil. Simmer gently, over low heat, for fifteen to twenty minutes. As always, keep the lid on. If the lid is not tight, valuable nutrients will be lost in the escaping steam. Remove from heat, strain, and drink.

❦ *Method 3* For a stronger medicinal tea, decoct according to Method 1 or Method 2. Remove from heat and let sit with the lid on overnight without straining.

Because the plant chemicals are so concentrated in roots and barks and are quite tenacious, you can decoct the same batch of herbs several times. With each subsequent decoction, the brew becomes milder. If you wish, you may add a little fresh herb mixture to each batch to maintain the strength. I generally brew my root mixtures three to four times before discarding. I not only appreciate the flavor as it becomes milder, but like the fact that I am not wasting valuable herbs.

What do you do if the tea formula contains both roots/bark and leaves/flowers? Does one decoct or infuse the tea? For beverage blends, where flavor is the most important aspect of the tea, it doesn't matter whether you decoct or infuse the herbs. But when making medicinal blends, proper preparation plays an integral part in how effective the tea is. If an herb tea formula is preblended and contains both roots/bark and leaves/flowers in the formula, you may wish both to decoct and infuse it to obtain the maximum benefits. Simply prepare the formula by first decocting the roots as instructed on page 47. Then turn the heat source off and add the herbs to be infused. Place the lid tightly on the pot and allow to steep for the appropriate length of time.

Dosage of Medicinal Teas

In order for herbs to be effective, they must be used with *consistency.* This is probably the most difficult aspect of herbalism for people of the twentieth century to adapt to. In our age of quick fixes and instant medicine, the old art of brewing and using herbal teas seems antiquated and time-consuming. In fact, it is quite simple. Brew a quart of tea in the morning (or at night), keep it on the stove or at room temperature during the day, and drink two to four cups by the end of the evening. If you aren't at home, the tea keeps quite well and travels easily in a thermos or quart canning jar.

The amount of medicinal tea to drink daily is determined by the health problem at issue and the herb(s) being used. For chronic health problems—those problems that are continual and/or recurring in nature and persist over a long period of time—make a quart of the medicinal tea(s) each day and drink three to four cups daily for three to four months. It is always appropriate to allow one to two days of rest each week from your tea schedule.

For acute health problems—those problems that are momentarily critical, severe, and/or reaching a crisis—drink the medicinal tea in *small, frequent* doses. For instance, for a high fever drink one-fourth of a cup of tea every half hour until symptoms are remedied. In acute situations, small doses served frequently are more effective than large amounts of tea taken infrequently throughout the day.

How Long Will a Tea Stay Fresh?

Though it is best to make teas fresh daily, they will last for several days if refrigerated or stored in a cool place. Because water has no preservative properties, the tea will soon become stale and may begin to ferment. If you notice a flat taste or bubbles forming, chances are your tea is no longer usable.

Making Medicinal Herbal Oils

Medicinal oils are among the most wonderful and beneficial herbal products. They are used for a variety of purposes, from massage to insect repellents, and they are remarkably easy to make. There are two distinct types of herbal oils available and there is much confusion between the two. Essential oils are the distilled, highly concentrated volatile oils of the plant. They are extremely concentrated and should be used with caution. It is virtually impossible to make high-quality essential oils in sufficient quantities at home unless you invest in a sophisticated distiller. On the other hand, infused herbal oils (fixed oils) are wonderfully easy and inexpensive to make. Though not as pure or as concentrated, they are completely safe to use. Generally recommended for external purposes, they can also be used safely internally. Once made, you can use them as is or make them into salves and ointments.

The Ingredients for Herbal Oils

Oil

The oil you use must be high-quality seed, nut, or vegetable oil. For medicinal purposes, olive oil is the oil of choice and preferred by most herbalists. Use the finest quality olive oil you can get for your medicinal herbal products. Olive oil is graded from "extra virgin," the first pressing of the olives and the finest and purest grade, to just plain "olive oil," the last pressing and, basically, an inferior quality. Olive oil makes a wonderful base for medicinal oils and seldom goes rancid. When making other than medicinal oils, lighter, less aromatic oils such as apricot, almond, canella or grape seed oil are recommended. These are considered cosmetic-grade oils and are excellent for massage, creams, and lotions.

I've frequently heard people say they were disappointed because their finished herbal oils do not have the strong concentration of scent that essential oils have. The essential oils of the plant are extremely volatile and difficult to capture. A fixed oil, such as a vegetable oil, does not capture the scent well. If you want your herbal oils to be aromatic, you will need to add a drop or two of essential oil to the finished product.

Herbs

There are many herbs suitable for making medicinal oils. (See the recipes in this book or refer to other herb books.) Either fresh or dried herbs can be used. If you've never made an herbal oil before, I recommend beginning with dried herbs because you will not have to be concerned with the growth of mold and bacteria. Should you decide to use fresh herbs, it is imperative to make sure they are *completely* free of any extra moisture. One method I've used quite successfully to eliminate extra moisture in fresh herbs is to wilt the herbs before using. Pick the herbs in the morning and allow them to wilt in a dry, shaded, warm place for several hours or overnight. This ensures that the excess moisture that causes bacteria to grow has evaporated.

Proportion of Herb(s) to Oil

The method I recommend for determining the proportion of herb to oil is the simplers' method. Place the herbs in a container and pour enough oil over them to cover the herbs. Then add one to two inches more oil so that the herbs are completely submerged. Exposed herbs can introduce bacteria and spoil your oil, so be certain the herbs are completely covered.

How to Make Medicinal Oils

There are four common methods used for making oils. Each of these methods is highly effective and is used professionally as well as for home use. I myself prefer the methods that employ a long, slow heating process, such as the solar, oven-extraction, or Crockpot or roaster-oven techniques, over the double-boiler method. But there are times when I've been thankful to be able to make a medicinal oil in the short time made possible by the stovetop method.

Solar Infusion Method

Using the simplers' measure, place the desired amount of herbs and oil in a glass jar. Cover tightly. Place the jar in a warm, sunny spot. In Europe and the Mediterranean the jars are placed in sandboxes to attract greater amounts of heat. When traveling in Switzerland, my daughters and I were fascinated and excited to find jars of St. John's wort flowers steeping in oil on the porches and balconies of many people's homes. The beautiful yellow flowers of St. John's wort turn the oil a bright red. It is truly beautiful and amazing!

Let the oil/herb mixture infuse for two weeks. People always ask why the oil doesn't go rancid sitting out in the hot sun. According to natural laws, it should. But for some magical reason, it seldom does. I believe it's because of the alchemical fusion of the sun, the herbs, and the oil. But once strained, the oil will definitely go rancid very quickly if left in the hot sun.

At the end of two weeks, strain the herbs, rebottle your beautiful herbal oil, and store it in a cool dark area. If you wish a stronger oil, add a fresh batch of herbs to the oil, and infuse for two more weeks. This will double the potency of your medicinal oil.

Using the solar method for making medicinal oils is my favorite method. I learned it from the wise old Gypsy herbalist, Juliette de Bairacli Levy. Though a bit more time-consuming than the other methods, it has the added benefits of the sun, the wisdom of the elders, and a delightful array of bottles sitting in a sunny spot in the garden or windowsill of your home.

Oven Extraction Method

Place the oil/herb mixture in a pan with a tight-fitting lid or in glass canning jars. Put the pan and/or jars in a larger pan with sufficient water to cover the bottom half of the container. Turn the oven on the lowest temperature possible and allow the herbs and oil to infuse for several hours. Check frequently to prevent the herbs and oil from overheating and burning.

Double Boiler Method

Place the herbs and oil in a double boiler, cover with a tight-fitting lid, and bring to a low simmer. Slowly heat for one-half to one hour, checking frequently to be sure the oil is not overheating. The lower the heat and the longer the infusion, the better the oil. This is a quick and simple method that appeals to many modern-day herbalists. One word of caution, however: oil heats up very quickly. Be mindful of the temperature. Your preparation can quickly go from a nice herbal oil infusion to deep-fried comfrey leaves!

Crockpot and Electric Oven Roaster Method

Both Crockpots and electric oven roasters allow for a long, slow cooking process. The roaster is most often used by small professional companies making quality herbal products. The herbs can macerate in the oil for a long period of time (two to four weeks) and the resulting oil is of a superior quality. Electric roasters can often be found quite inexpensively at bargain shops and second-hand stores. They are in hot demand by herbalists!

Place the herbs and oil in the Crockpot or roaster and turn to the lowest heat. Place the lid on and let the mixture steep for the desired length of time. The heat is generally higher in the Crockpot and usually two to four hours is sufficient to prepare good-quality herbal oils. Check frequently to protect against overheating and burning. In the roaster, the herb/oil mixture can steep for two to four weeks. It gives a superior, dark-green herbal oil.

Straining and Storage

Strain the herbal mixture thoroughly. Line a large stainless-steel strainer or potato ricer with cheesecloth or muslin. Pour the mixture through. Reserve this oil. In a separate container, press the remaining oil from the herbs. Do not mix the oils from the two pressings. The oil from the second pressing will have a higher percentage of water and sediment in it and will not be of as good quality as the first. It is still usable, however.

Rebottle the oil and store in a cool, dark area. It does not have to be refrigerated, but heat will deteriorate the quality quickly, so keep it in a cool place.

What to Watch Out For

Though herbal oils are extremely easy to prepare and will last for several months or longer, there are some possible "trouble spots" to watch for when preparing and storing them:

❦ If your herbal oil grows mold, there is either too much water content in the herb itself or there was moisture in the jar. Use dry herbs or wilt the herbs before using. Be absolutely certain the container is completely dry. Check the inner lid; if it has a circle of cardboard in it, discard it.

❦ If there is a large air space in the jar, this may encourage the growth of mold. Use jars that are the correct size for the amount of oil you wish to make and fill to the top with oil to discourage bacterial growth.

❦ Sometimes when the jar is left in the sun or other heat source, condensation from the heat forms inside the jar, providing the moisture needed for mold to grow. This rarely happens but if it does, try placing the container in a different heat source or temperature. I've also been told that if you take off the lid and wipe it and any "head room" inside the jar with a clean cloth every day or so, it decreases the risk of mold.

❦ You may notice small bubbles forming in your oils as they infuse. This is from the gas that some herbs naturally release during preparation. This does not indicate spoilage.

❦ Do not overheat your oils. You do not want deep-fried herbs. Oil goes from warm to burning very quickly. When macerating, keep the oil warm, the heat low, and use a double boiler or other system that doesn't apply direct heat.

Sample Recipes for Medicinal Herb Oils

MULLEIN FLOWER OIL

Mullein flower oil is the remedy par excellence for ear infections. Warmed to body temperature and dropped down both ears, it quickly relieves the pain of earaches. Because of its antiviral and antibiotic properties, it helps eliminate the infection as well. (Be sure to use wild mullein flowers, *Verbascum thapsus,* not one of the ornamental cultivated varieties which do not have the same medicinal properties.)

¼ cup dry (or fresh wilted) mullein flowers
½ cup extra virgin olive oil

To Make:
Though any of the methods listed above can be used to make mullein flower oil, the solar method is the one most often employed. Place the mullein flowers in a glass jar and cover with olive oil. Place the jar in a hot, sunny window or outside in the direct

sunlight and let sit for at least two weeks or longer—the longer the better. To make the mullein flower oil extra potent, do a double or triple preparation; remove the flowers, add fresh flowers (dried or wilted), and repeat the process.

Please note:

Mullein Flowers are often difficult to purchase, so gather some in the summer and fall. Mullein, a stately plant, grows wild throughout the United States and is found in many other parts of the world. The long, fragrant flowering stalk is a virtual insect condominium; insects love to live in it. So when picking mullein blossoms, put them in a basket or on a newspaper laid on the porch or lawn and allow time for the insects to depart.

INSECT REPELLENT OIL

1 part bay leaves   2 parts rosemary
4 parts pennyroyal   1 part eucalyptus leaves

Enough olive oil or other high-quality vegetable oil to completely submerse herbs. Top off with another inch or two of oil.

To Make:

Wilt the fresh leaves or used dried herbs. Cover with enough oil to completely submerse herbs, plus one to two inches more. Follow any of the methods listed above for making medicinal oils. Strain. Add a drop or two of essential oil of pennyroyal and/or eucalyptus essential oil to strengthen the scent. This is an excellent insect-repellent oil. It is quite safe for human and animal use and as effective as anything can be for keeping those pesky insects away.

SPORTS MASSAGE OIL

2 parts St. Johns wort
1 part hops
1 part arnica
1 part mullein leaves
2 parts camphor oil or camphor crystals (available in some
herb stores and some pharmacies)
Essential oil of wintergreen
Enough olive oil or other high-quality vegetable oil to completely
submerse herbs. Top off with another inch or two of oil.

To Make:

Wilt the fresh leaves or use dried herbs. Cover with enough oil to completely submerse the herbs, plus one to two inches more. Follow any of the instructions listed above for making medicinal oils. Strain. Add the camphor oil and enough wintergreen oil to give it a strong pungent odor.

PREGNANT BELLY OIL

½ cup coconut oil
½ cup cocoa butter
1 cup almond oil
¼ ounce roses

¼ ounce lavender
¼ ounce chamomile
Essential oil of lavender

To Make:

Warm the oils together until thoroughly melted. Let herbs macerate in the oil over a very low heat for about one hour. Strain the herbs from the oil while still warm. Add enough essential oil of lavender to scent. 10,000 I.U. of vitamin E oil may also be added. Vitamin E may be purchased in capsules of 1,000 I.U. each. Prick with a pin and squeeze out the oil. You can also purchase liquid vitamin E with the percentage of the vitamin it contains.

Salves and Ointments

The pharmacy shelves are lined with salves and ointments. Many of the most famous of these contain herbs: Vick's Vapor Rub, Bag Balm, and Tiger Balm. Do you remember Bag Balm; that marvelous ointment that's still sold in the original spring green can with a big milking holstein cow on it? Some of the older commercial preparations are among the best ointments you can buy because they still contain many natural products. But no matter how excellent, none will compare with the herbal salves you can make quickly and inexpensively at home. Things mass-made, those things manufactured by machines, are devoid of heart and lack the healing touch that only the hands and heart of the living can instill.

Once you've successfully made a medicinal herbal oil, you are only one step away from a salve. Salves, ointments, and balms (all names for the same basic preparation) are comprised of wax, herbs, and vegetable or animal oils. The oil is used as the solvent, a substance that extracts the medicinal properties of the herbs, and provides a healing, emollient base. The wax gives firmness to the salve. The herbs provide the healing medicinal properties.

Easier than making cookies and just about as fun, salves are deeply rewarding to create. They require little time and the finished product looks so professional and works so effectively that many people have been inspired to start small businesses with their favorite salve recipes.

The Basic Recipe for Salves and Ointments

Step 1 · Prepare a medicinal oil following any one of the methods given on pages 50–1.

Step 2 · Strain the oil. To each cup of herbal oil, add one-fourth cup beeswax. Heat the oil and beeswax together over very low heat until the beeswax is completely melted. Check for proper firmness by placing one tablespoon of the mixture in the freezer for just a minute or two. Test the firmness and adjust if necessary. If you wish a harder salve, add more beeswax. If you wish a softer salve, add more oil.

Step 3 · When you are satisfied with the consistency, remove the salve mixture from heat and immediately pour into small glass jars or tins.

Store any extra salve in a cool dark place. Stored properly, salves will last for months, even years. Some people recommend adding natural preservatives to the mixture (for instance, vitamin E or tincture of benzoin) but I've never found them necessary or particularly effective. Salves kept in cars or in the hot sun will lose their properties after a short length of time. You will notice the color looks faded and it will smell rancid. But that happens even with the addition of so-called preservatives.

Some of My All-Time Favorite Salve Recipes

ST. JOHN'S WORT SALVE

This is an excellent, all-purpose salve that is especially beneficial for rashes, cuts, wounds, and diaper rash. I first made this salve back in 1974 and was so pleased with the results that I have been making it ever since. I still haven't found another formula more effective as an all-purpose salve.

1 part St. Johns wort flower　　　　1 part calendula flowers
1 part comfrey leaf

To Make:
Follow the instructions for making oil (pages 50–1) and salve (page 55).

GOLDENSEAL SALVE

This salve is excellent when an astringent, disinfectant action is needed. It serves both as an emollient and a disinfectant.

1 part goldenseal　　　　　　1 part echinacea
1 part myrrh gum

To Make:
Follow the instructions for making oil (pages 50–1) and salve (page 55).

comfrey

ANTIFUNGAL SALVE

I have used this salve successfully for athletes foot, fungus infections, and for mange on animals.

2 parts chaparral　　　　　　1 part myrrh
2 parts black walnut hulls　　　1 part echinacea
1 part goldenseal
A few drops of essential oil of cajeput or tea tree oil

To Make:
Follow the instructions for making oil (pages 50–1) and salve (page 55).

SEVEN

How to Make Herbal Pills and Capsules

Herbal Pills

Herbal pills are simple and practical to make. You can formulate your own formulas for individual problems and make them taste so good that even children will eat them. Made with herbs that are especially good for sore, irritated throats, homemade pills can be formulated to taste good enough to suck on, keeping the medicine in the mouth where it belongs. Depending on your technique, these little pill balls can look quite professional. I've had students who can roll perfectly round, tiny little balls. Mine start off as perfectly round little balls but get larger and larger as the rolling goes on. Eventually, I make one big wad and store it in a glass jar in the refrigerator, telling people to roll their own as needed! You'll develop your own technique as you roll your balls and observe some interesting things about yourself in the process.

Step 1 • Place powdered herbs (see recipe below) in a bowl and moisten with enough water and honey (or maple syrup) to make a sticky paste.

Step 2 • Add a tiny drop of an essential oil, such as peppermint or wintergreen, to the mixture and mix in well. Too much essential oil will ruin the recipe, so be conservative.

Step 3 • Thicken with additional slippery elm or comfrey root powder. Add enough of these herbs to form into a nice smooth paste. Knead until the mixture is the consistency of bread dough.

Step 4 • Roll into small balls the size of pills. You can roll them again in carob or slippery elm powder for a nice finished look.

Step 5 • Place on a cookie sheet and dry in a very low oven (the pilot light will work) for several hours, or sun dry for a day. These pills, once dried, do not need to be refrigerated and will last indefinitely. If you choose not to dry them, they must be stored in the refrigerator.

Sample Herbal Pill Recipe

THROAT BALLS

These are excellent for a sore and/or strep throat

1 part licorice root powder   ½ part echinacea powder
1 part comfrey root powder   ⅛ part goldenseal powder
1 part slippery elm powder

Adjust flavors to suit your taste.

Herbal Capsules

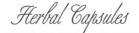

Capsules are a popular way to take herbal medicine. An herbal capsule seems non-threatening and innocuous. However, though herbal capsules have some advantages and are certainly easy to administer, they are not always the best form for taking herbal medicine. In order for the medicine in the capsule to be utilized, it must first enter the digestive tract, where it is acted upon by digestive enzymes before being distributed throughout the body. If the digestive process is not working efficiently, which is often the case when one is ill, the action of the medicine may be delayed or inefficiently used by the body. Herbs in liquid form, such as tinctures and teas, enter the bloodstream quickly and are more efficiently used by the system. The advantages of herb capsules are that they are easy, quick, and tasteless. Also, people are familiar with medicine in this format and are often more willing to take their herbs in capsulated form rather than as teas or tinctures.

Encapsulating herbs is a delightful, rather mediative process. And, like the other processes of herbal medicine making, it is quite simple. Though you can easily encapsulate herbs by hand, there are wonderful little home encapsulating machines available now that are inexpensive and very efficient. My favorite is the Capsule Machine, made by Pure Planet Products, 3635 N. 68th Street, Scottsdale, Arizona 85251.

The herbs must be finely powdered to encapsulate well. You can purchase them already powdered or powder your own in a coffee or seed-and-nut grinder. Empty gelatin capsules, which are used for encapsulating the powdered herbs, can be purchased at pharmacies and natural food and herb stores. They come in a variety of sizes, from tiny, baby-size capsules to giant horse-size capsules. The size generally used for adults (and used in most encapsulating machines) is "00." Two "00" size capsules are considered a standard adult dose. It takes approximately one ounce of powdered herb to fill thirty "00" capsules. Each "00" capsule holds about one-half teaspoon of powdered herb. For years, the only capsules available were made from gelatin, a by-product of the meat industry. But nongelatin capsules are now available in most natural food and herb stores. They are made from plant cellulose and are an excellent alternative for vegetarians.

When encapsulating herbs with a strong physiological action, such as cayenne or goldenseal, it is always best to formulate the active herb with other, less potent herbs. The addition of such herbs as slippery elm, marshmallow root, and comfrey root can serve both to enhance the formula and to temper or buffer the effects of the stronger herbs.

There are really only two steps to encapsulating herbs by hand. (If using an encapsulating machine, you simply follow the directions that come with it.)

Step 1 • Powder the herbs and mix together well.
Step 2 • Open the capsule and fill both ends with the powdered herbs. Stick the capsule back together.

I always work over a small shallow dish. This makes the capsulating go quickly and eliminates spillage. Make sure your hands are completely dry when working with capsules, as any moisture will make them stick together. Store capsules in glass jars away from heat and moisture. Moisture will ruin the capsules.

EIGHT

Syrups

Syrups are the most yummy of all herbal preparations. Because they are sweet, children often prefer their medicine in this form and for those people who are unfamiliar with the bitter taste of medicinal herbs, syrups prove a good introduction to the world of herbal medicine. Though syrups are great tonics and are excellent for sore throats, coughs, and digestive problems, they are not the medicine of choice for all health problems. It requires a lot of cooking and a lot of sweetener to make an herbal syrup. Both cooking and sweetening tend to disturb the medicinal action of most herbs. However, syrups do have their place on the medicine shelf and are quite fun to make. This is my favorite method for making syrup:

Step 1 · Use two ounces of herb mixture (see sample recipes, pages 61–62) to one quart of water. Over low heat, simmer the liquid down to one pint. This will give you a very concentrated, thick tea.

Step 2 · Strain the herbs from the liquid. Compost the herbs and pour the liquid back into the pot.

Step 3 · To each pint of liquid, add one cup of honey (or other sweetener such as maple syrup, brown or white sugar). Most recipes call for two cups of sweetener per pint of liquid (a one:one ratio of sweetener to liquid). Sugar was added in such large quantities in the days before refrigeration to help preserve the syrup. Though this does aid in preserving the syrup, I find it much too sweet for my taste. Since most people these days do have refrigerators, I generally suggest adding less sweetener.

Step 4 · Warm the honey and liquid together to mix well. Most recipes suggest cooking the honey and tea together for twenty to thirty minutes longer over high heat to thicken further. It does certainly make a thicker syrup, but I'd rather not cook the living enzymes out of the honey so I suggest warming them only enough to mix them well.

Step 5 · When finished heating, you may wish to add:

Brandy for flavor, to preserve, and for its relaxant properties. Brandy is also excellent to add to cough syrups because it does relax the throat muscles and calms spastic coughing. An appropriate amount would be three to four tablespoons per cup. A good-tasting fruit brandy adds a pleasant flavor as well.

A few drops of an essential oil such as peppermint, wintergreen, or spearmint. The essential oils add a refreshing flavor and additional medicinal properties.

A fruit concentrate for flavor and for added vitamins and minerals.

Step 6 · Remove the syrup from the heat and bottle for use. Syrups will last for several weeks, even months, if refrigerated. In the olden days when refrigeration wasn't available, a higher percentage of sugar/honey was used because it helped to preserve the syrup. Alcohol was often added both for its preservative properties and for its relaxant qualities.

A couple of years ago, one of the big wild cherry trees that grow abundantly on our land was blown down in one of those infamous New England windstorms. Though I was sad to experience the death of such a beautiful old tree, I was delighted with the amount of cherry bark I was able to strip off her old limbs. I spent an afternoon singing to myself in the woods and working those lengths of inner bark into three- and four-inch strips. I collected enough wild cherry bark to last several seasons and promptly cooked a large portion of it into a sweet, delicious syrup. It's been an effective cough medicine for two winters worth of coughs and colds. Wild cherry bark is still a widely used herb in current U.S. pharmacopeias and is found in several cough formulas.

Sample Herbal Syrup Recipes

COUGH AND SORE THROAT SYRUP

2 parts slippery elm bark
2 parts valerian
2 parts comfrey root
1 part wild cherry bark
2 parts licorice root

1 part ginger root
1 part cinnamon bark
4 parts fennel seeds
⅛ part orange peel

To Make:
Follow the directions for making syrup (page 60).

HOPS/VALERIAN COUGH SYRUP

This is an excellent syrup for spasmodic, dry coughs. Because valerian loses much of its effectiveness when decocted, prepare the other herbs first. When finished decocting, add the valerian to the liquid and let the tea sit overnight.

1 part hops
1 part valerian

1 part coltsfoot
1 part comfrey root

To Make:
Prepare a decoction of the coltsfoot, comfrey, and hops. Add the valerian and allow to steep overnight. Follow the instructions for making syrup (page 60).

This is an excellent formula for women of all ages to take for adding easily digestible vitamins and minerals to their diet. Iron-Plus is high in iron, calcium, vitamin A, and a host of trace minerals. With the addition of concentrated fruit extracts and sweetener, it is a tasty liquid vitamin/mineral supplement.

3 parts nettle

3 parts dandelion leaf

3 parts dandelion root

3 parts raspberry leaf

2 parts watercress

2 parts alfalfa leaf

1 part hawthorn berries

1 part yellow dock root

1 part dulse

¼ part horsetail

To Make:

Follow Steps 1–4 listed above for making syrup (page 60). After removing from heat, stir in two teaspoons of spirulina powder and two teaspoons of nutritional yeast for each pint of syrup you've made. Add one-fourth cup brandy and one-fourth cup fruit concentrate. Fruit concentrates, available at natural food stores, are concentrated extracts of fresh fruit and add additional vitamins and minerals as well as a delicious fruity flavor. Do not add juice, as it will dilute the syrup and encourage possible fermentation. The suggested dosage of iron-plus syrup is four to six tablespoons daily.

How to Make Herbal Tinctures and Liniments

The most popular form of herbal medication available today, tinctures are highly concentrated liquid extracts of herbs that are easy to prepare, simple to administer, and have a prolonged shelf life. They are perfectly adapted to the busy life-styles of modern herbal enthusiasts.

The Advantages of Tinctures

❦ **Longevity and Stability** Once tinctured, an herb will retain its medicinal properties far longer than most other preparations. Alcohol tinctures will last for many years. Tinctures made from vinegar have a shorter shelf life.

❦ **Ease of Storage** Unlike bulky raw botanicals, tinctures store compactly. They are excellent for car first-aid kits and for traveling. They also fit compactly into the standard metal medicine chest found in most American bathrooms.

❦ **Ease of Administering** Once made, tinctures are ready to administer with no further preparation. The tinctures are dispensed directly under the tongue or mixed with warm water, tea, or juice. They are very helpful when a person is very ill with an acute illness such as a flu or fever. It takes much less effort to take a few drops of tincture than it does to get up and make a pot of tea.

❦ **Ease of Preparation** Anyone is capable of making high-quality tinctures. There is no mystery or complicated process involved in preparing them. What is required is good-quality herbs, a high-quality solvent, a measuring cup, and a little time.

❦ **Cost Efficiency** Though tinctures are fairly expensive to purchase (you are paying for the quality time and expertise of the herbalist and wildcrafter who collected the herbs), they are relatively inexpensive to make yourself. If you need to take a tincture over a long period of time for a chronic situation or as a tonic, you should consider making your own. Commercially prepared bottles of tinctures can get quite costly.

Selecting the Herb(s)

Almost all herbs tincture well with the correct mixture of alcohol and water. Herbs can be tinctured as a ready-made formula comprised of two or more herbs, or tinctured as single herbs and combined later into formulas. Most herbalists prefer to tincture herbs as single extracts. This allows control of the water/alcohol ratio for individual herbs and their constituents. It also allows them greater flexibility when creating formulas from single-herb extracts. Though I appreciate the reasoning behind single-herb extracts, I prefer tincturing my formulas together. I find there is a union, a fusion as it were, that happens as the herbs macerate and merge together. Instead of being single components, they become one, and thus enhance the effects of one another. But there really is no single right way. Experiment and discover which method you like best. Or use them both.

Selecting the Menstruum

The menstruum is the solvent, or liquid substance, used to extract the chemical constituents of the herbs. There are basically three menstruums commonly used in tincture preparation: alcohol, glycerin, and vinegar. As with any approach, there are pros and cons to each.

Alcohol As a Menstruum

Alcohol is a potent, effective menstruum that extracts fats, resins, waxes, most alkaloids, and some of the volatile oils, as well as many other plant components. Furthermore, alcohol serves as an excellent preservative, maintaining the integrity of the herb for many years. Alcohol tinctures are rapidly assimilated by the body and their effects are quickly felt.

When using alcohol, water is a necessary component of the menstruum because both solvents are needed to extract the different plant chemicals. The ratio of water to alcohol determines the actual menstruum. This alcohol/water ratio is either included within the actual alcohol content or is added to the alcohol, depending on the type of alcohol being used. A standard menstruum is one part alcohol to one part water, though this varies depending on the herbs being used and whether the herbs are fresh or dried. Any good 100-proof alcohol naturally supplies this ratio without you having to do anything, because it is 50 percent alcohol and 50 percent water. "Proof" represents the alcohol/water ratio in the alcoholic beverage and is represented as twice the percentage of alcohol. An 80-proof brandy is composed of 40 percent alcohol and 60 percent water. However, if you use a pure grain alcohol (190 proof) the actual water content is low—5 percent—while the alcohol content is very high—95 percent. Water would have to be added to the menstruum in this case in order that the water-soluble substances in the herbs can be extracted.

There are several kinds of alcohol used for tincture making. Brandy, vodka, and gin are favorites because each can be purchased as 80–100 proof. For preservative properties and extraction purposes, you must use at least 25 percent alcohol (50 proof) by volume. Wine is unacceptable for tincture making because of its low alcohol content, though you can make delicious herbal wines. When making tinctures, don't scrimp on quality; buy the best alcohol you're able to afford.

Glycerin As a Menstruum

Glycerin is a sweet, mucilaginous constituent of all fats and oils of both animal and plant origin. A highly nutritious substance, glycerin is very sweet, sweeter than sugar. Because of the sweet flavor and because it does not contain alcohol, it is especially useful in making tinctures for children. Alcoholics and other people averse to drinking alcohol also find glycerin a good menstruum for tincture making. It is considered somewhere between alcohol and water in its potency as a solvent. Though it has good preservative properties and dissolves mucilage material, vitamins and minerals, it does not dissolve resinous or oily plant constituents.

Glycerin is sold in natural food stores and herb shops. Be certain to use only pure 100 percent vegetable glycerin. Not only is the quality higher, but glycerin made from animal fat is usually intended for cosmetic purposes and not for human consumption.

Different ratios of glycerin to water are used in the menstruum. I have heard herbalists recommend anywhere from one part glycerin to four parts water to a one:one ratio. As you can see, there is lots of room for flexibility. I prefer a glycerin tincture using two parts glycerin to one part water (a two:one ratio). The amount of herb remains the same and the preparation is the same as that described below.

Vinegar As a Menstruum

Though alcohol is the menstruum of choice these days because of its potency and effectiveness, vinegar is also a suitable menstruum and may be preferable in certain situations. Though it is not as potent a solvent as alcohol and does not break down the plant constituents as efficiently, there are advantages to using vinegar. Vinegar is 100 percent nontoxic and can be tolerated by almost everyone. It helps regulate the acid/alkaline balance in our bodies and is an excellent tonic for the digestive tract. It also tastes good and can be used as a food. Vinegar tinctures are a fine alternative for alcohol-sensitive people and can be used for children, alcoholics, and others averse to drinking alcohol.

I recommend using vinegar as a menstruum for *tonic* tinctures, those tinctures that are to be used over a long period of time to strengthen and build the system. Vinegar is preferred as a base for tonic formulas that become part of our diet and daily fare. When possible, select organic apple cider vinegar. Add a little honey to the formula and it tastes delicious—almost like a tasty salad dressing. You can use vinegar tinctures with your vegetables and salads or sip a small amount just by itself. Though vinegar tinctures may not be as concentrated as alcoholic tinctures, the body has an inherent ability to discern what it needs in food and to use it efficiently.

For a stronger medicinal tincture, alcohol is a more effective menstruum. Alcohol tinctures are extremely potent and quick-acting in the body. But for tonic formulas, vinegar is the menstruum of choice. Vinegar draws out many of the plant constituents and is especially valuable for extracting alkaloids, vitamins and minerals. Because vinegar is acidic, it is not an effective menstruum for plant acids.

There is some controversy as to the shelf life of vinegar tinctures. Most literature reports that vinegar tinctures have a short shelf life, six to eight months, then quickly begin to deteriorate. My personal experience and that of many other practicing herbalists is that vinegar tinctures, if stored in a cool dark place, last for many years. I have vinegar tinctures that are two, three, and four years old and are still very viable.

My friend, Cascade Anderson Geller, who taught the botanical medicine courses at the National College of Naturopathic Medicine for many years, says that vinegar tinctures last indefinitely so long as 100 percent vinegar is used (5–7 percent acetic acid). She has experimental jars of vinegar tinctures that are ten years old. But if even a small amount of H_2O is added, or if the fresh herbs used are too moist, fermentation problems will result.

How to Make Tinctures in the Traditional Method

There are basically two methods used for making tinctures. One, the standard method, involves lots of calculations, math, measuring cups, scales, and so forth. You spend about as much time doing math as making the tincture and the end product is basically the same as the simpler's or traditional method. Needless to say, the traditional method of tincture making is what I prefer. Over hundreds of years, the kinks have been worked out of this method, and the result is an extremely simple and unfussy system. All you need to make a tincture in the traditional method is the herbs, the menstruum, and a jar with a tight-fitting lid.

Step 1 · Chop your herbs finely. I recommend using fresh herbs whenever possible. High-quality dried herbs will work well also, but one of the advantages of tincturing is the ability to preserve the fresh attributes of the plant. Place the herbs in a clean, dry jar.

Step 2 · Pour the menstruum over the herbs. *Completely cover* the herbs with the menstruum and then add an additional two to three inches more liquid. The herbs need to be totally submersed by the menstruum. I like to leave a couple of extra inches of liquid above the herbs. This allows room for the herbs to swell as they soak up the liquid. If the herbs do swell and start to emerge above the liquid, just add more menstruum. Cover with a tight-fitting lid. If using vinegar as the menstruum, warm the vinegar first before pouring it over the herbs to facilitate the release of herbal constituents.

Step 3 · Place the jar(s) in a warm, dark place and let the herbs and liquid soak (macerate) for four to six weeks. In Western herbology the suggested time to allow the tinctures to macerate is two weeks. In Chinese herbology and several other more indigenous traditions, herbs are left to macerate for months, even years. I have found that the longer the herb is allowed to tincture, the better. I like to let them steep for at least six weeks.

Step 4 · I encourage the daily shaking of the bottles of tinctures during the maceration period. This not only prevents the herbs from packing down on the bottom of the jar, but is also an invitation for some of the old magic to come back into medicine making. During the shaking process, you can sing to your tincture jars, stir them in the moonlight or the sunlight, wave feathers over them—whatever your imagination inspires you to do. It adds a special magic to your preparations (and lets your neighbors know that you really are crazy).

Step 5 · At the end of the appropriate length of maceration time, strain the herb(s) from the menstruum. Use a large stainless-steel strainer lined with cheesecloth or muslin. A potato ricer works very well for straining the herbs also, but it, too, must be lined with fine cheesecloth or muslin. Use the cloth to wring out every drop of herbal essence. Reserve the liquid, which is now a strong potent tincture, and compost the herbs. Rebottle and label.

Storage

Store your finished tinctures in a cool, dark closet and/or in dark amber bottles. They should be kept away from light and heat. You may wish to keep a small supply of the tincture ready for use in a one- or two-ounce dropper bottle (available from natural food stores and pharmacies). The remainder of your tincture can be stored in larger jars. Often, in their enthusiasm for making tinctures and because the process is so easy, people go overboard and make gallons of tinctures. Remember, tinctures are concentrated extracts; a little goes a long way. It's better not to make too much of any one kind. Usually a pint is a sufficient amount of any one tincture, unless it is a particular formula you will be using often.

Dosage

The dosage of tinctures varies and is really dependent on the individual herb/formula being administered and the size/condition of the person being treated. Often, I've noticed, the dosage recommended on a bottle of tincture ranges from as much to fifteen to sixty drops. This doesn't help the person who knows nothing about herbs and is used to a prescription that very clearly states "one pill three times daily." The wide range suggested for tinctures wisely takes into account the vast differences in individuals as well as the nature of the disease, but may be confusing to the novice. Usually, you will find it safe to use one-fourth to one-half teaspoon of tincture three times daily for chronic imbalances. For acute situations use one-eighth to one-fourth teaspoon every hour or two. It is best to begin with a smaller amount and to increase the dosage as necessary.

Tinctures can be administered directly under the tongue or diluted in water, tea, or juice. If you are using an alcoholic tincture, and prefer not to have the alcohol, add the tincture to boiling water. Remove the water from the heat source and let it sit for five to six minutes uncovered. Alcohol evaporates rapidly in high temperatures, leaving only the herbal essence in the water.

Herbal Liniments

A liniment is an external application that is rubbed into the skin. Liniments are generally used as disinfectants and/or for soothing strained muscles and ligaments. There are many recipes for making various types of liniments. Either oil, alcohol, or vinegar can be chosen as the menstruum. Essential oils are often added to the liniment to increase its potency. My very favorite recipe (see below) is for a liniment that is both an excellent disinfectant and an excellent treatment for tired, strained muscles.

Liniments are made *exactly* the same as herbal tinctures. However, a liniment is for *external* purposes only, while tinctures are chiefly for internal purposes. Be sure to label your liniments "For External Use Only" if using a solvent that is inedible.

Liniments are excellent for disinfecting wounds and cuts. My all-time favorite liniment is one that's been passed down from the famous herb doctor, Jethro Kloss. I have made and used this liniment for over twenty years and find it the very best disinfectant for external use. It is also excellent for poison oak and ivy, though you may wish to dilute it, as it will sting. It also helps heal wounds and infections in animals, though it should always be diluted when used to treat them. This liniment is very simple and inexpensive to make and is a valuable herbal preparation to have on hand.

GOLDENSEAL/MYRRH LINIMENT

1 ounce goldenseal powder   ¼ ounce cayenne powder
1 ounce echinacea powder   1 pint rubbing alcohol
1 ounce myrrh powder

To Make:
Follow the instructions for making a tincture (pages 66–67).

The Herbal Medicine Chest

It's a wonderful feeling to stock your medicine chest with herbal products you have made yourself. And it's such a good feeling to know you're helping carry on an ancient tradition of healing. As I mentioned earlier, making products may not be your forte, but give it a try at least; you may get hooked and become a lifelong medicine maker. Because each of these herbal products is simple and easy to make, success in your medicine-making career is almost guaranteed. If, however, you have neither the time nor the desire to make herbal products, most natural food and herb stores carry an excellent selection of herb products, many of which are made by small companies using the same methods described above. (See Appendix II for resources.)

Whether your products are made by your hands or someone else's, find a suitable place in your home to store them. The traditional medicine chest found in the bathroom of most homes is a wonderful place. Take out the outdated bottles of pills, the old ointments, and the half-used syrups and replace them with your herbal medicines. They will be in place and available when you need them. Sewing baskets and fishing-tackle boxes also make good storage containers. Or if you're lucky enough to have an empty closet or shelf in your home, you can start your own herbal pantry. The idea is to organize your herbal products so that they are available for use whenever you need them.

Though jars of herbs and herbal products look quaint in sunny windows, herbs store best in a cool, shaded area. Remember, heat, light and air will deplete the quality of herbal products rapidly. Take this fact into account when choosing a place to store your products. It is not necessary to store herb products in the refrigerator, but if you do have extra space in your fridge, salves, and oils will last longer there.

A good herbal medicine chest includes one or two salves, a disinfectant liniment, a liniment for sore muscles, a syrup for coughs and sore throats, and several tinctures for different medicinal purposes. The tinctures you choose to have in your medicine chest will vary, depending on the health issues you and your family deal with most frequently. I generally recommend a tincture for stress, a formula for colds and flus, and an immune stimulant formula to help ward off infections. There are also several excellent formulas found throughout this book that are recommended for specific women's problems. These formulas can be tinctured and stored in your first-aid kit for use as needed. A nice selection of herbs will round out your first-aid supplies.

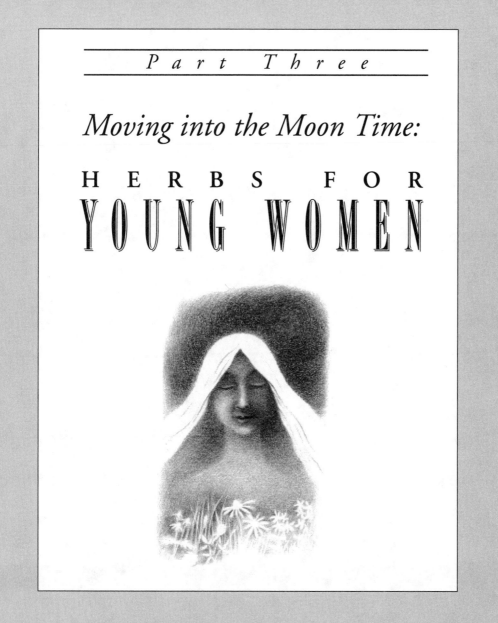

Part Three

Moving into the Moon Time:

HERBS FOR YOUNG WOMEN

ELEVEN
New Beginnings

I have a vision of the Earth made green again through the efforts of children. I can see children of all nations planting trees and holding hands around the globe in celebration of the Earth as their home and all children, all people as their family.

—R. St. Barbe Baker

At an early age we learn from our culture that, at best, our menstrual cycles are just a messy interference in our daily lives. There is little joy or wonder expressed at the onset of the first spots of blood that initiate girls into the powerful stages of womanhood. Instead, young women often encounter their first menstrual flow with fear and apprehension. Though these feelings are normal, healthy responses to the new phenomenon occurring in a young woman's life, they are seldom balanced by positive reactions and the support of family and friends.

My mother was a beautiful countrywoman and had a powerful influence on me when I was growing up. She was strong—alive with the warmth of a fire burning deep inside her. She had birthed five children, worked hard, laughed easily, and loved my father dearly. Certainly she was not ignorant of the cycles of a woman's life. Yet, my introduction to my first menstruation lacked any depth of understanding. That I was making the first dramatic shift into the cycle of womanhood was never mentioned. Like most young women, I was ill-prepared to handle the changes that seemed to happen almost overnight in my body, mind, and spirit. Handing me a box of Kotex, my mother seemed a little embarrassed, a little pleased. She asked me if I knew how to use them. I, of course, answered yes, not caring that I didn't. And so I was launched into my menarche years, the major life cycle of my womanhood, the life cycle that would occupy most of my adult years.

I thought little about this odd introduction, or lack of it, until many years later. By the time it occurred to me what an odd and incomplete introduction it had been, I had already been experiencing my moon cycle for many seasons and had weathered the "normal" patterns of menstrual pain and discomfort. I had experienced heavy bleeding from a short and unsuccessful bout with an IUD, had had a severe PID infection after giving birth to my son, and had suffered a "normal" amount of cramping and irregular menstrual cycles. Though once in a while I felt concern about the amount of clotting and bleeding that sometimes accompanied my moon cycles, I didn't think any of this differed from the "norm." Like most young woman, I had never really learned what the "norm" was.

In 1978 I began organizing women's Healing Ways retreats in Northern California. These were large, heartwarming gatherings that sparked a holy fire and carried our women spirits high. Many well-known teachers would come and share healing techniques for women. One year a close friend and fellow herbalist, Jeannine Parvati Baker, offered a workshop in "Women's Moon Time." It opened my eyes to menstruation in ways I had never been taught in sex education class and changed my entire view of this cycle of womanhood. It also made me painfully aware of how ill-prepared young women in our culture are to enter their moon time.

Jeannine spoke very little during the entire three-hour workshop. Instead she had the participants sit in a circle and pass around a speaking stick, a long, gracefully carved piece of wood that granted each woman in turn a chance to talk without interruption. It was a large circle of well over fifty women. As the stick passed from woman to woman, each shared her story of her first moon cycle. What teachings flowed from these women! It was a marvelous sharing of intimacy and secrets, of feelings sequestered in the moon time energy of each of us.

One beautiful young Italian woman told of how she was staying with her grandmother near the beach. She had ridden her bike down to the water and was playing in the sand when she first started to bleed. The bright blood stared up at her from where it pooled in the very white sand. Having never been told about menstruation, she concluded she was bleeding to death. She frantically rode her bike the long distance back to her grandmother's, thinking all the while that she wouldn't make it before all her blood was gone. Fortunately, her grandmother was very sensitive and supportive.

Another woman told of her anger and frustration at the way her family had treated her at the beginning of her menstrual years. Her tomboy relationship with the neighborhood guys and her wonderful sense of freedom were sternly criticized by her parents, and especially by her father. At the onset of her moon time, she was no longer allowed to play randomly with her buddies, the neighborhood boys. A stricter curfew was imposed. She felt like she was always being watched. Feeling like a jailed princess, she deeply resented the restrictions she believed were caused by her moon time.

Though there are women whose memory of their first moon cycle is of an exciting and memorable event, they are by far in the minority. For most women the first menstrual cycle is an awkward and embarrassing time, made worse by the dramatic hormonal shift of adolescence. Negative preconditioning ensures that the onset of the menstrual cycle in young women is often met with physical and emotional discomfort. There is little positive feedback for the contemporary adolescent and little information available about how to make this important transition smoothly.

Often a young woman's body is not prepared to handle the added stress that dramatic hormonal changes are demanding. In one short month they metamorphose from girls to women. Overnight they enter the realm of fertility. They can become pregnant and be mothers. It is a memory instilled in the genetic encoding of our beings. We have changed. Though mostly unaware of these changes, they change us.

In other major cycles of a woman's life, such as pregnancy and menopause, there is greater understanding and support for the roles that changing hormones play in the system. Herbs, vitamins, nutrition, and psychological counseling are often recommended to support the woman's system through these times of internal stress. But when a young woman enters puberty, the new hormonal demands on her system receive little attention. For unexplored reasons the physical needs of the young woman are seldom considered.

At the end of the twentieth century, women have come of age and are finding their voices, and the collective voice of women of the "middle years" is often the loudest. After years of enduring menstrual difficulties in silence, their voices are often angry. Women undergoing menopause—women who have been a quiet minority for so long—are also finding their voices and are speaking out. In the last few years they have formed support groups to assist one another in understanding this new stage of womanhood. Books are being written to support the process of the aging woman. But the young woman just entering menarche continues to be ignored. The changes she goes through are hardly recognized by those around her. Her voice is still quiet and shy. Her needs remain unknown. However, until we recognize and honor those needs, we do the ensuing cycles of womanhood a grave injustice.

The biggest single factor in our ease or dis-ease as we enter the early years of our moon time is our society's attitude toward menstruation. We live in a society that still ignores or denies the powerful changes that occur each month in the menstruating woman. Instead, we support the myth of the lady in white, Kotex's tennis star. Dressed in virgin white, our heroine continues to play tennis as if nothing extraordinary is happening. In truth, there are dramatic changes occurring in our menstruating bodies and psyches that are hardly recognized or honored by our society. It is difficult to initiate a rite of passage, the initiation from one cycle to the next, when the society one lives in hardly recognizes that there is a transition at all.

Nonetheless, I have several friends who, very aware of our culture's lack of initiation rites for their daughters, have sought to create their own rituals or rites of passage for them as they entered their moon time. Having no village rituals that are a cultural heritage passed down through generations, these brave mother/daughter teams are attempting to create meaningful ceremonies pertinent to the twentieth century. Most of the time, these celebrations/ceremonies are beautiful as well as meaningful experiences. But sometimes they have proved to be awkward and embarrassing situations for the daughters. Usually this has happened when the mother planned a "surprise" for her daughter, or created a ceremony based on her own desires and needs, not on those of her daughter. A young woman should always be asked if she would like to participate in such a ceremony and be involved in planning the event so that it is tailored to her needs. Often a daughter's initial response is one of horror and self-consciousness that her mother would even think to call attention to this "embarrassing" matter. Her mother should be honest with her and explain why a joyful, celebratory event could change her daughter's entire relationship with her moon time experience. But her mother should be prepared to back down if the young woman chooses not to mark the occasion with a ceremony. Just knowing that her mother regards this as a special moment in her life and will be "there" for her, supporting and encouraging her as she moves into this new phase, will give her something that most young women continue to be denied.

Celebrating the Rites of Moon Time

Following are some simple suggestions that have worked as passages into the moon time for young women. Unlike the elaborate celebrations and feasts of primitive cultures at initiatory rites, these are simple contemporary ceremonies honoring the young women of menarche years.

❧ Invite a *small* group of older women who have known your daughter for several years. Serve a dinner of your daughter's favorite foods. She might like to help plan the menu and prepare the food. After dinner, create a circle and have the guests share stories of their first moon cycle. It is nice if each woman brings a small gift that is symbolic of womanhood. When the circle is completed, toast your daughter with a special lunar tea, following the infusing instructions on page 47. Have each woman guest make a wish for your daughter and drink to her womanhood.

❧ Your daughter and you might have a special moon time ceremony involving just the two of you. You could start by making a special lunar tea. Place it in a fine crystal bowl in full moonlight. You and she might take turns speaking your wishes for her woman-hood. The next morning, the two of you go out together and drink from the crystal, making a toast to your daughter and her life.

❧ Carry out a "Blessing Way" ceremony adapted from Native American traditions. It is lovely to create if your daughter is open for the experience; you can freely adapt it to fit your daughter's needs. Invite a few friends to join you or do it just with your daughter. The rest of the family may be invited if she feels comfortable about including them. It's nice when a young woman's father can be present and even participate in this ceremony. It may be done indoors, but is especially empowering when done in a natural setting.

Begin by washing your daughter's feet. This is a symbolic act of cleansing away old energy and inviting new energy to come in. It is also a way of humbling oneself to an-other. In this ceremony, you are honoring your daughter for her emergence as a woman. When you have finished washing your daughter's feet, anoint them with a scented mas-sage oil. Next, brush her hair and rearrange it in a new style. If your daughter wears her hair down, braid it and weave flowers into it. If she wears her hair up, let it flow loosely. This rearranging of hair is symbolic of the changes she is undergoing and reflects a new beginning. It's fun to use flowers to decorate her hair, or to surprise your daughter with a fancy new hair clip. (If her father is participating, have him be the one to wash and anoint your daughter's feet before you rearrange and decorate her hair.) For the last part of the ceremony, have each person present take a sip of Lunar tea and offer a wish or prayer for the young woman.

TWELVE

The Raging Hormones of Adolescence

One of the major causes of physical discomfort in the early years of menstruation is hormonal imbalance. "Raging hormones" can cause all kinds of havoc, from dysfunctional menstruation to dramatic, uncontrolled mood swings. Acne and other skin problems can also be caused by hormone imbalances. Generally, the cause of the problems is not the total amount of hormones circulating in the system, but rather the abrupt fluctuations in hormone levels and the consequent disruptions in the flow of energy throughout the system.

Just what are hormones and what do they do? Why are they so vitally important to our well-being? Hormones are biochemically diverse substances produced by the endocrine glands. Carried through our system via the bloodstream, they continuously send messages to the other organs, influencing virtually every activity of our body.

The word "hormone" comes from the Greek word "to excite." And all hormones do in fact stimulate the body in one way or another. There are over fifty known hormones produced by the body. Estrogen and progesterone, along with FSH and LH, are the main female sex hormones and are essential to the health of the reproductive system and its monthly cycle.

Estrogen governs the first half, or the follicular phase, of the menstrual cycle. It is produced in the ovaries in various amounts during the entire menstrual cycle and plays a major role in preparing the body for conception. Estrogen is responsible for the growth of the endometrium tissue that forms in the uterus in preparation for a fertilized egg. Estrogen helps relax the blood vessel walls, improving circulation and vascular tone in the genital tract which, in turn, stimulates the secretions of the cervix, creating a more hospitable environment for sperm.

But estrogen's role is not limited to just creating a healthy home for every egg that's delivered from the fallopian tubes. It is also essential in developing the young female fetus into a fully mature woman. From the very beginning of our existence estrogen plays a major role in our development as women. In the absence of the male hormone, testosterone, estrogen helps shape our secondary sex characteristics, giving us the physical characteristics—enlarged breast glands, specific hair patterns, higher voices and broader hips—that distinguish our bodies from those of men.

As well as aiding the circulatory system by relaxing the blood vessel walls, estrogen is important to the skeletal system. It is one of the major factors in helping retain bone calcium, thus reducing the likelihood of osteoporosis. It is also known to have a profound effect on our emotions. During the first half of the menstrual cycle, when estrogen output is highest (and if it is well balanced), many women experience a mild euphoria. A good flow of estrogen in the system stimulates the libido and our zest for life. Not only does estrogen secrete special cervical juices for the sperm to live in, it also stimulates the sensual energy of women and gets our emotional and sexual juices flowing. An estrogen imbalance, on the other hand, can cause a host of problems, such as fibrocystic breast condition, endometriosis, dramatic mood swings, infertility, and painful, cramping menstruation.

Progesterone is the other major sex hormone and governs the second half, or luteal phase, of the menstrual cycle. Progesterone is also produced by the ovaries and serves a vital role in fertility and creation. Its major role in fertility is to prepare for and support pregnancy. In Latin, progesterone means "supporting gestation." If progesterone is lacking in the system, spontaneous abortion can occur within the first few weeks of conception. Low progesterone levels may cause depression, sluggishness, and a feeling of lethargy. Sexual and sensuous energy is often at a low at the height of the progesterone cycle.

Though there are certainly other hormones at play in our reproductive cycles, progesterone and estrogen claim the main stage. The pituitary gland, respectfully called the "master gland," is responsible for the production of FSH and LH, important hormones that stimulate the growth and development of the follicle. The pituitary also secretes prolactin, a hormone that initiates and maintains the flow of breast milk during lactation. Interestingly, prolactin suppresses ovarian function during lactation, and in some instances may decrease fertility during lactation. However, this is not a foolproof method of birth control—as has been proven many times!

Healthy hormonal activity is dependent on both the liver, which provides the precursors or building blocks needed for the production of hormones, and the enigmatic endocrine system. In Eastern practices such as yoga, the endocrine glands are called chakras and are considered to be the major energy centers of the body. A group of small glands situated in prime areas throughout the body, the endocrine glands secrete minute but powerful hormones. Each of the endocrine glands works in close relationship with the others. Any alteration in the chemical patterns of one gland will affect others throughout the system. The endocrine glands play a major though little understood role in the transitional periods of womanhood.

For the young woman, nourishing and strengthening the endocrine glands ensures an easier transition into the menstrual years. When the endocrine glands are healthy and well nourished, many of the so-called symptoms of adolescence are eliminated or lessened. Painful, cramping menstruation, heavy bleeding, irregular cycles, and teenage acne can often be completely eradicated.

The liver also plays a major role in hormone balance. Many of the sex-related hormones are produced directly by the liver. Hormones produced elsewhere rely on hormonal precursors, the necessary building blocks of the hormones manufactured by the liver. When the hormones are balanced properly and supplied in sufficient amounts, many of the problems associated with menstruation can be eliminated.

Often referred to as the master detoxifier, the liver is also responsible for removing toxic substances from our bloodstream. Toxins produced as a result of our own metabolism and those absorbed environmentally are successfully removed from the bloodstream by a well-functioning liver. However, if the liver is not functioning up to par, these substances circulate longer in the system, causing all manner of imbalances, including painful, irregular menstruation, heavy bleeding, low energy, acne, allergies, digestive disturbances and general poor health.

For young women just entering their moon time, both a healthy liver and endocrine system are imperative for an easier transition into womanhood. Their good health ensures a smooth, regular menstrual flow, acne-free skin, and a radiant, vital flow of energy. Erratic mood swings are generally far less noticeable as well.

Herbs for the Liver and Endocrine Glands

The following list of herbs are those that are generally used for strengthening both the liver and the endocrine gland systems. All of these herbs are safe to use, producing no known toxicity or side effects, and are readily available in most herb stores. (See Appendix II for a list of sources of high-quality herbs.)

Astragalus (Astragalus membranaceous) Astragalus is an herb from China and, though not specifically indicated for liver and endocrine imbalances, is such a wonderful tonic herb for the entire system that I feel it appropriate to include it here. Astragalus builds and strengthens the entire system and gives energy to the internal organs. It is used for wasting diseases, for strengthening the immune system, and for improving digestion and the assimilation of nutrients. A valuable tonic herb, it is especially recommended for those under thirty-five. Astragalus is pleasant tasting and can be used daily in tea or tincture form. In China, it is often cooked in soup or served with vegetables and grains to improve the health of the entire family.

Burdock root (Arctium lappa) Burdock is a nourishing herb, excellent for building and strengthening the entire system of young women. It is high in a variety of minerals, especially iron, thus enriching the life force of the blood. It is specifically recommended as a tonic and a cleansing herb for the liver and the lymph system. Burdock is also useful for all skin problems and often clears persistent teenage acne if taken regularly for three to four weeks. It is slightly bitter, but the flavor is easily masked with sweet-tasting herbs like licorice and fennel seed. Burdock is often combined with dandelion root as a liver cleanser and endocrine tonic tea. It is completely nontoxic and is frequently served as a food *(gobo)* throughout the Orient.

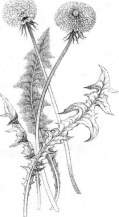

Dandelion root (Taraxaeum officinale) Both the root and the leaf of this plant are excellent for young women. But the root is considered one of the

Dandelion

"herbs supreme" for the liver. It both detoxifies and nourishes this important organ. Though dandelion root is powerful in its action, it is both safe and gentle. Used as a tea for several weeks, it will help cleanse and stimulate the liver. It aids in digestion, has an excellent reputation for clearing skin problems, and acts as a tonic on the endocrine glands. Because it has a bitter taste, it is more palatable when mixed with pleasant-tasting herbs such as licorice, ginger, sassafras, and sarsaparilla. This combination of herbs makes a root beer–like tea that is both nourishing and tasty. (See Materia Medica for more information.)

Licorice root (Glycyrrhiza globra) This is one of the primary herbs used as an endocrine gland tonic. It contains chemical substances that are similar to adrenal cortical hormones and is beneficial for adrenal deficiency and other glandular imbalances. Licorice also contains estrogenic and other steroidal properties and is used to regulate and normalize hormone production. It is commonly included in formulas for women. Both as a tonic and a detoxifier, it is an excellent herb for the liver. Sweet in taste, licorice helps to mask the flavors of more bitter herbs and is often included in formulas to soften the medicinal tastes. It is not recommended for those suffering from hypertension and high blood pressure. (See Materia Medica for more information.)

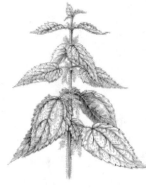

nettle

Nettle leaf (Urtica urens, U. diocia and related species) I consider this one of the best liver and blood tonics for young women. It is a powerfully effective herb, yet completely benign, and can be used over an extended period of time. In many cultures nettle is considered a delicious and wholesome food. It is extremely high in minerals, especially in iron and calcium, and thus enriches the blood and nourishes the nervous system. Young women especially benefit from its blood-enriching properties. It is also an excellent cleanser and aids the liver in its functions. Its mild diuretic properties are helpful for young women who experience bloating and/or dramatic mood swings during the menstrual cycle. It is an excellent endocrine-gland tonic and is used both as a cleanser and as a nourisher. Nettle has a rather "green" taste that most teenagers don't find particularly good. The flavor is easily improved with peppermint, spearmint, lemon balm and/or lemon verbena. (See Materia Medica for more information.)

Oregon grape root (Mahonia repens and Berberis aquifolium) This lovely holly-like plant is found growing throughout the Pacific Northwest and is considered the West Coast counterpart of goldenseal and bayberry, both of which grow on the East Coast. It is an excellent herb for the liver and is used for liver congestion and sluggishness. It stimulates bile production, thus enhancing the entire function of the liver. It is a primary herb used to aid the digestion of fats and oils and is useful in weight-loss plans when a sluggish system is suspected. Combined with dandelion root, it is an excellent herb for skin disorders and is helpful for teenage acne. Combined with ginger and dong quai, it stimulates hormonal production in young women and aids in regulating the menstrual cycle. It has a bitter taste and should be combined with sweet herbs like licorice in formulations for young women.

Pau d'arco (Tabecuia impetiginosa, and related species) Also known as lapacho or taheebo, pau d'arco has long been recognized as an important herb for treating cancer, autoimmune diseases, glandular disorders, candida, and other serious health problems. The history of its use can be traced back to the Mayans and Incas, who regarded it as an important healing herb. It is currently used by doctors in Argentina and Brazil for treating leukemia and other types of cancer. Impressive findings have been recorded on the success of these treatments, and modern researchers are exploring possibilities of its use in cancer treatments in the United States.

Pau d'arco is an aid to the health of the liver and endocrine gland system. Though a strong herb, it exhibits no harmful side effects and can be mixed with a variety of other herbs to make a pleasant-tasting tea. It is used both as a curative for specific health problems and as a tonic to build and strengthen the system.

Because it is found growing in the rain forests of South America, care must be exercised when purchasing it. Many herbs purchased from Third World countries are heavily contaminated with pesticides, so purchase only organically grown plants. The harvesting of many jungle plants for medicinal purposes is contributing to the rapid destruction of the rain forests. Only *woods-grown* pau d'arco should be purchased. It is available in herb and natural food stores.

Seaweed (Hizike, kelp, arame, and related types) Seaweeds are exceptionally high in minerals and are considered one of the best foods for nourishing the endocrine glands. They are far higher than most other food sources, both animal and plant, in concentrated minerals and vitamins. For most endocrine gland imbalances, seaweed is highly recommended. Because of its unfamiliar flavor and texture, it is often hard to get people to try it, though in many parts of the world it is enjoyed as standard fare. (See page 85 for more information on seaweed.)

Wild yam (Dioscorea villosa) This is an important herb for the health of the liver and the endocrine system. Its active constituents include steroidal saponins (mainly diosgenin) which are important hormone precursors, especially of progesterone. It is also an excellent digestive aid. Wild yam is commonly used in formulas for the liver, the endocrine glands, and the female system. Its rather insipid flavor can be blended with other, more pleasant-tasting herbs for tea. It is commonly tinctured. Wild yam is safe to take over an extended period of time and has no residual side effects. (See Materia Medica for more information.)

Yellow dock root (Rumex crispus) Another tonic building herb for the liver, yellow dock root is rich in minerals, especially iron. It is excellent for young women who are chronically tired and stressed, as yellow dock supplies a rich source of easily digestible iron. This herb is considered one of the best liver detoxifiers and cleansers and enriches the blood, thus improving overall health. Young women who have stubborn skin problems will find yellow dock root especially beneficial. It is also aids in the digestion of fats and oils and can facilitate weight loss when the problem is due to sluggish elimination.

The following herbal formulas have been developed specifically for the young woman entering her moon time. In order for most of these formulas to be effective they must be taken over a period of several days to weeks. Herbs do not generally work overnight, so there needs to be a personal commitment to using them daily. All of these formulas can be prepared as tinctures and capsules for ease in administering. A simple herbal tea, however, is often the most powerful medicine. These teas have been formulated to taste fairly good, but can be adjusted to personal taste.

HEPATONIC TEA

This is a tasty blend of herbs and is recommended as a tea. A mild formula, it is best used as a tonic to help gently regulate hormones and nourish the system. The suggested dosage is three to four cups daily.

2 parts raspberry leaf	1 part dandelion leaf
1 part nettle leaf	1 part licorice root
1 part alfalfa leaf	1 part motherwort leaf
2 parts spearmint (or peppermint)	1 part lemon grass

A pinch of stevia for sweetness

To Make:

Use one teaspoon of mixture per cup, or four to six tablespoons per quart. Bring water to a boil. Place herbs in a quart jar and pour boiling water over them. Cover tightly. Infuse for at least twenty minutes. Strain and rebottle the tea. The tea can be poured into a thermos to keep warm during the day.

LIVER/ENDOCRINE TONIC TEA

This is another excellent tonic formula recommended for toning the liver and endocrine glands. It helps prepare the body for the vast hormonal changes it undergoes during adolescence. It is a fragrant-tasting, full-bodied blend and can be served iced or hot as a nice beverage tea. The suggested dosage is three to four cups daily.

3 parts sassafras root bark	½ part wild yam root
2 parts sarsaparilla root	½ part cinnamon bark
1 part dandelion root	½ part ginger root
1 part licorice root	Pinch of stevia (optional)
½ part yellow dock root	

To Make:

Use one teaspoon of mixture per cup or four to six tablespoons per quart. Add herbs to cold water and bring to a slow boil over low heat. Simmer gently for twenty minutes. Strain. Store in a quart jar or thermos.

ENDOCRINE STRENGTHENER

This strong, rooty blend is bitter and rather unpleasant-tasting, and is therefore best when used as a tincture or when powdered and capsulated. It is indicated for the more serious signs of hormone imbalance in young women such as acne, painful menstruation, delayed menstruation, and heavy bleeding. The suggested amount is two "00" capsules morning and evening or one-fourth teaspoon of tincture three times daily.

1 part licorice root	1 part vitex
1 part black cohash root	¼ part ginger
1 part pau d'arco bark	½ part echinacea root
1 part cramp bark	½ part kelp powder

To prepare as a tincture, see instructions on page 66.
To prepare as capsules, see instructions on page 58.

LIVER/ENDOCRINE CAPSULES

This potent formula is an excellent medicinal formula. It cleanses and strengthens both the liver and the endocrine glands, while nourishing and building the entire system. It is recommended for serious hormonal imbalances that manifest themselves in depleted energy levels, dramatic mood shifts, painful and irregular menstrual cycles, and/or lack of menstruation. Because of its bitterness, this formula is also recommended for use in tincture or capsule form. The suggested amount is two "00" capsules morning and evening or one-fourth teaspoon of the tincture three times daily.

1 part yellow dock root	2 parts hops
2 parts dandelion root	1 part kelp powder
1 part pau d'arco	1 part licorice root
1 part vitex berries	1 part wild yam root

To prepare as a tincture, see instructions on page 66.
To prepare as capsules, see instructions on page 58.

Dietary Recommendations

It seems most adolescents thrive on snack foods and soft drinks and have an aversion to anything green. This is not true of all teenagers, but it's certainly true of most. Expecting teens to make major dietary changes is unrealistic. However, not making any dietary changes is very detrimental to *any* health program one chooses to follow. I have found a simple solution that seems to work for my twin teenage daughters and many of the teenagers I have counseled.

Ask your teenager to follow a simple, wholesome diet for four weeks. Have her eliminate white sugar, soft drinks, salty and fried foods, and all sweets. The rest of her diet can remain basically the same, though I do recommend eating more fresh fruits and raw salads than usual. In addition to eliminating nonnourishing types of food, the young person should add the appropriate herbal formula(s) and several of the dietary suggestions listed below. At the end of four weeks, evaluate her response to the program. Usually the physical results are so pronounced that without much coaxing she will be willing to stay with the program. Sometimes modification will be required after the initial trial period. It doesn't matter how perfect a health program is, it won't work if the person isn't willing to follow it. So allow your teenager to tailor her program so that it's suitable to her taste buds but still healthful enough to be effective. It is necessary during the initial trial period to be fairly strict in order to see desired results.

Eliminate from the diet:
White sugar and sugar products
Refined, processed food
Salty snack items such as chips, pretzels
Sodas and soft drinks
Fried food
Caffeine

Add to the diet:
Fresh fruit
Raw vegetables and salads
High-quality protein, such as fish, fowl, soy protein
Appropriate herbal formula(s)
Appropriate dietary supplements
Fresh squeezed vegetable and fruit juices. It is a worthy investment to buy a juicer.
  Fresh juice is such a potent food, alive with nutrients. It is especially useful during
  the teenage years, when the tendency to eat convenience foods is so great.

Suggested Dietary Supplements

High-Calcium Protein Shake

This is a delicious, nourishing breakfast for all teenage girls. It takes only a few minutes to mix up and ensures an adequate supply of calcium, protein, vitamins, and minerals. After going through a difficult time getting my daughters to eat a hearty breakfast before school, we settled on this morning shake. (The following proportions make enough for two hearty servings.)

1 cup milk
1 cup nonsweetened juice (experiment with different flavors)
1–2 bananas (I often freeze ripe bananas for a thicker, creamier shake)
¼ cup frozen strawberries (or fresh fruit when it's in season)
¼ cup yogurt
1 teaspoon bee pollen
protein powder (follow the proportions listed on the container)
2 teaspoons spirulina
½ teaspoon pure vanilla extract

There are infinite varieties to this basic shake. Sometimes I add frozen orange juice for an Orange Julius–like shake. Sometimes I use juice in place of milk. I've found a dash of pure vanilla extract always enhances the flavor of the shake. One big glass of this in the morning and I know my daughters are off to school with a nourishing, sustaining breakfast.

Spirulina Tablets

I can't overstress the value of adding spirulina to a teenager's diet. A simple blue-green algae, spirulina has been used for thousands of years as a high-power food source. Some 60–70 percent protein by weight, it is considered the highest source of digestive plant protein and is second only to dried whole eggs when compared with animal forms of protein. It is also a remarkable source of vitamin A, calcium, the B vitamins, and chlorophyll. Convincing people to try this green algae in powder form is often an ordeal, though it's easily camouflaged (except for the unmistakable dark green color) when blended into fruit and vegetable juice. Spirulina is also sold in easy-to-take tablet form. The general dose is two tablespoons of powdered spirulina, or six tablets daily. Your daughter, I'm sure, will find the capsules much more appealing than the powdered form.

Seaweed

Though seaweed is a popular and common food in many cultures, it is considered either weird or "gourmet" in the United States. Most adults adapt fairly quickly to the flavors and textures of seaweed, but I've seldom met a teenager who will readily eat it. Yet seaweed is an excellent food source and a wonderful supplement to the diet, especially for young women suffering hormonal imbalance. Seaweeds provide concentrated trace minerals and are a marvelous source of the natural biochelated iodine so necessary to the function of the thyroid gland. Most seaweed provides the building blocks needed by the endocrine glands to manufacture necessary hormones. Seaweed is also generally high in calcium (one tablespoon of hizike provides more digestible calcium than an eight-ounce glass of milk).

Though the taste of these rather exotic sea plants may not excite the palate of the normal teenager, it is worth an attempt to get your teen to try seaweed. Seaweed can be incorporated into many foods or the capsules/tablets can be worked into a daily health program. The dosage varies, depending on the type of seaweed. Kelp is the most common seaweed available and easily found in capsulated form. However, kelp is also the "fishiest" and strongest-tasting of the seaweeds. Many of the other, lesser-known seaweeds are very mild and pleasant-tasting. All are easily found in natural food stores, gourmet shops, and groceries stores featuring Oriental and Asian foods.

When taking seaweed in tablets or capsules, a dosage of ten to twelve capsules a day is generally suggested. Though this may seem like a lot of capsules, remember that eating seaweed this way is like eating salad in capsules. You would have to ingest a lot of those capsules to get all your greens!

Liquid Floradix Iron with Herbs and/or NatureWorks Herbal Iron

Floradix (distributed by BioForce) is a liquid vitamin mineral formula made from organic herbs and vegetables gathered in the high mountains of Europe. It is available in natural food stores throughout the country. I have recommended it for years because it is such a highly concentrated and effective formula and is readily available. It is also pleasant-tasting, so people find it enjoyable to take. Liquid Floradix with Iron is often recommended for women low in iron, for pregnant and nursing mothers, and for women who are chronically tired. I have also found it an excellent tonic formula for teenage girls. It is an excellent source of digestible vitamins and minerals and biochelated iron. It helps stabilize energy, and mood swings, and regulates the menstrual cycle. Follow the recommended dose on the bottle, but for severe menstrual problems and/or low energy, I suggest doubling the amount recommended on the bottle.

NatureWorks Herbal Iron is another liquid vitamin/mineral formula frequently found in natural food and herb stores. It is quite tasty and is comparable to Floradix in quality.

You can also make an excellent vitamin/mineral formula by following the recipe for Iron-Plus Syrup on page 62.

Bee Pollen

Another of the bee's little gifts, bee pollen is a concentrated source of nearly all known nutrients. It is a complete protein, containing all twenty-two amino acids, and it has high levels of twenty-seven different minerals, enzymes, and coenzymes, including vitamin B_1, B_2, and B_6, pantothenic acid, folic acid, vitamin C, and the fat-soluble vitamins A and E. I find the pollen delicious, but not every teenager does. It is easy to camouflage it by mixing it in blender drinks or by stirring it into cereal. The suggested dosage is about one-fourth teaspoon daily. Because there is a small percentage of people who are allergic to bee pollen, it is best to test your teenager's sensitivity to it by having her take just a small dose to begin with and then increasing it with time. If she suffers from allergies, you may wish to have her consult an allergist before she takes the bee pollen.

Dong Quai

This is one of nature's gifts to women. A lovely herb that looks like delicately carved pieces of ivory, dong quai grows in China and is one of the most widely used herbs in the Orient. A wonderful tonic herb for the female reproductive system, dong quai can be used over an extended period of time to tone, nourish, and feed the reproductive organs. It is wonderful for helping young girls regulate their menstrual cycles, especially if there are early signs of imbalance in the menstrual cycle. When used as a tonic herb, the general dose is one-fourth teaspoon of tincture twice daily. If taken in capsule form, the suggested amount for teens would be two capsules twice daily. Dong quai is a bittersweet herb and blends well in tea. Some women enjoy the rather unusual flavor of the root and choose to take their daily dose by chewing a small piece (about one-fourth inch) of the root each day. (See the Materia Medica for more information on dong quai.)

Menstrual Discomfort

There really is no such thing as a "normal" menstrual cycle. Each young woman begins her moon time in a manner unique to her and experiences it each month thereafter in her own way. There also may be changes from one month to the next. Some young women may begin their menstrual cycle one eventful month and from then on have a monthly cycle as regular as clockwork. This is no more "normal" or "abnormal" than the young woman who experiences her early menstrual cycles as sporadic and irregular. The patterns of menstruation are as varied as the women who have them.

Some cultural traditions hold that women menstruate on the full of the moon; other cultures believe that all women bleed together on the new moon. The moon's phases do exert a powerful influence on the fluid bodies of the earth and on the psychic energy of women. I'm certain that the moon's transit does have a marked influence on our menstrual cycles. I've noted this for many years at women's gatherings—many of which were held on the full moon.

Just as influential as the moon's energy are the relationships women form with one another when living in a community together. Often women who live in the same household, go to school together, or who work together share similar menstrual cycles. Menstruating women emit chemical secretions called pheromones that actually stimulate hormonal activity and elicit a sympathetic response in other women in close proximity.

Another important topic concerning "normal" menstruation is what comprises an "average" amount of bleeding. My response is, "any amount that is usual for *you* and that doesn't constitute a problem." In other words, if a young woman bleeds lightly, doesn't experience cramps, is on a "regular" schedule (no matter how unique it may be), and has no other related menstrual difficulties, her light bleeding is *not* a problem for her. The same is true of a young woman who experiences heavy menstrual flows. If the flow feels healthy, the blood is bright, the cycle is not accompanied by heavy cramping or excessively low energy, and she doesn't feel "wasted" or worn out from her cycle, her heavy bleeding does not signify an abnormal menstrual cycle.

What *does* constitute an abnormal or problematic menstrual cycle? How would one detect the early signs of potential menstrual difficulties in a young woman? These are the signals to look for:

Pain and cramps (dysmenorrhea)
Dark brown blood
Lingering cycles: several days of spot bleeding before or after
Clotting

Excessively heavy bleeding (menorrhagia)
No menstrual cycle (amenorrhea)
Serious acne and skin problems
A feeling of exhaustion following the menstrual cycle

I would not become alarmed if any one of the above problems occurred occasionally. Our reproductive systems are highly sensitive to emotional fluctuations. Sometimes painful cramping or delayed menstruation is due to an excessively taxing month—final exams, breaking up with a boyfriend, or social problems—but if the problem recurs regularly, it is a definite sign of physiological imbalance. To be sure that there is nothing seriously wrong, it is wise to consult with a health care professional, preferably one who is holistically minded.

For Painful Cramping Menstruation (Dysmenorrhea)

The following teas are excellent for relieving cramps and painful menstruation.

CRAMP BARK TEA

2 parts cramp bark (or black haw)
1 part pennyroyal leaf
½ part ginger root (fresh-grated is best, though the dry root will do)

To Make:
Add four to six tablespoons of the herb mixture per quart of cold water. Place on low heat and slowly bring to a slow simmer. Keep pan covered tightly. Simmer only two to five minutes, then remove from heat. Drink in small amounts (one-fourth cup) every fifteen minutes until cramps subside.

CINNAMON GINGER TEA

1 part valerian root
1 part cramp bark

1 part ginger root (fresh grated is best)
½ part cinnamon bark

To Make:
Use four to six tablespoons of the herb mixture per quart of water. Place cramp bark, ginger root, and cinnamon in cold water and slowly bring to a simmer. Simmer gently for about fifteen minutes on low heat, keeping the pot tightly covered. Remove from heat and add valerian root. Let the mixture infuse for one-half hour or longer. Drink small amounts (one-fourth cup) every fifteen minutes until cramps have subsided.

2 parts pennyroyal leaf and flower 1 part motherwort
1 part oat straw ½ part yarrow leaf and flower
1 part raspberry leaf

To Make:

Add four to six tablespoons of the herb mixture to one quart of cold water. Keep pot covered. Over very low heat, bring just to the simmering point. Remove immediately. Drink small amounts (about one-fourth cup) throughout the day until cramps subside.

Other Helpful Hints

❦ Oil of pennyroyal, *though extremely toxic if used internally, provides excellent temporary relief for cramps when used—externally—*as a massage oil over the pelvic and lower stomach area. My daughters and I have used this oil directly on our skin with excellent results. However, the essential oil is extremely strong; you may wish to dilute it in a little olive oil, especially if you have sensitive skin. *Do not get the oil near the vulva or lip openings. Pennyroyal oil will irritate and burn the delicate membranes of the vagina.* Used sparingly and wisely, it is a very helpful healing substance. (See Materia Medica for more information on pennyroyal and pennyroyal oil.)

❦ Place a heating pad over the lower back while simultaneously putting a poultice made of fresh grated ginger over the pelvic area. This is a wonderful soothing remedy that usually brings quick relief. It's quite easy to make this effective poultice. Make a pot of strong ginger tea by grating fresh ginger and adding it to cold water. Bring the ginger tea to a low boil and simmer (with the lid kept on tight) for ten to fifteen minutes. Allow to cool just slightly. Dip a clean cotton cloth in the tea and wring out any excess liquid. Put a dry towel over the pelvic area, and then place the hot poultice over it. Cover with a thick towel to keep the heat in and leave in place for fifteen to twenty minutes or until the poultice begins to cool. Repeat until the pain is eased. To keep the poultice hot for a longer length of time, place a heating pad over the outer towel.

❦ Nervine tinctures are very helpful for alleviating cramps. They are also handy preparations for young women to use while at school. Both Jennifer and Melanie, my stepdaughters, have found that using tinctures at school stimulates interest in, rather than aversion to, herbal medicine among their friends. Because tinctures are very concentrated and are quickly absorbed into the bloodstream, results are often speedy. Any of the tea formulas on page 89 may be made into tinctures for quick assimilation. I've also found a simple tincture of equal parts cramp bark, valerian root, hops, and ginger root to be very effective. (See pages 66–67 for instructions on how to make tinctures.)

In young women cramps are generally caused by a lack of blood calcium, poor nutrition, stress, and nervous system disorders. They can usually be eliminated by good dietary habits and by removing stress factors. Neither of these are easy to accomplish, however, especially for a young person. It requires a dedicated sense of commitment and self-empowerment. The following measures have helped many teenagers considerably. I generally suggest that a young woman follow the program rigorously for two months and note any improvement. Usually, the improvement is so noticeable and welcome that a teenager will of her own volition continue following the program until the problem is corrected.

On a Daily Basis

❦ Take evening primrose oil, borage oil, or blackcurrent seed oil (available in capsules in most natural food stores). Take 500 milligrams twice a day, or follow the suggested dosage on container. These natural plant oils are rich in GLA (gamma linolenic acid) which regulates and controls prostaglandin production in the body. Excess prostaglandins circulating in the bloodstream are often responsible for menstrual discomfort, mood swings, and cramps. Eating foods rich in GLA and taking supplemental oils like these has resulted in marked improvement for many young women.

❦ Take two to three cups daily of Hepatonic Tea. (See page 82.) This tea may be made every three days, stored in the refrigerator, and drunk cold.

❦ Take liquid Floradix with Iron (or another liquid vitamin/mineral formula) daily. Follow the dosage recommended on the bottle.

❦ Follow the dietary guidelines listed in Chapter 12, pages 83–84.

❦ Take two capsules of dong quai daily. (However, discontinue dong quai capsules one week before the menstrual cycle begins and do not begin again until all bleeding has stopped. Dong quai is not recommended during the actual menstrual cycle as it can stimulate bleeding by directing energy and heat to the pelvic area).

One Week Before the Menstrual Cycle Begins

❦ Make Endocrine Strengthener (see page 83) or Liver/Endocrine Capsules (see page 83) into a tincture. (For directions on making tinctures, see pages 66–67.) Take one-fourth teaspoon tincture three times a day.

❦ Drink two to three cups Cramp Bark Tea daily. (See page 89.)

❦ Take a biochelated calcium supplement and pay special attention to eating a calcium-rich diet during the week before your menstrual cycle is due to begin.

During the Menstrual Cycle

Follow any of the suggestions given above for relieving menstrual stress. Oftentimes, if one has been following the program faithfully, there is a noticeable improvement after the first menstrual cycle. One is tempted to believe the problem has been corrected. But, usually this isn't the case, especially for long-standing problems. A pattern frequently seen in healing is for the body to respond quickly at first, as though it is "hungry" for the good treatment. Then the effects taper off and the progress is slow but sure. It generally takes at least *three full menstrual cycles* or longer to fully correct long-standing problems.

For Irregular or Delayed Menstruation

As young women begin their journey into womanhood, their hormones take several months or even years to regulate and develop a smooth rhythm or cycle. A similar hormonal metamorphosis occurs at the completion of the fertile years of a woman's life. As women enter the menopausal years, their cycles often take months, even years, to completely stop. During this time, irregularity is often the norm. I find nothing unusual about this, nor do I become alarmed unless there are accompanying problems. Frequently, irregular menses can be regulated by simply drinking mugwort tea. Mugwort belongs to the wonderful artemisia family and is ruled by the Goddess Diana. (Artemis or Diana is the goddess of the moon.) All of the artemisias are of particular interest to women, but especially mugwort. Its peculiar name simply implies it was the herb (wort) of the mug, thus mugwort. It has long been used as an herb for young women to help regulate their menstrual flows. It is *very* bitter, however, and will need to be blended with more pleasant-tasting teas or made into a tincture.

If a young woman has not only an irregular cycle but cramps, heavy bleeding, spot bleeding, or any other of the problems listed above, I would suggest following this program:

On a Daily Basis

❦ Take Hepatonic Tea (see page 82) or Liver/Endocrine Tonic Tea (see page 82). Drink two to four cups daily.

❦ Take evening primrose, black current seed or borage oil in capsule form. These oils are available in capsule form in natural food and herb stores. Take 500 milligrams twice a day or follow the dosage recommended on the bottle.

❦ Take Endocrine Strengthener (see page 83) or Liver/Endocrine Capsules (see page 83) as a tincture. (For directions on making tinctures, see pages 66–67.) Take one-fourth teaspoon two to three times daily.

❦ Take two capsules of dong quai daily. Don quai is available in herb and natural food stores in capsule form. Or you can purchase the powdered herb and encapsulate your own. (See page 58 for directions.)

❦ Take liquid Floradix with iron daily (or another liquid vitamin/mineral formula). Follow the dosage recommended on the bottle. Floradix is available in natural food and herb stores. Or you can make a similar formula by following the recipe for Iron-Plus Syrup on page 62.

❦ Take a biochelated calcium supplement daily. Follow the recommended dosage on the bottle.

❦ A young woman's menstrual cycle will often be delayed or stop altogether due to a lack of nutrients in the diet. A lack of protein, in particular, can cause this. Be certain that there is an adequate supply of good-quality protein in a young woman's diet, especially if she is active in sports. The High-Calcium Protein Shake (see recipe on page 84) is an excellent nutritional snack and can be drunk a couple of times daily by an active young person.

When the Menstrual Cycle is Due

If the menstrual cycle has been delayed for a long time, you may wish to establish a speculative "menstrual time" to follow the ensuing suggestions. It generally requires two, and often three, full cycles to see results. When establishing your hypothetical menstrual cycle, it is best to choose a time right before the full moon to begin. I can't tell you for sure why this time works best—though I have my theories—I have just observed that it does.

❦ Drink two to three cups of pennyroyal leaf tea daily. To prepare, use four to six tablespoons of herb per quart of water. Pour boiling water over the herbs, cover, and infuse for twenty minutes. Strain.

❦ Rub a little pennyroyal oil over the pelvic area in the evening before bedtime. (But please apply it sparingly and do *not* get the oil near the sensitive vaginal opening as it may irritate delicate vaginal tissue.)

❦ One of the oddest (and oldest) suggestions of all for establishing a regular period is to wear red (red underwear, red pants, red slip, and so forth) when your period is due, and just hang out with menstruating friends. Go to the movies with them, eat lunch with them, sit next to them. Catch those pheromones! It frequently works (not always, but enough times to make one believe there is something to it).

For Excessive Bleeding

When the flow is truly excessive and not just a heavy cycle, it should be attended to as soon as the problem is detected. A very excessive menstrual flow may indicate an extreme hormonal and/or endocrine imbalance. It may also indicate a more serious physiological problem. It is definitely a sign that things are not functioning properly. I have found the following treatment program very effective in treating a heavy menstrual flow.

On a Daily Basis

Include sufficient amounts of high-quality trace minerals—iodine, in particular. Include seaweeds in the daily diet. Though definitely not a favorite of any teenager I know, seaweeds are one of the most specific "medicines" and remedies for this problem. If a teenager isn't willing to eat seaweed, have her take sixteen to twenty capsules of kelp daily. (Kelp, as well as other seaweeds, is available at natural food stores and in shops that specialize in Asian food). Have her start slowly and build up to the total amount to give her system a chance to adjust to this onslaught of minerals. Frankly, I think learning to like seaweed is far more tolerable than eating so many capsules daily. There are some very fine-tasting dishes that can be prepared from seaweed and even some where you'd have difficulty knowing there was any seaweed in the dish.

Adhering to a good diet is imperative in this situation. I would suggest incorporating the dietary suggestions on pages 83–84 fairly religiously into the health program. Pay special attention to the "What to Eliminate" list. Do not use pennyroyal herb or oil, as pennyroyal can stimulate bleeding.

Include the following in the daily diet:

❦ Take capsules of dong quai daily. (Discontinue use during actual bleeding stage.)
❦ Take Floradix, NatureWorks Herbal Iron, or Iron-Plus Syrup (see page 62) daily. Double the suggested dosage on the bottle.
❦ Take one-fourth teaspoon vitex tincture twice a day. Vitex tincture can be purchased at herb stores, or you can easily make your own by following the directions on page 66.
❦ Drink two to three cups of Moon Time Tea (see below) every day.

MOON TIME TEA

2 parts raspberry leaf   1 part alfalfa leaf
2 parts nettle leaf   ½ yarrow

To Make:
Place four to six tablespoons of the herb mixture in a quart canning jar and cover with boiling water. Cover tightly and allow to infuse for at least twenty minutes (though the longer the better). Strain.

You may make several days' worth and store in a closed container in the refrigerator for ease of preparation. Though it's best to drink this liquid warm or at room temperature, it's fine to drink it cold.

During the Menstrual Cycle
❦ One week before the menstrual cycle begins, discontinue the dong quai tablets. Dong quai may stimulate bleeding if taken during the actual menstrual cycle.
❦ One week before the menstrual cycle begins take one-fourth teaspoon three times daily of a tincture made of equal amounts of shepherd's purse and yarrow. You can purchase shepherd's purse/yarrow tinctures at herb stores or make your own by following the tincture instructions on page 66. Take this tincture consistently during the week before your menstrual cycle is scheduled to begin.
❦ Once bleeding starts, continue taking the shepherd's purse/yarrow tincture, but in more frequent dosages, one-eighth teaspoon of tincture every hour or even every half hour if bleeding is profuse.
❦ Make the following tea and drink throughout the day:

2 parts nettle
1 part shepherd's purse leaf/flower
¼ yarrow leaf/flower

To Make:

Use four to six tablespoons of herbs per quart of water. Place herbs in quart jar and cover with boiling water. Cover tightly and allow to infuse for at least twenty minutes (though the longer the better). Strain.

Success in correcting excessive menstrual bleeding depends on following the above program during the entire month and sticking to the regime through several cycles. The regime during the actual time of bleeding is designed to treat the symptoms and, though it may lessen the flow of blood, will not bring lasting results. Because excessive menstrual bleeding can sometimes signify more serious problems, it is best to consult your family physician, preferably a holistically oriented woman doctor.

F O U R T E E N
Acne and Skin Problems

Though we don't often think of it as such, our skin is our largest organ of elimination and assimilation. It reflects the state of our entire system and is a good barometer of our internal health. When a teenager manifests chronic skin problems it is a sign that something is amiss. It can be as simple as poor eating habits—an excessive intake of chips, chocolate, sodas, colas, coffee, and candy—or can be an indication of hormonal imbalance, nervous system disorders, or allergies. Severe teenage acne is not normal. It can leave the skin scarred for years, and can emotionally affect the young person in a very negative manner.

The following herbal skin care program offers a natural and gentle way to correct acne and skin problems. You can purchase most of these natural cosmetic products in natural food and herb stores. Read the labels to be sure that these "natural" products don't contain synthetic or unnecessary ingredients such as fragrance, coloring agents, or chemical preservatives. These items frequently exacerbate the problem. I've also included my favorite recipes for those of you who would like to make your own natural products. They are some of the best, most natural, and least expensive cosmetics available. And, as you've already learned, making your own products can be a lot of fun.

Dietary Suggestions for Teenage Acne and Related Skin Problems

❧ Cut back on sugar, chocolate, fried foods, and sodas. Most teenagers find it easier to completely eliminate sugar and chocolate from their diet rather than try to regulate the amount. It's almost more torturous to eat small amounts of something than to completely eliminate it for a time.

❧ Drink up to four quarts of water a day.

❧ Take black current seed oil, borage, or evening primrose oil in capsulated form daily. (These encapsulated oils are available in natural food stores.) Take 500 milligrams daily or follow the recommended dosage on the container. These oils are high in GLA (gamma-linoleic-acid) and have proven very helpful in treating teenage acne. Black current seed oil and borage oil are both less expensive than evening primrose oil and higher in GLA.

❧ Drink two to four cups of herbal tea daily. Choose the appropriate tea and drink at least two cups daily for several weeks.

When a young woman's skin problem is related to nervous tension and stress, she should drink the following formula for several weeks.

2 parts chamomile
1 part oat straw
1 part lemon balm

⅛ part valerian
½ part skullcap

To Make:

Use four to six tablespoons of herbs per quart of water. Place herbs in a quart jar and cover with boiling water. Cover tightly and infuse for at least twenty minutes. Strain.

Another excellent tonic formula that is highly nutritious and feeds the skin on a cellular level is Hepatonic Tea. (See page 82.) This is good as a general, all-purpose tea for the skin.

Still another fine possibility is the Liver/Endocrine Capsule. (See page 83.) This is especially good for cleansing and strengthening the liver. It also helps to balance and regulate the hormones. If the skin problem is related to hormone imbalance, poor eating habits, allergies, or general poor health, this formula is highly recommended.

A Five-Part Program for Radiant Skin

To achieve a healthy, radiant skin, the following daily, weekly, and monthly program should be carefully followed.

Daily Wash with cleansing grains. (See below.)
 Close pores with a tonic astringent. (See pages 98–99.)
 If the skin is dry, massage with a light, nonoily cream. (See pages 99–102.)
Weekly Use a facial mask and herbal steam. (See pages 102–3.)
Monthly Treat yourself to the entire program.

Daily: Miracle Grains

These cleansing grains, a perfect soap replacement, are mild and nourishing. They are suitable for all skin types and can be used daily. Lightly cleanse your face and neck with Miracle Grains (see recipe below). To use, mix one to two teaspoons of the grains with water, stir into a paste, and gently massage into the skin. The grains massage off dry, dead skin, increase circulation to the surface, and provide a nourishing "meal" for your face. After thoroughly cleansing, rinse the grains off with warm water.

MIRACLE GRAINS

1 cup finely ground oats
2 cups white clay
¼ cup finely ground almonds
⅛ cup finely ground lavender
⅛ cup finely ground roses
lavender, peppermint, orange *pure* essential oils (optional)

valerian

To Make:

Step 1 · Grind all ingredients to the desired consistency. You may wish to grind the oats very fine. The almonds are nice with just a touch of "grit" left in them. Grind the roses and lavender into a fine powder; there will always be a bit of coarseness or graininess left in the herbs which serves as the cleansing "grains." The clay is already finely powdered. I have found that blenders and electric coffee grinders work best for grinding small amounts of herbs, flowers, and spices. However, a word of wisdom: do not use the same grinder for coffee and herbs. If you do, your coffee will forever smell and taste like roses and lavender.

Step 2 · Mix all ingredients together. You may wish to add a drop or two of essential oil(s) to enhance the scent and the effect of the grains. Do not add too much! The oils must be *pure* essential oils, such as lavender, peppermint, or orange. Do not use synthetic oils, as they can possibly burn and irritate the skin.

To make moist miracle grains, add honey and a small amount of pure distilled rose water (or plain distilled water) to the dried powdered mixture to make a paste. The honey serves as a natural preservative for the grains as well as adding its wonderful moisturizing quality. Mix only enough moist grains to last for a week or two to prevent spoilage. Store the remainder of the grains in powdered form and mix as needed.

Step 3 · Store grains in a pretty glass container. A shell makes a nice scoop and mixing receptacle as well. You can also store the grains in spice jars with shaker tops.

As with each of my recipes, you are not only invited, but encouraged, to be creative. You can add cornmeal, seaweed, vitamin E and A, and numerous other substances to your cleansing grains.

Daily: Tonic Astringent

Each night after rinsing off the cleansing grains, give your face a final rinse with a light astringent to tone and close the pores. If you have dry skin use rose water, a very light, gentle astringent. Rosewater is available at some pharmacies, gourmet food stores, and at natural food and herb stores. Be certain to purchase only pure food-grade rosewater or make your own using the recipe below. If your skin is medium to oily, use Queen of Hungary's Water (see recipe below).

QUEEN OF HUNGARY'S WATER

6 parts lemon balm (also known as melissa)
4 parts chamomile
1 part rosemary
3 parts calendula
4 parts roses
1 part lemon peel
1 part sage
3 parts comfrey
witch hazel extract to cover (part vinegar may also be used).
rosewater

To Make:

Step 1 • Place all the herbs in a wide-mouthed jar and cover with witch hazel extract (and/or vinegar). Be sure there is about one to two inches of witch hazel/vinegar above the herb mixture. Cover tightly and let sit in a warm spot for two to three weeks.

Step 2 • Strain. Set the liquid aside and compost the herbs.

Step 3 • To each cup of herbal extract add one-half cup rosewater.

Step 4 • A drop or two of essential oil, such as lavender or rose, can be added to enhance the scent.

Step 5 • Rebottle. This product does not need to be refrigerated, as it is naturally preserved.

R O S E W A T E R

Though rosewater is technically produced by distilling fresh rose petals, the following recipe is a simple, effective method that ensures perfect rosewater each time.

Fresh unsprayed rose petals (It is best to use the petals just as the roses are opening; they are at their prime then and will yield the strongest "water.")
Witch hazel extract (vodka or gin can be substituted)
Distilled water

To Make:

Step 1 • Place fresh rose petals in a quart jar. The more fragrant the roses, the stronger the scent of the rosewater.

Step 2 • Make a mixture that is three-fourth parts witch hazel extract and one-fourth part distilled water. Pour the mixture over the rose petals, completely covering them and leaving an additional two to three inches of liquid above the flowers. Cover tightly and place in a warm, shaded area. Let the mixture sit for two to three weeks.

Step 3 • Strain and rebottle for use.

Daily: Cream Massage

The finishing touch of your daily skin care program is to treat yourself to a light, delicate facial massage, using a special cream formulated for your skin type. Not all teenagers need to use facial cream on a regular basis. Dry skin is not often a big problem among younger women. In fact, oily skin is more often a concern. However, a light facial cream used in the evening, after facials, and after exposure to wind and sun prevents dry skin later in life.

The following recipe is by far the most wonderful face cream I have ever used. It is made with only natural ingredients. A *real* moisturizer, it provides nourishment, moisture, and food for the skin, and it is relatively easy and inexpensive to make. Hundreds of my students have used this recipe. Almost all agree it is the best skin cream they have ever used. Many people have further personalized the recipe for their own unique skin types. This basic formula, though excellent as it is, can be further embellished.

Unlike many commercial creams that only coat the surface of the skin, this cream penetrates the epidermal layer and moisturizes the dermal layer of the skin. Because it is extremely concentrated, a little goes a long way. A common mistake when using this cream is to use too much of it. You need no more than one-sixth of a teaspoonful. Take a tiny amount and gently massage into your face and skin. There will be a temporary feeling of oiliness that will, within a few minutes, disappear as the cream is quickly absorbed. Though I recommend just a small amount on your face, you can be generous on the rest of your body. Because you make this cream yourself, you can afford the luxury of using your richest face cream on your entire body.

Though this recipe appears easy, it is also a bit challenging. You are attempting to mix (emulsify) oil and water—and they don't normally mix. Follow the recipe closely. If it doesn't turn out the first time, don't be discouraged: try again. It is well worth the effort.

ROSEMARY'S FAMOUS FACE CREAM

Group I Ingredients
¾ cup grape seed oil (Other natural oils such as apricot oil and almond oil can be used, but grape seed oil is the lightest and least oily and therefore the best suited for most teenagers' skin.)
⅓ cup coconut oil and/or cocoa butter (I use both.)
1 teaspoon lanolin (Omit if you have an allergy to lanolin.)
½ ounce grated beeswax

Group II Ingredients
⅔ cup distilled water (You can also use distilled rosewater or orange flower water. If the skin is oily, witch hazel extract or Queen of Hungary's Water can be substituted for part of the distilled water in the recipe.)
⅓ cup aloe vera gel
a drop or two of essential oil for scent

Optional Ingredients (to be added to Group II before Group I is blended in)
Vitamins A and E as desired (To be effective in the cream, at least 10,000 units of vitamin E and 150,000 units of vitamin A should be used.)
Black current seed oil (Use 1000 to 2000 milliliters per cup.)
If making the cream for someone with acne, add Evening Primrose Oil or Black Current Seed Oil to the recipe.

Please note before blending Group I into Group II:
❦ The basic proportions of this cream recipe should be about one part Group I (oils) to one part Group II (waters).
❦ In Group I, the oil proportions should be approximately two-thirds cup liquid oil (such as grape seed, almond, or apricot) to one-third cup solid oil (cocoa butter, coconut oil, beeswax, lanolin).
❦ The Group II water mixture can include distilled water, rosewater, lavender, orange,

and other flower waters. It can also include tap water, but tap water may introduce bacteria into your cream that can result in the growth of mold. The water mixture also includes an essential oil for scent, aloe vera gel, and any optional ingredients such as vitamins. If using aloe vera gel, your cream will be a little heavier but very moisturizing. When using aloe, it is important to use the gel and not the fresh plant. The fresh plant may introduce bacteria to your cream and cause it to mold. It is also important not to use aloe or cream made with aloe in it on staph infections. Though aloe is excellent for many skin infections, it provides a perfect medium for staph to grow in and will actually spread the infection.

There is a lot of flexibility and room for creative input in this recipe. The basic formula can be embellished with any number of ingredients: vitamins A, D, and E; elastin, collagen, and avocado oil; various combinations of essential oils, herbs, and so on. There is just one caution: Experiment in small batches. You don't want to waste a lot of costly ingredients in a large, less-than-perfect batch.

What is essential to the success of this cream recipe is *proportions* and *temperature*. The proportions of Group I and Group II must be similar, and everything must be at room temperature when the cream is made.

To Make:

Step 1 · Melt Group I ingredients over low heat in a double boiler. Heat the ingredients just enough to melt them.

Step 2 · Pour mixture into a glass measuring cup and let cool to room temperature. I usually let it sit overnight in a cool room. Oils should become thick, creamy, semisolid, and cream-colored. This cooling process can be hastened in the refrigerator, but keep an eye on it so that it doesn't get too hard. When it is completely cool, you are ready for Step 3.

Step 3 · Place Group II ingredients in the blender. Turn the blender on to the highest speed. In a *slow, thin* drizzle (just as in making mayonnaise) pour Group I oil mixture into the center vortex of the blender.

Step 4 · When most of the oil mixture has been added to the water mixture, *listen* to the blender and *watch* the cream. When the blender "coughs and chokes" and the cream looks as thick and white as buttercream frosting, turn the blender off. *Do not overbeat!* If there is still a little liquid left, hand-beat it in or carefully blend for a second or two longer. You should have a beautiful, rich thick cream. It will continue to thicken a bit as it sets up.

Step 5 · Pour the blend into cream or lotion jars and store in a cool place. This cream will not go bad stored at room temperature. However, if you make more than you can use in a month or two, it will keep longer if the excess is stored in the refrigerator.

Please note, if you are not successful the first time:

❧ Followed as above, the cream recipe should work for you. If it doesn't, and the water mixture and oils separate, it is most likely because of improper temperatures. The water mixture has to be room temperature and the oils completely cooled. Another possible explanation for failure is that the blender speed may have been set too low. It must be set at a high speed in order for the cream to properly emulsify.

❧ If the water and oil separate, let them separate entirely and then begin the process over again. Or put a little note on your package that says "Shake Before Using." I've actually re-emulsified creams that have separated by either hand-shaking them or beating them for a few minutes with an electric beater.

Weekly: Facial Mask

Facials are used to draw a fresh supply of blood to the skin and stimulate circulation to the facial area. They are excellent for cleansing the pores and healing blemishes and acne. Facials also help tone and firm the skin—something that teens don't have to concern themselves with but that their moms might like to know.

There are several kinds of facials available. My favorites are made with a base of clay and/or honey. I find clay particularly suitable when one wants a drawing, firming facial. It is also very high in minerals and nourishes the skin. Clay is composed of mineral deposits that are thousands of years old; these unique deposits have witnessed untold numbers of sunrises and sunsets, rain and windstorms; they have been the soil of ancient forests and been walked upon by dinosaurs. We mix that clay with a little water and put it on our faces in the name of Cosmeos. Now that is pretty powerful medicine! Various types of cosmetic grade clays are available in natural food and herb stores.

Honey, too, has its magic. A natural, nonoily moisturizer, it both nourishes and cleanses the skin. It is a marvelous cosmetic aid. Honey is a natural disinfectant. Bacteria cannot survive in it, so while honey nourishes, it also cleanses the skin. It may take a little getting used to its stickiness, but the effects are so noticeable that it is well worth it. Any type of honey will do, though it is easiest to apply if it is somewhat liquid.

Select the facial for your skin type. If choosing a clay facial, mix it with just enough water to make a nice paste. The thicker the clay/water mix, the more drying the facial; the thinner, the less drying. Apply and leave on until completely dry.

If choosing the honey pack, apply a fingerful to *completely* dry skin. Be sure all your hair is out of reach; it gets very sticky when full of honey! I usually turban-towel it out of sight. Gently massage the honey into the skin. Use upward strokes. Massage, pat, and rub onto your face. Let your senses tell you what strokes to use. The skin becomes so invigorated it fairly glows. Rinse honey off with warm water. It comes off very easily, but be sure to rinse off completely or you will feel sticky for the rest of the day. The fresh flow of blood brought to the surface of the skin by the honey facial will create a deep, warm, lasting glow.

How to Determine What Type of Facial to Use

For dry skin, choose a white cosmetic grade clay. White clay, though lightly drawing, is very gentle to the skin. For a more nourishing facial, mix with yogurt and/or avocado.

For oily skin: choose either green, red, or yellow clay. These clays are much more drying than the white variety. They are also very high in minerals, thus feeding and nourishing the skin. They are excellent for such problems as acne, pimples, and oily skin. In natural therapeutics, these clays are often used for poison oak and poison ivy, bee stings, and insect bites.

For all skin types: honey makes an excellent facial. It brings fresh blood to the surface, removes impurities, and soothes and softens the skin.

Weekly: Herbal Steam

Select an herbal steam that is best for your skin type (see recipes below). Bring the herbs to a boil in a large pot of water. Remove from the heat source. Completely cover the pot and your head with a large thick towel. It should be *very* hot under that towel—*almost* uncomfortably hot. Try to steam for at least five to eight minutes To regulate the heat, raise or lower your head or lift a corner of the towel to let in a little cool air. If you need to come out to catch a breath of cool air now and then, do so. It is best to stay under the towel for as long as possible. Your face should be rolling with steam.

It really does feel fabulous. A facial steam is the best possible way for deep-pore cleansing. Each of the herbs used is rich in nutrients that feed and tone the skin. The aromatic cleansing oils of the plants are released by the heat and absorbed by the skin. And best of all, it feels so good!! Your face will glow with radiance. Immediately after you complete your facial steam, rinse your face with *cold* water and mist with rosewater. Then, *gently* pat dry.

Below are some of my favorite recipes for facial steams. Everybody who makes these steams has their favorite recipe, which is, I suspect, based on whatever herbs they have on hand. When blending your own formulas, use herbs that have been traditionally used for the care of the skin. You may wish to check your choice of herbs in a good herbal resource book. (See Appendix I.) Know the action of the herb; is the herb slightly drying/astringent or moisturizing/mucilaginous? Add flowers for color and texture. It's a lovely feeling to steam your face over a fragrant pot of simmering roses, marigold, chamomile, and lavender blossoms—very nourishing for the soul!

FACIAL STEAM FOR DRY-TO-NORMAL SKIN

1 part lavender	2 parts calendula
2 parts chamomile	3 parts comfrey
2 parts roses	

FACIAL STEAM FOR NORMAL-TO-OILY SKIN

1 part witch hazel	2 parts calendula
1 part sage	¼ part rosemary
3 parts comfrey	

To Make:

Mix all the herbs together, adjust amounts to suit you, and store in dry, airtight glass bottles.

To Use:

Bring two to three quarts of water to a boil in a large pot. Add a healthy handful of the herb mixture and let simmer with the lid on for just a couple of minutes. Remove the pot from the heat source. With a large towel, completely cover your head and pot of steaming herbs. Enjoy this minisauna. It does wonders for the skin.

For Skin Blemishes

"Don't squeeze that pimple!" Parents have been telling their kids this forever and kids still squeeze pimples as if doing so were just irresistible. But squeezing pimples prematurely leads to scarring and also prolongs the healing process. Instead of squeezing, teens should try the following treatment. As often as possible during the day, they should apply Pimple Juice (see below) directly on the blemish, using cotton balls. In the evening, they should apply a dab of Face Mud (see below) directly on the blemish and leave it overnight.

PIMPLE JUICE

½ ounce goldenseal root powder
½ ounce echinacea root powder
½ ounce black walnut hull powder

½ ounce myrrh powder
1 pint rubbing alcohol

To Make:

Mix the powdered herbs together and place in a wide-mouthed jar. Pour the rubbing alcohol over the herbs and cover with a tight-fitting lid. Place the mixture in a warm spot in the house and shake once a day to keep the herbs from packing together at the bottom of the jar. Let sit for two to three weeks. Then strain and rebottle. Do not shake the herb mixture for a couple of days before straining. This allows the herbs to settle on the bottom of the jar and makes straining easier.

Pimple Juice does not need to be refrigerated and will last indefinitely. Be sure to mark *For External Use* only. To make it even more effective, add a drop or two of tea tree oil (an essential oil available at natural food and herb stores) to the finished juice.

FACE MUD

For this recipe, use either green or red clay. These clays tend to be stronger and more potent than the white, cosmetic grade clay. Mix into a thick paste with Pimple Juice. Store in a small jar with a tight-fitting lid. If the lid is left off, the clay will dry out. To reconstitute, mix with water or more of the above mixture. Tea tree oil is a wonderful addition to this healing "mud." Add just a tiny drop or two.

In the evening, after washing the face well with cleansing grains and warm water, dab some of the Pimple Juice on the blemish. Next, apply a dab of the Face Mud directly on the pimple(s). Leave it on until it's completely dry—or better yet, leave it on overnight. Rinse off with warm water.

Women of the
CHILDBEARING
YEARS

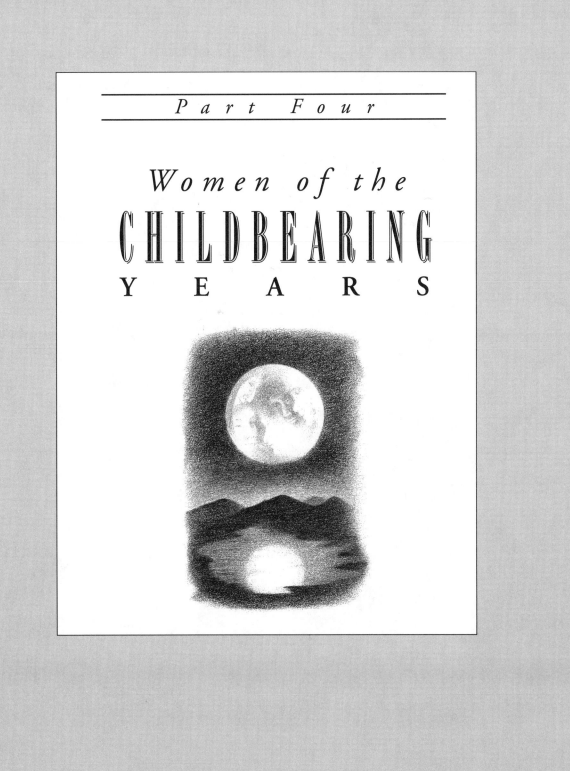

F I F T E E N

Women's Health

CHILD-
BEARING
YEARS

·

107

The wise woman within us remembers our goodness. She speaks to us in our dreams, through the rustling of leaves, the singing of a stream, the aroma of herbs and the call of the whippoorwill. She encourages us to heal our wounds. She asks us to remember our connection to all that is beautiful and sacred. She asks us to remember that we are a part of all beauty.

—Deb Soule of Avena Botanicals

Our fertile years, those years that begin at the onset of the first menstrual cycle and end at the completion of the last cycle, occupy the greatest percentage of our adult life. No longer the child beginning on the long journey of life, not yet the crone, the older woman who has earned her right to wisdom through the experiences of living life, we enter our fertile years, the years of creative endeavor and the manifestation of life purpose. These are generally the years when we form lasting relationships, experience love and lovers, raise families, and transform our deepest dreams into reality.

For many women these fertile years, though empowering and creative, also mark a period of intense physical discomfort. The natural processes of ovulation, menstruation, and childbearing are often beset with pain and physical difficulties. Such common problems as infertility, menstrual discomfort, hormonal imbalances, breast tumors, cervical and vaginal inflammation, endometriosis, and vaginal infections often surface during these years. The problems may often be deep and old, tracing back to childhood fears and angers, traumas buried but not forgotten in the souls of our being. We frequently accumulate emotional aches and pains gathered in the bittersweet process of experiencing life. These old sorrows are stored deep in the moist hidden recesses of our reproductive organs, in the source of our feminine beings, composting there until they either turn into fertile soil or, more often, ferment and decay. These hidden pains, feelings, and emotions are often the root cause of many of the physical problems that surface during our adult years as growths, blockages, or obstructions in our reproductive systems.

When I was just beginning my career as an herbalist, I was perplexed by the vast number of women who had problems in their reproductive organs. For a long time, I accepted the commonly held belief that this was because the female body was a more complex organism than the male body. We gave birth, mothered, menstruated, passed through menopause; there were more "parts," it seemed, to break down. Although this view certainly doesn't give credit to the equally complex male system, the myth continues to be perpetuated by many women.

One thing I've learned for certain as I've walked the Medicine Wheel of Time is that there are no simple answers. It's true, our bodies are wonderfully complicated and intricate. But unlike machines, this marvelous human system has evolved over countless eons and is an incredibly capable organism. I hardly think that the problems concerning menstruation, fertility, birthing, and menopause are due to faulty evolution. Instead, I question the environment we live in and our current cultural attitudes and beliefs. Is it possible that our human bodies, accustomed to a much slower process of maturation, have not developed the ability to assimilate this radical chemical and psychological onslaught?

It may be that the vast array of chemicals introduced daily into our environment are contributing to the rise in women's health problems. But the roots of this plague go even deeper, embedded in the very core of our beings. We have lost touch with our feminine source of power, that place that nourishes and sustains us. Instead, we continue to support and perpetuate those myths, including that of radical feminism, that lead us further down the road of imbalance and ill health. In order to reclaim our health and our Wise Woman tradition, we must begin to nourish that center of power that feeds our life force. The power stems from the very organs that make us unique.

An extremely responsive system of our bodies, our reproductive organs act as sensors for our inner feelings. Our wombs are our centers and do far more than produce babies: they give birth to the power in us. They help create our dreams; they birth our own vital juices. The rhythms of the universe, the ebb and flow of the tides of life, the energies of the earth and moon are mirrored in the cycles of womanhood.

Deeply wounded, our feminine organs are much like the spirit of the female earth we live upon; powerful but abused. They are crying out for healing. We have the same indomitable spirit within us as the earth that nourishes us. We have the same amazing strength and force, and the same ancient wisdom implanted in our bones. It is learning to listen to that wisdom and respond to it that is our current task. And it is happening in a collective way right now.

To understand our feminine imbalances and find the paths to wellness, we must return to simple truths and learn again the message of the rhythmic earth and the corresponding moon cycles. In many native cultures, the earth is considered feminine in gender. She is the mother, the nourisher of all life. The moon is considered the grandmother, wise, elusive, and dreamlike. These two great feminine luminaries are part of us, encoded in our psyches. What happens to the earth, happens to *us*. We feel it in our bones and flesh. "If," as Sister Miriam McGillis so eloquently says, "we humans are the sense organs of the earth, and the place where the earth dreams, then perhaps our bodies are also the place where she weeps." Feminine pain is often not just personal pain, but a reflection of the earth and humanity. What the earth feels, *we* feel. As we learn to heal ourselves and speak to our feminine needs, then we also begin the process of healing the earth, our families, and our sisters.

Herbs connect us to the heart of the earth and to her ancient healing power. Herbs awaken our Wise Woman selves. They help restore the balance deep within us because the plants themselves embody wholeness. Herbs feed and nourish our entire systems and instill within our hearts the spirit of life and beauty.

Herbs for Women

There are many remarkable healing herbs used specifically for the female system. They serve as tonics, feeding and nourishing the reproductive system, and many are also used for healing specific ailments. The following herbs are some of my favorites, the ones I most often use in my herbal work with women. (For a detailed description of each of these herbs see the Materia Medica in Part VII.)

Angelica *(Angelica archangelica)*
Black Cohash *(Cimicifuga racemosa)*
Black haw *(Viburnum prunifolium)*
Blue Cohash *(Caulophyllum thalictroides)*
Comfrey *(Symphytum officinale)*
Cramp Bark *(Viburnum opulus)*
Dong quai *(Angelica sinensis)*
False unicorn root *(Chamaelirium luteum)*
Ginger *(Zingiber officianle)*
Licorice root *(Glycyrrhiza globra)*
Motherwort *(Leonurus cardiaca)*
Mugwort *(Artemisia vulgaris)*
Nettle *(Urtica dioica)*
Pennyroyal leaf *(Hedeoma pulegioides* and related species)*
Raspberry leaf *(Rubus idaeus, R. strigosus)*
Squaw vine *(Mitchella repens)*
Vitex *(Vitex agnus casus)*
Wild yam root *(Dioscorea villosa)*
Yarrow *(Achillea millefolium)*

raspberry

Though all the above herbs are used frequently for the female system, they each have different properties and physiological actions and are indicated for different needs and specific actions. It is important to have a basic understanding of the primary actions of these herbs on the reproductive system. This will help you chose the most appropriate herb(s) for each situation and also give you a rudimentary understanding of how and why each herb is working. The following categories characterize the major physiological action of herbs used for the female system. Since herbs are multifaceted and have many actions, most will fit into one or more categories.

Uterine Tonics

These herbs are specific for toning and strengthening the whole female reproductive system. They are generally extremely potent in vitamins and minerals. They feed and nourish the reproductive organs, are used for restoring vitality and balance, and give general tone to the system. They are generally recommended for use over long periods of time and have little or no known side effects. Some examples of uterine tonics are: black cohash root, comfrey root and leaf, dong quai root, ginger root, licorice root, motherwort leaf, nettle leaf, squaw vine, strawberry leaf, and vitex (chaste berry).

Emmenagogic Herbs

These herbs help stimulate and promote normal menstrual flows. They are very beneficial for relieving menstrual cramps and for bringing on suppressed or delayed menstruation. While many emmenagogues are also uterine tonics, some promote menstruation by irritating or stimulating the uterine muscles. Be sure you know whether the emmenagogue herbs you are using primarily promote menstruation through a tonic, nourishing action or through a stimulating or irritating action. Some examples of emmenagogic herbs are: angelica root, black haw, blue cohash, cramp bark, dong quai root, false unicorn root, ginger root, motherwort leaf, mugwort leaf, pennyroyal leaf, squaw vine, and yarrow flower and leaf.

Hormonal Balancers and/or Regulators

These are herbs that balance and normalize the functions of the endocrine glands. They balance estrogen and progesterone production and regulate the activity of these and other hormones. Hormonal balancers are useful in all aspects of menstrual dysfunction. Contrary to popular opinion, they do not actually contain hormones, but are considered hormone precursors. They provide the necessary elements or building blocks to produce hormones. Most are also considered prime "liver" herbs, since much of the activity of hormonal production is dependent on the health of the liver. Some examples of hormonal balancers are: black cohash, black haw, dong quai root, false unicorn root, licorice root, vitex (chaste berry), and wild yam root.

Uterine Contractors

These herbs promote uterine contractions and are used for stimulating delayed menstruation, stimulating contractions during prolonged labor, and as abortifacient agents. Some of these herbs contain oxytocin, which encourages the production of prostaglandins in the body. High levels of prostaglandins in the system stimulate uterine contractions. Some uterine contractors work by stimulating blood flow to the uterus. Other uterine contractors cause contractions by irritating and activating the uterine membrane. A few of the herbs considered uterine contractors are actually toxic and should be avoided. Though these herbs are a potentially helpful group, you should be sure to understand *them and their particular function well before using them in your herbal work.* Some examples of uterine contractors are: angelica, blue cohash root, cotton root bark, parsley root and leaf, pennyroyal leaf and flower, rue leaf, and tansy leaf.

Herb Teas for General Health

There are many nourishing and tasty teas that serve as general tonics for the reproductive system and the endocrine glands. The following are two of my favorite female tonic teas. When using them as a tonic for the reproductive system, it is necessary to drink two to four cups daily for an extended period of time (two to three months). Herbs work surely and steadily, but not overnight. To make it easier to prepare and drink your tonic teas, make at least a quart at a time. I suggest making your tea in the evening and letting it infuse overnight in a quart canning jar. The next morning, warm it, strain, and pour it into a thermos. It will be hot and ready to drink whenever you wish.

FEMALE TONIC TEA

This is an especially nice tonic formula for the reproductive system. It is rich in vitamins and minerals, and contains uterine tonic herbs. It has a nice refreshing "green" taste.

2 parts raspberry leaf
1 part strawberry leaf
2 parts nettle
2 parts peppermint and/or spearmint

2 parts lemon grass
1 part squaw vine
stevia to taste

To Make:
Use four to six tablespoons of herb mixture per quart of water. Add herb mixture to cold water and bring to the simmering point. Remove from heat and allow to infuse for twenty minutes. Strain. Drink three to four cups daily.

WOMEN'S "ROOT" TEA

This is one of my favorite "root beer" teas. It has a flavor reminiscent of homemade old-fashioned root beer. It is a wonderful tonic for the endocrine glands, contains liver cleansing herbs, and is useful for gently regulating hormone production.

3 parts sassafras bark
2 parts dandelion root
1 part licorice root
1 part pau d'arco
1 part vitex (chaste berry)
1 part wild yam root

1 part ginger root
½ part cinnamon
¼ part orange peel
¼ part dong quai root
Optional: a pinch of stevia

To Make:

Use four to six tablespoons of herb mixture per quart of water. Add herb mixture to cold water and simmer for twenty minutes. Strain. Drink three to four cups daily.

The Liver

Our largest and most metabolically diversified internal organ, the liver performs more functions than any other single organ of the body. It is believed that the word liver derives from an Anglo-Saxon word "to live," and certainly, no one could live long without one. In traditional Chinese medicine the liver was believed to house the soul and be responsible for the flow of chi, or energy, in the body.

The liver is the body's master detoxifier and cleanses the system, not only of environmental toxins, but of metabolic wastes. It is also a major organ of digestion; every ingested substance must be processed by the liver before being distributed through the body. The health of the entire body is directly related to the well-being of the liver.

Our reproductive organs are also dependent on the health of the liver for their vitality and well-being. The liver is directly responsible for manufacturing many of the building blocks necessary for hormonal production. It also helps regulate hormonal activity. When a women does not respond well to an herbal therapy based on uterine tonics or feminine tonic herbs, the emphasis of the herbal program should be shifted to the liver. I've seen many tenacious cases of reproductive problems respond well to liver tonic herbs. It is also interesting to note that many of the herbs used for the reproductive system are specifically indicated for the liver as well. When an herbal program includes the liver as well as the reproductive system, recovery is often much quicker and more thorough.

The following two formulas are excellent examples of liver tonic teas that are also specific for the reproductive system.

BITTERROOT BLEND

This rooty bitter blend includes herbs that are excellent, both for the reproductive system and for the liver. The flavor may need to be enhanced by adding sassafras, cinnamon, lemon or orange peel, and ginger.

1 part yellow dock root   1 part wild yam root
2 parts dandelion root   ½ part oregon grape root
1 part vitex (chaste berry)

To Make:

Use four to six tablespoons of herb mixture per quart of water. Add the herb mixture to cold water and simmer over a low heat for twenty minutes. Keep pot tightly covered. Strain. Drink three to four cups daily.

A nice-tasting tea, this includes leaves and flowers that are tonics to the liver.

3 parts nettle leaf
2 parts dandelion leaf
1 part alfalfa leaf

1 part chamomile flowers
2 parts red clover flowers
2 parts lemon balm (melissa)

To prepare:
Use four to six tablespoons of herb mixture per quart of water. Add the herb mixture to cold water and heat over low heat to the simmering point. Keep pot tightly covered. Remove from heat and let infuse for twenty minutes. Strain. Drink three to four cups daily.

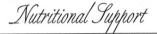

Nutritional Support

Diet is essential to most health programs. But it is easy to get fanatical about diet and attempt to establish guidelines you can't possibly adhere to. Be reasonable and responsible in your own eating needs. Establish a balanced, healthy diet designed for your personal needs, based on simple guidelines that are constructive to follow. The female system by its very nature is *yin* (inward, sweet, moist, expansive) and generally needs balancing with a diet that is more *yang* (outward, solid, dry, contractive). Concentrate on whole natural foods: whole grains, dark green leafy vegetables, root vegetables, high-quality protein, and natural oils from seeds, nuts, and grains. Avoid as much as possible all refined processed food, sweets (natural sweets as well as candy bars and ice cream), coffee, and alcohol. An excellent, well-written book that provides sensible dietary guidelines is Food and Healing by Annemarie Colbin. (See Appendix I for other suggestions.)

In cases of severe reproductive disorders, I suggest seeing both a holistic health care professional and a nutritional consultant. A nutritional consultant will help you set up a dietary program aimed at your needs and help you establish guidelines for following it. Unless you are already informed about diet and are an extremely disciplined person, you will find the consultant's guidance not only helpful but necessary.

Sitz Baths

A wonderful and very effective therapy for restoring the health and vitality of the reproductive system, sitz baths can be enjoyed weekly as a tonic treatment or used more frequently as part of a more rigorous health program. Sitz baths apply the principles of hydrotherapy to draw fresh blood to the pelvic area. Using applications of hot and cold water, you alternately dilate and constrict the blood vessels in the pelvic area. When the blood vessels are dilated, a fresh flow of blood is carried to the area. When they are constricted, the blood is forced away. This pumping action serves to concentrate energy in the area and aids in removing stagnation and blocked energy. At one time sitz baths were used extensively in medical practice, but are now largely ignored even though they have been proven beneficial in treating many female problems.

To do a sitz bath you will need two large buckets. They need to be big enough to hold your buttocks comfortably, yet must fit inside your bathtub or shower. Plastic buckets are more comfortable than metal ones. Fill one bucket with hot, hot water. For added benefit you can make an herbal tea, such as nettle or raspberry tea to add to the hot water. The other bucket needs to be filled with the coldest water possible. You might need to drop a few ice cubes into the cold water to keep it really icy cold.

Now, get ready. Carefully ease your buttocks into the hot water. The water should be almost uncomfortably hot, but not so hot that you burn! Sit for several minutes and just when it starts to get comfortable, transfer your hot, pink buns to the cold bucket. It will be shocking. Force yourself to sit there for several minutes. And just when it begins to feel tolerable—you've got it—back into the hot bucket. Repeat this process five to six times, several times a week. Just in case it sounds too torturous, it really doesn't feel that uncomfortable, and the benefits are certainly worth it.

Rest

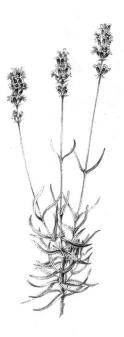

lavender

As in any program of health, a fine balance of rest and nonstressful activity must be maintained. I mention this very simple fact because in years of practice I have seen that many of the causes of reproductive imbalance stem from just being tired out from trying to keep up with a social structure that demands that women be "superwomen." Sometimes, just slowing down and finding the inner strength to admit we cannot/do not have to do everything is the only medicine needed.

If you've been experiencing recurring health problems, look seriously and deeply at the level of stress that characterizes your life-style and the business of your days. The remedy for your health problem may be just to slow down. Granted, this can be a very difficult prescription to fill. Allow plenty of time to sleep. Try sleeping all you want. This is a marvelous luxury that most women never allow themselves, yet it is one of those simple remedies that can achieve miracles. Allow time for massage, for exercise, for quiet reflection. Do only what is absolutely necessary during your day. Although it sounds easy, this can be an immensely difficult decision to stick to; it requires taking back control of your life. But while it may lose you your "superwoman" title, it will do wonders to help you regain your power and health.

Ceremonies

Develop ways to empower your Wise Woman self. Ceremonies are wonderful ways to do this. Developing a relationship with the earth is another way. Garden! Dance! Sing! Dream! Create the space in your life to enjoy those activities that enrich your soul and strengthen your inner woman. It is by nourishing the wellspring of our creativity that our power returns to us and the richness of our life unfolds.

Ceremonies can be as simple as making lunar teas on the full moon. Or bleeding into the earth during your menstrual cycle (a very empowering experience, by the way). Or enjoying a weekly herbal bath replete with bubbles, candles, and incense. I have always enjoyed celebrating life with ritual. One of my favorite annual ceremonies is to camp out on our mountain alone on my birthday, an especially magical rite because I'm a December child and the mountain is deep in snow. When I come down from the mountain I feel empowered by my Wise Woman self and ready to enjoy another year of life.

Supplements

There are several concentrated food substances that revitalize the reproductive organs. I would suggest incorporating these into your daily health program. (Further information on these food supplements is provided in Part III and Part VI of this book.)

❦ Take two dong quai capsules three times daily. Or eat a small piece of dong quai root about the size of the pink portion of your small fingernail daily. This truly is a wonder herb for women. But do not take dong quai during your moon cycle as it may stimulate bleeding. (For more information, see the Materia Medica in Part VII.)

❦ Take one-fourth to one-half teaspoon of bee pollen daily. (Those with allergies should use bee pollen with caution.)

❦ Take one to two teaspoons spirulina daily.

❦ Take liquid Floradix with Iron daily, in the dosage suggested on the bottle. This liquid herbal vitamin/mineral formula is an excellent source of iron, calcium, and other minerals and vitamins. You can also make a vitamin/mineral formula similar to Floradix by following the recipe on page 62.

❦ Take 200–400 I.U. of Vitamin E daily. Vitamin E is essential to the health of the reproductive system.

❦ Consume adequate amounts of calcium and magnesium each day. Though most people think they get enough calcium by eating large amounts of dairy food (milk, cheese, cottage cheese, ice cream, butter, etc.), dairy is not the best source of dietary calcium. Many vegetables, including seaweeds, have a far greater concentration of assimilated calcium/magnesium. Also, seeds and nuts are good sources of these minerals. Many herbs are excellent sources of calcium/magnesium: nettle, comfrey, watercress, parsley, oat straw, horsetail, seaweed, and yellow dock. It may be necessary to back up your diet with a high-quality calcium/magnesium supplement as well.

Menstrual Problems: Cramps, Light or Heavy Bleeding, PMS, and Endometriosis

We romanticize that in centuries past a woman's moon time was an honored event and that women were held in high esteem during their monthly bleeding. Moon lodges were built especially for this purpose some distance from the rest of the village. Each month, menstruating women were assured a week's vacation from the daily routine of life. Other women would cook and bring them food. Menstruating women had no contact with the children or men of the village. There was a list of taboos that prohibited them from doing many of the everyday tasks of life, but left them free to dream and rest and gossip with the other village women in the same "condition."

This is a belief that imagines once way back in history people were freer and more liberated about menstruation than they have been in recent days. I believe that somewhere, back in an obscure and remote time, a time buried deep in the recesses of our memories, this may have been true. But in more recent times, it is likely that the actual reason for separating women from the rest of the group while they were bleeding was less out of honor and respect for menstruation than out of fear and aversion to an "unclean" act. The fact that the practice did give women a needed rest and an opportunity to relax from daily chores was simply a by-product of the restrictions and taboos placed on women in earlier times.

In truth, I feel we are far more open and have greater opportunities to change existing patterns and myths about menstruation today than ever before. The menstruating woman sequestered away in a moon lodge is a thing of the past (though moon lodges can be lovely places to empower your Wise Woman self). Likewise, the lady in white playing tennis while wearing a tampon is rapidly becoming an image of the past. Today we can consciously recreate our menstrual myths and our sense of womanhood as it is born again each month in the womb of our moon time.

This reformation is dependent on the younger generation of women, as most change is. But it depends also on the older generation of women who will teach and guide their daughters through the early stages of womanhood. As young women are introduced to their menstrual cycles in a positive and empowering manner, the negative images surrounding menstruation will naturally metamorphose. It is this cultural process of change that ensures lasting transformation. And as our images and ideals of menstruation change, the health problems associated with it will begin to disappear as well.

Painful/Cramping Menstruation (Dysmenorrhea)

Cramps can be very debilitating and can force a menstruating woman into bed during the entire duration of her menstrual cycle. The usual medicine offered is aspirinlike medication. Though this may very well suppress the pain, it will never correct the problem. Herbal therapies offer a wonderful alternative to symptom-suppressing medication and have an excellent success rate when used over a period of time.

About ten days before menstruation begins, the level of blood calcium begins to drop and continues to drop until about three days into the cycle. Blood calcium deficiency is characterized by muscle cramps, headaches, water retention, achiness, depression, and insomnia. These are not only symptoms of cramping and painful menstruation but are also the symptoms associated with PMS.

To Prevent Monthly Cramps

❦ Increase your intake of calcium ten days prior to your period to ensure that you have an adequate supply of blood calcium. Include in your diet foods high in easily digestible calcium, such as sesame seeds, tahini, sesame butter, yogurt, kelp, hizike (and other seaweeds), dark green leafy vegetables such as kale, parsley, spinach, fresh sprouts, and herbs such as comfrey, raspberry, and nettle.

❦ Take Floradix and/or some other biochelated calcium supplement daily. (To make your own calcium/iron supplement, see page 62.) Do not depend entirely, however, on a supplement to supply the necessary amount of calcium. You must include calcium in your diet as food. A supplement is just that—a supplement—and not a substitution for proper nutrition.

❦ For three weeks each month, drink three to four cups of the following tea every day.

HORMONAL REGULATOR TEA

1 part wild yam	2 parts licorice root
1 part ginger	2 parts sassafras
2 parts dandelion root (raw)	1 part yellow dock
2 parts burdock root (raw)	¼ part vitex

To Make:

Use four to six tablespoons herb mixture per quart of water. Add herbs to cold water and bring to a slow simmer. Keep pot covered. Simmer for twenty minutes. Strain. Drink three to four cups daily.

For ten days before your menstruation begins, drink three to four cups of the following tea formula.

HERBAL
HEALING
FOR
WOMEN
•
118

HIGH-CALCIUM TEA

2 parts oat straw

1 part horsetail
   (also known as shavegrass)

2 parts comfrey

2 parts nettle

4 parts peppermint

2 parts pennyroyal

4 parts raspberry leaf

To Make:

Use four to six tablespoons herb mixture per quart of water. Add herbs to cold water and being to a slow simmer. Keep pot covered. Remove from heat and let infuse twenty minutes. Strain. Drink three to four cups daily.

❦ If, during your moon cycle, cramping does occur, do not eat or drink anything cold. Place a warm compress and/or a heating pad over the pelvic area and drink the following tea every fifteen minutes until the cramps cease. This blend is also very effective when made into a tincture.

CRAMP-T

1 part cramp bark (or black haw)

1 part pennyroyal leaf

1 part valerian root

½ part ginger

To Make:

Use four to six tablespoons of herb mixture per quart of water. First decoct the cramp bark and ginger root for twenty minutes, simmering slowly over low heat. Turn off the heat and add the pennyroyal and valerian root to the mixture. (Valerian and pennyroyal lose their herbal essence if decocted and are best prepared by infusing.) Steep an additional fifteen to twenty minutes. Strain. Drink one-fourth cup every fifteen minutes until cramps cease.

❦ Valerian root tincture is very helpful for relieving the pain of cramps. A wonderful nervine tonic, valerian has specific remedial actions on the muscles and ligaments. It is excellent for relieving cramps, muscle spasms, and backaches due to tired muscles. Valerian is dose dependent: its effectiveness is determined by the dosage administered. Though it is wise to begin with small amounts, do not be concerned about taking too much. Valerian is most effective when taken in fairly large dosages. I generally recommend taking one-half teaspoon every twenty minutes until the pain subsides. I've taken up to one-half ounce myself during insomnia attacks, with excellent results. Unlike the drug Valium, whose name sounds vaguely similar, valerian is not addictive.

❦ Another remedy for cramps that I've found very helpful is rubbing pure pennyroyal oil over the pelvic area. *Be careful not to get too close to the sensitive vaginal lips; because the oil is extremely concentrated, it can burn or irritate the sensitive skin around the vulva. If you have sensitive skin, dilute the pennyroyal oil in a small amount of vegetable oil.* And in any case, use only a small amount of pennyroyal oil. A few drops should be sufficient. I was experiencing mild cramps the first time I tried this remedy. I had decided that pennyroyal oil might be useful and rubbed a small amount on my hands, then proceeded to massage my pelvic muscles. It felt wonderful and was very warming and soothing. Since a little worked so well, I thought I'd try more. By the time I was finished with my pelvic "massage," I had probably used a teaspoon or two of oil. I was feeling fine. Shortly afterwards, I had to run to the local store. I was standing in line with a cart full of fruit and vegetables when I felt a gush of warm blood. I promptly excused myself and rushed to the nearest bathroom. I must have expelled my entire menstrual blood in that one strong outburst. It was amazing and taught me a good lesson. I have since employed this treatment successfully, but have never used more than a few drops.

Pennyroyal oil is a powerful uterine contractor and will help ease menstrual cramps. It also stimulates and encourages the menstrual flow. But the oil (not the whole plant) is extremely toxic if taken *internally*. So one must be careful when working with it.

Unfortunately, though pennyroyal is a lovely little healing mint, it has acquired a bad reputation. In the 1970s two young women who thought themselves pregnant, decided to self-abort. Ignoring warnings that pennyroyal oil is extremely toxic when taken internally, they each drank a full ounce of distilled pennyroyal oil. Both young women died as a result. Because of this tragic accident, an herb that had always been valued by midwives for its healing properties came to be thought of as highly poisonous.

The good news about pennyroyal is that you can still use the herb in tea (which is totally nontoxic). The oil is available for external use only. (NEVER, NEVER USE THE OIL FOR MAKING TEA!) But the herb is a wonderful aid for menstruating women, helping to alleviate cramps, and bring on delayed menstruation.

If you follow the above suggestions for three to four months, you should notice a significant improvement in your menstrual cycle. Do not expect much change the first cycle or two. The herbs may take several cycles to make a significant difference. It generally requires a commitment and several moon cycles before one begins to notice the changes; but once begun, those changes are deep and enduring. It may also be beneficial during this period to evaluate your relationship to your moon cycle. Joining women's support groups, doing dream work, and finding other ways to explore the inner threads of your being often provide the tools necessary to aid in the process of healing the feminine.

Excessive Menstruation (Menorrhagia)

The usual suggestion for women suffering from menorrhagia is to be placed on birth control pills. If birth control pills do not control the excessive monthly bleeding, another "cure" sometimes offered is a hysterectomy. One day when I was working at my herb store, I got a call from a very worried mother. Her daughter had suffered from the onset of her menstrual cycle with severe menorrhagia. Her concerned parents had followed their doctor's advice and put her on an early program of birth control pills.

Though this helped some, the young woman continued to bleed excessively and on several different occasions had to be treated with blood transfusions at the local hospital. Though she was barely eighteen, her doctors felt there was little hope for ever establishing a normal menstrual cycle and were suggesting a hysterectomy to correct the problem.

When I first saw Marie, she was pale, drawn, and obviously very anemic. But her spirits were good. She was an exceptionally bright, enthusiastic young woman. She had determined that she did not want a hysterectomy and was willing to try anything to avoid one. I knew my "prescription" was strange to her: eat seaweed, take tinctures, sitz baths, drink tea; no potato chips, soda pop, or candy. Because of the extreme nature of her disorder, I suggested a fairly rigorous program for her to follow and asked for her full commitment in following it.

Within the first three months her menstrual cycles improved dramatically. By the sixth month she began experiencing the first "normal" flows in her life. Several years later when I saw her again, she was happily married and the mother of a healthy baby girl. She reported that her menstrual cycles continued to flow normally, although she had to be careful of what she ate and used extra precautions with her diet. Though she no longer had to follow as rigorous an herbal or dietary program, she continued to use herbs to help regulate and normalize her menstrual flow.

There are several causes for menorrhagia. It may be caused by endometriosis (see page 128) or by blockages in the pelvic area, such as fibroids, cysts, or tumors (see Chapter 19). Menorrhagia is often a result of imbalances in various organ systems of the body. There are two systems of the body that seem to have a direct influence on the amount of bleeding that occurs each month, the endocrine gland system (especially the thyroid) and the liver. By nourishing and strengthening the endocrine glands and the liver and by correcting the underlying causes, excess bleeding during menstruation can often be reduced to a comfortable flow.

Diet plays an essential role in correcting menorrhagia and one should incorporate many of the suggestions below. Not only do diet, herbs, and supplements help correct the problem, they are also essential in restoring the excess minerals and vitamins lost during the course of a heavy menstrual flow. The following suggestions are recommended, both to correct the problem and to restore energy to the body.

To Curb Excessive Menstrual Flow
❧ Include seaweed in your diet each day. You can take seaweed in capsule form, but preferably incorporate the seaweed into your diet as food. Try some of the milder-tasting seaweed, such as hizike (hijike) and dulse. (Kelp, though excellent, is strong-tasting and has a very fishy aftertaste.) Seaweeds may be eaten with cooked grains, in soups, casseroles, and salads. They are incredibly high in trace minerals and vitamins and feed and nourish the endocrine glands. They are specifically recommended for the health of the thyroid gland, which plays a major role in regulating menstrual flow.
❧ Take a liquid-iron mineral supplement each day. I generally recommend liquid Floradix Iron with herbs or other, similar preparations. (To make your own liquid iron supplement, see recipe on page 62.) If the menorrhagia is severe, you may wish to double

the dosage normally recommended. Floradix Iron and Herbs is available in most natural food/herb stores and is an excellent natural iron/mineral tonic. Liquid iron supplements help build the blood and restore depleted vitamin and mineral reserves in the body. After an excessive menstrual flow, it is not uncommon to feel completely worn out and drained. So it is important to rebuild the system with foods rich in iron, vitamins, and other minerals.

❦ Eat plenty of dark green leafy vegetables, root vegetables, high-quality protein foods, and whole grains. (Avoid red meat.) Eat for well-being and wholeness.

❦ Take the following two herb formulas throughout the month. Both are excellent teas for both the liver and endocrine gland system.

VITA-ROOT TEA

2 parts wild yam root

2 parts sassafras and/or birch bark for flavor

2 parts licorice root

1 part cinnamon

1 part burdock root

1 part vitex

3 parts dandelion root

2 parts pau d'arco

1 part comfrey root

1 part ginger root

Optional: ginger, cinnamon, orange peel, licorice, or other pleasant-tasting herbs to taste.

To Make:

Use four to six tablespoons of the herb mixture per quart of water. Place in cold water over a low heat and slowly bring to a simmer. Simmer gently for twenty minutes, keeping the pot covered all the while. Strain. Drink three to four cups daily for at least four months.

WOMEN'S POWER CAPSULES

1 part dong quai powder

2 parts burdock root powder

1 part astragalus powder

4 parts dandelion root (raw) powder

1 part yellow dock root powder

2 parts spirulina powder

To Make:

Mix the herb powders together and capsulate in "00" size capsules. Take two capsules three times daily during the month. Discontinue taking the capsules when you start to bleed and begin them again at the completion of your menstrual flow.

❦ Avoid all refined foods, sweets, alcohol, caffeine, and nicotine. These will only exacerbate the problem you are trying to correct.

❦ Do not use dong quai or angelica during menstruation, as these herbs can promote bleeding.

❦ One week before menstruation begins drink three cups of the following tea daily.

HERBAL
HEALING
FOR
WOMEN
•

122

FLOOD GATES TEA

2 parts shepherd's purse leaf　　　1 part nettle leaf
1 part yarrow flowers/leaf　　　　2 parts white oak bark

To Make:

Use four to six tablespoons of herb mixture per quart of water. Place herbs in cold water and slowly heat to a simmer. Simmer over low heat for twenty minutes. Strain.

❧ When bleeding begins, continue drinking this tea frequently in small amounts (about one-fourth cup every half hour. Flood Gates Tea can also be made into a tincture (for directions, see page 66). If taking it in tincture form, take one-fourth teaspoon every hour, or more frequently if needed.

As with the program for painful menstrual cycles, do not expect to see dramatic changes in the first month or two. Give the body a chance to progress slowly and steadily. Though this requires a commitment to your personal well-being and the courage to make life-style changes, the process is generally empowering and the results long-lasting.

Lack of Menstruation (Amenorrhea)

Many women experience partial or total amenorrhea: their menstrual cycles just stop. There can be many causes for this complete lack of menstruation in women. Emotional stress, blocked or hidden traumas, lack of adequate nutrition (especially the lack of high-quality protein and fats), hormonal imbalances, an overly rigorous exercise program, or a negative outlook toward menstruation—each can result in amenorrhea. One of the most common causes is the use of birth control pills. Many women have waited for months, even years, for their menstrual cycle to return after having been on birth control pills for an extended period of time.

If a treatment program is followed conscientiously, the menstrual cycle will almost always reestablish itself and return. I have found the following measures effective in helping to restore menstrual cycles.

❧ Drink Female Tonic Tea (see page 111) or Women's "Root" Tea (see page 111) every day to restore hormonal balance and cleanse and strengthen the liver. You can either alternate these teas or drink the one that tastes the best to you.

❧ Take Liquid Floradix Iron with Herbs or a similar liquid iron vitamin mineral formula daily. Follow recommended dosage on the bottle. (For directions on how to make a liquid vitamin mineral supplement, see page 62).

❧ If you can remember the days of the month when you used to menstruate, establish that as your current menstruating cycle. If you don't remember when your menstrual cycle occurred, choose a new menstrual cycle for yourself. The full moon can be an excellent reference point and is an especially powerful time for most women. The fluid energies of the earth are strong. Our bodies seem to respond to the great magnetic forces set in motion by the energies of the moon. Observe the cycles of the moon and their effect on you and, if possible, establish your menstrual cycle in harmony with the rhythmic flow of the moon.

If working with these forces may seem foreign to you, think about the powerful influence the moon has on our lives. When the moon waxes full, the tides of the earth are at their highest. At the waning of the moon, the tides are at their lowest. All the fluid energy of the earth responds to the moon cycles. Animals and plants are also directly affected by the cycles of the moon. Though there have been numerous scientific studies conducted on the effects the moon has on life on earth, the mystery has not been lessened. The magic of the moon's influence on our lives cannot be explained in rational terms. It can only be felt and experienced.

❦ Drink three to four cups of the following formula during your envisioned menstruating time.

BRINGING ON THE MOON TEA

2 parts pennyroyal herb	½ part yarrow
2 parts peppermint	½ part mugwort
1 part ginger	

To Make:

Use four to six tablespoons of herb mixture per quart of water. Place herbs in cold water and bring slowly to a simmer over low heat. Keep covered tightly. Take off the heat immediately and allow to steep for twenty minutes. Strain.

❦ During this period surround yourself with other menstruating women. This may sound like a strange suggestion, but it certainly works. And it has actually been proven successful by scientific studies. Women who work together, go to school together, or live together often establish a similar menstruating rhythm. Menstruating women secrete a chemical called pheromone. This enzyme triggers a hormonal reaction in other women which can stimulate the menstrual cycle. Many of us who have attended the large women's conferences held in northern California have been amazed to find out how many women actually get their periods during the course of the gathering. We would have to bring in truckloads of sanitary pads! And watch out if the moon was full! This triggered the response even more.

Find out who the menstruating women are in your circle and when their cycles occur. Whenever possible, make time to be with them during their menstrual cycles. Invite them over for lunch, go to the movies together, work next to them. Though this may seem like an odd suggestion and may be difficult to implement within your circle of associates, it's an idea that works well and is worth experimenting with.

❦ Several days before menstruation is scheduled to begin according to the schedule you've set up, take pennyroyal herbal baths each evening. Herbal baths are wonderfully therapeutic; it is like emerging your entire body in a giant cup of tea. Your pores will be wide open and receptive in the warm water, and the herbs will readily permeate the epidermal layer.

Pennyroyal herb is a powerful uterine contractor and has been highly valued by many women to bring on delayed menstruation. It is useful both as a tea and an herbal bath for amenorrhea. To prepare for a bath, fill a large cotton handkerchief with a handful of pennyroyal *herb*. (Never use pennyroyal *oil* for this purpose!) Tie the herb bag onto the nozzle of the bathtub and let the hot water pour through it for a few minutes. Adjust the temperature of the tub and immerse yourself in the water. Untie the herb bag from the nozzle and use it as a refreshing washcloth. For a nice treat, light a candle and some incense. While relaxing in this wonderfully fragrant herb bath, drink a cup of pennyroyal tea. (For further cautions on the use of pennyroyal, see page 118–9 and the Materia Medica in Part VII.)

❦ Ceremonies are great for helping to reestablish your menstrual rhythm. Many years ago, I was told this story by my very close friend, Dyana. She had been on birth control pills since high school and had continued to take them for their efficiency and convenience. When she finally decided to discontinue the pill, her menstrual cycle did not return—as is often, though not always, the case. For several years Dyana did not have a menstrual cycle and, at first, enjoyed the freedom from her monthly bleeding. But as time went by, she became concerned and wanted to reestablish her connection with her moon cycle.

At that time Dyana had recently been introduced to ceremony. And being the wonderfully creative, wild, and artistic woman she was, she decided to choreograph a ritual for the return of her moon cycle. It was quite an elaborate affair. She invited a small group of women to join her for an all-night ceremony by the ocean at full moon. Exactly what they did I still don't know but it involved dancing to the moon, crushing ripe red berries in the place of the "third eye"—that point on the forehead's center, right above the eyes—drinking moon tea, and sharing stories around the fire. In truth, the actual steps in their ceremony weren't important. The results were: Dyana started her menstrual cycle within a few days.

I make these suggestions, strange though some may seem because I have seen them work for so many women over the years. If I knew of one magic pill or a single cure-all, I would suggest it, too. Perhaps *the Great Cure-all* is our ability to honor ourselves and to accept responsibility for taking care of what is most precious in ourselves. Most people are not willing to take *that* "pill." It requires too much conscious effort and dedicated commitment. One drinks it down with hard work, not just a glass of water.

Premenstrual Syndrome (PMS)

Until recently PMS was regarded by the medical community primarily as an imaginary dis–ease. I wonder if men were to suffer monthly from severe debilitating cramps, joint pain, bloating, headaches, and excess bleeding if PMS would be so easily dismissed as imaginary or "all in the head." It is estimated that over half the women in the United States suffer PMS symptoms every month. PMS is both a general term used to describe many of the problems already mentioned and a specific term used to describe a particular set of symptoms that occur around and during menstruation. Symptoms of PMS are varied but generally include water retention, nervousness, depression, tension, swollen, tender breasts, cramps, menstrual pain, joint pain, acne, intense craving for sweets, and a range of other symptoms that all stem from an oversensitization to the sex hormones produced by our bodies.

PMS creates a recurring monthly anxiety for many women and certainly inhibits some women from enjoying this cycle of womanhood. Instead of their moon time being a special moment to enjoy their unique "womanness," it marks a period of stress, pain, and discomfort. Though there are certainly physical causes for PMS, the root of the problem can often be traced to how we view our woman self and the negative images of our menstrual cycle that have been imprinted in our subconscious. Often this recurrence of monthly pain around our menstruation is a result of childhood abuse (not always remembered) or pain suffered in our reproductive organs.

The physical manifestations of PMS indicate an imbalance of estrogen, prolactin, adrenal, and thyroid hormones. The potentially detrimental estrogen components known as estradiol and estrone are normally converted by the liver into estriol. Estriol's function is to decrease the activity of the detrimental effects of estradiol and estrone. This process is dependent on the health of the liver and the endocrine glands (primarily the adrenals and thyroid). The liver is responsible for breaking down hormones and for cleansing the system of metabolic and environmental toxins. If the liver is not in good working order, it becomes overburdened and inefficient and is not able to handle the peak levels of sex hormones released during menstruation and ovulation. The system, in effect, becomes self-poisoned, congested with too many of its own hormones. These hormones, most notably estrogen components, can wreak havoc within the system, causing the symptoms of PMS and other potential reproductive problems.

To Prevent PMS

PMS is helped greatly by diet, exercise, and healthy living. Many women have decided to use their PMS symptoms to help them get in touch with their inner selves and, in the process of doing so, have corrected the problems associated with their menstrual cycles.

Follow these dietary suggestions to encourage the health of the liver and support its role in reducing sources of exogenous estrogen:

❧ Increase your intake of complex carbohydrates, which are found in vegetables, whole grains, beans, and fruit.
❧ Increase your intake of eggs, garlic, onions, and beans, all of which are rich in sulfur-containing amino acids.
❧ Increase your intake of antioxidants (foods rich in vitamins C and E and selenium) to increase the detoxification of estrogen.

❦ Decrease your intake of fats, especially saturated animal fats, and use unsaturated fatty acids, such as those in cold-pressed vegetable oils, instead.

❦ Decrease your intake of milk and dairy products, which are sources of exogenous estrogens. (Yogurt is acceptable.)

❦ Decrease your intake of members of the cabbage family (cabbage, brussels sprouts, cauliflower and broccoli). (Though considered excellent for our general health, these vegetables are found to be thyroid antagonists and may contribute to exogenous estrogen.)

❦ Eliminate sugar, white flour, and refined foods.

❦ Eliminate all methyl-xanthines, such as caffeine, theophylline, theobromine (coffee, tea, chocolate, and cola).

❦ Eliminate red meat and fowl, which are sources of exogenous estrogens. (Organic fowl is acceptable.)

❦ Once a day, drink a "smoothy" made of the following ingredients.

NUTRITIONAL SMOOTHY

1 teaspoon kelp	1 tablespoon spirulina
2 tablespoons granulated lecithin	1 raw egg
2 tablespoons nutritional yeast	

To Make:

Blend these ingredients in a blender with fruit juice and yogurt to taste. Bananas, frozen strawberries, and other frozen or fresh fruit help to disguise the taste of the kelp, yeast, and egg. You may have to experiment with the flavors before you are satisfied that this is a drink you not only should, but want to drink each day.

When You Have PMS

❦ Since diet plays an extremely important role in correcting PMS, it is important to work closely with a holistic practitioner and/or to follow the dietary suggestions listed above.

❦ The primary systems of the body to focus on when working with PMS are the liver, endocrine system, and nervous system. The following teas support these three major systems of the body. Drink one or more of them daily for two to three months. You may alternate the teas to suit your taste and moods.

ENDO-LIVER TEA

1 part yellow dock root

3 parts dandelion root

2 parts burdock root

1 part wild yam root

1 part astragalus

3 parts licorice root

1 part ginger

2 parts pau d'arco

1 part fo-ti

½ part vitex

½ part dong quai

Optional: cinnamon, orange peel, stevia, more licorice root, roasted dandelion root, to taste.

To Make:

Use four to six tablespoons of herb mixture per quart of water. Add herbs to cold water and bring to a slow simmer over low heat. Keep pot covered. Simmer gently for twenty minutes. Strain.

NERVOUS SYSTEM TEA

1 part oat straw leaf, stem

3 parts chamomile flowers

3 parts raspberry leaf

1 part squaw vine leaf

1 part motherwort leaf

3 parts melissa leaf

3 parts peppermint leaf

2 parts nettle leaf

2 parts red clover flowers

1 part horsetail leaf

To Make:

Use four to six tablespoons of herb mixture per quart of water. Add herbs to cold water and over low heat slowly bring to a simmer. Keep pot covered. Immediately remove from heat and let infuse twenty minutes. Strain.

red clover

❦ For the water retention often associated with PMS, drink Natural Diuretic Tea (below) for seven to ten days before your menstrual cycle begins.

NATURAL DIURETIC TEA

2 parts dandelion leaf

1 part pipsissewa leaf

3 parts nettle leaf

1 part chickweed leaf

To Make:

Use four to six tablespoons of herb mixture per quart of water. Add herbs to cold water and over low heat slowly bring to a simmer. Keep pot covered. Immediately remove from heat and let steep twenty minutes. Drink three to four cups of tea daily. For convenience and ease of administering, this formula may also be made in tincture form. (See page 66 for instructions on how to make a tincture.)

☙ Take one to two teaspoons spirulina daily. (Or take capsules of this rich green algae if its taste is unappealing to you.)

☙ Take evening primrose oil, borage, or black current seed oil (500 milligrams twice a day or follow dosage recommended on the container). These three oils are high in gamma-linolenic acid (GLA), which has a marked positive effect on PMS symptoms. It is especially beneficial for breast tenderness.

☙ Take two capsules of dong quai three times a day. Discontinue the capsules a couple of days before your menstrual cycle begins and start up again only after you have completely stopped menstruating.

☙ Take ginseng during the month. It is especially valuable for those women who lack vitality and energy or who are excessively "yin" in nature.

☙ Take a liquid vitamin mineral tonic such as liquid Floradix Iron with Herbs or NatureWorks Herbal Iron each day. (If you wish to make your own mineral tonic, follow the instructions on page 62.)

☙ Take at least two sitz baths a week. (See page 113 for instructions.)

☙ There are many herbs that are exceptionally high in calcium, such as nettle, comfrey, boneset, borage, oat straw, horsetail, watercress, seaweed, lamb's quarter, amaranth. These, along with calcium-rich foods, should be incorporated into your daily diet. Also, a good natural biochelated calcium supplement is recommended. But do not depend on a supplement to supply your calcium needs. Incorporate plenty of calcium-rich herbs and foods in your diet as well.

☙ Breast tenderness is often associated with PMS and is usually due to water retention and an imbalance of hormonal activity. Using Female Tonic Tea (see page 111) and/or Women's "Root" Tea (see page 111) during the month and incorporating several of the other suggestions will greatly reduce breast tenderness. PMS is definitely correctable. It develops, however, over a long period of time, perhaps even from the traumas of childhood, and it generally takes a commitment to life-style changes. Be patient. Using the suggestions listed here, develop a health program that works for you. Follow your program for at least four to six months. Make adjustments when necessary, but be faithful to it. Remember that lasting change is often slow in occurring. The quick change we long for is most often short-lived. Herbal remedies, though quite capable of offering short-term relief, are best when used over long periods. Only then do they ensure lasting health benefits.

Endometriosis

Though I have only a little to add to the small body of knowledge already collected on natural remedies for endometriosis, I've included it because so many women suffer from this disease and so little is known about it. Any bit of helpful advice that might bring relief to the hundreds of women who suffer from endometriosis should be readily shared. It is estimated that upwards of 15 percent of American women have endometriosis and it has rapidly become the most common cause of infertility in the United States.

Endometrial tissue lines the uterus, where it normally builds up each month. During menstruation the excessive tissue is shed. For unknown reasons, this tissue sometimes detaches from the uterus wall and spreads to other parts of the body where it can cause severe problems. This abnormal tissue has been found on the ovaries, fallopian tubes, bladder, and occasionally in such diverse places as the lungs, elbows, head, brain, and nasal passages. Though no longer attached to the uterus, the endometrial tissue continues to respond to the hormonal fluctuations in a woman's body. Whether it is attached to the uterus or the ovaries, fallopian tubes, etc., it still bleeds during the menstrual cycle. This abnormal bleeding has no way to flow out of the system. It collects and stagnates, causing serious inflammation, pain, and occasional formation of cysts and scar tissue.

Little is known about what causes endometriosis. I have heard several hypotheses, but most of them seem little more than educated guesses. There is some speculation that women who develop endometriosis have an immune system deficiency. Whether this is the cause or the result of endometriosis is questionable. Endometriosis tissue has even been found in the pelvic areas of infant girls, leading to the theory that the disease could be related to genetic defects or is possibly the result of toxic chemicals in the environment. Since endometriosis is a hyperestrogenic disease (produced by an oversecretion of estrogen), the abusive use of hormones in the raising of dairy, beef animals, and chickens could very well stimulate the overproduction of these hormones in our own bodies. The most accepted theory, however, is of "retrograde menstruation." During menstruation, especially if accompanied by excessive cramps, endometrial tissue is forced out of the uterus cavity and back up through the fallopian tubes. This "retrograde flow" carries with it endometrial tissue, which attaches itself to other organs and proceeds to grow. Since it can be found in different places throughout the body, it is believed that the disease is transported both through the lymph nodes and the blood. But all of the above are just hypotheses at this point. The cause of endometriosis has not yet been determined with any certainty.

Regardless of what causes endometrial tissue to migrate outside the uterus, estrogen stimulates its growth. Most treatment protocols focus on lowering estrogen levels in the body. Orthodox treatments include birth control pills, ERT (estrogen replacement therapy), surgery, or pregnancy. Though pregnancy offers temporary relief from endometriosis, it does not give lasting results, and can hardly be considered a remedy. A recent drug, Danazol, has been used "successfully" for some cases of endometriosis. It is a male steroid that creates a scary scene of symptoms such as bleeding between periods, growth of facial and chest hair, acne, bloating, weight gain, decrease in breast size, and symptoms associated with decreased estrogen such as hot flashes), but it does decrease pain for some months.

Natural therapies offer help through diet, herbs, vitamin therapies, and stress-reduction techniques. Seeking to establish balance in the entire system, holistic therapies are based on the belief that given the right tools, the body can heal itself. Though there is little data available in this country about the long-term effects of natural therapies, what evidence does exist is supportive and encouraging. Dr. Catherine Kousimine of Switzerland has had many years' experience in successfully treating endometriosis with holistic therapies. Likewise, the well-known women's health clinic in France, Dispensaire des Femmes, also reports favorable results using natural therapies. Several woman I have known personally have also reported excellent progress following a holistic program. These good results include reduction of estrogen in the system and relief from both menstrual pain and excessive bleeding.

Though there is little information available to document the long-term success of either holistic or orthodox treatments, relief *is* in sight for endometriosis suffers. Noninvasive herbal therapies offer long-term building, cleansing, and fundamental support. The results of these herbal programs are not felt overnight. It may take several months for the benefits to be truly appreciated. The orthodox treatments for endometriosis—which include strong drugs, pain killers, hormones, and/or surgery—offer more immediate relief, but fail to correct the problems that caused the endometrial tissue to relocate in the first place. Combining both allopathic and natural treatments may be the most holistic choice to make. We still know very little about endometriosis and must ultimately make our choices based on our belief systems and what feels right to us.

Though the cause of endometriosis and the cure still remain something of a mystery, the pain and discomfort it causes is very real. Frequently the early symptoms go unnoticed or are dismissed because of their close association with the menstrual flow. The primary symptoms of endometriosis include:

Severe pelvic pain around menstruation and ovulation
Excessive or irregular menstrual flows
Bleeding between menstrual cycles
Painful intercourse
Infertility (endometriosis has become the leading cause of infertility in young
  women)
Intestinal discomfort
Painful bowel movement and urination
Backache

Not all painful menstrual cycles, backaches, and intestinal discomfort indicate endometriosis by any means. However, if you are experiencing several of the above symptoms and they are getting progressively worse, it is possible that abnormal endometrial tissue may be involved. Oddly, some women experience no symptoms whatsoever, except perhaps infertility, and may never discover they have endometriosis except by chance in connection with another operation or test.

Unfortunately, healing endometriosis is not a simple matter. Reducing estrogen levels in the body and regulating hormonal production is the specific goal in most forms of natural treatment. To accomplish this, the primary focus is on the health of the liver and the endocrine system. The liver takes the raw estrogen secreted by a woman's ovaries and fat cells and breaks it down into estriol, a safer form of estrogen. Estriol doesn't cause the tissue proliferation that raw estrogen (estradiol) does. A high ratio of estriol to estradiol not only limits the amount of endometrial tissue produced and decreases the painful symptoms of endometriosis, but also protects against breast and uterine cancer.

❦ Drink three to four cups of Endo-Tea (see below) daily for a period of three to four months. This tea specifically helps strengthen and cleanse the liver so that it can function at its optimum.

ENDO-TEA

3 parts dandelion root   1 part oregon grape root
3 parts wild yam root   1 part vitex (chaste berry)
2 parts burdock root   ½ part dong quai root
2 parts pau d'arco bark
Optional: sassafras, cinnamon, ginger and orange peel to taste.

To Make:

Use four to six tablespoons of herb mixture per quart of water. Add herbs to cold water and bring to a slow simmer over low heat. Decoct for twenty minutes. Strain. Drink three to four cups daily. This formula is also very effective as a tincture. (See page 66 for directions on how to make tinctures.)

❦ Take pau d'arco tincture three times a day for six weeks. Stop for a week and then repeat cycle.

❦ Take vitamin E supplements. Vitamin E is a natural antagonist to estrogen and helps to break down excess estrogen in the body. It normalizes hormone production and is essential to the health of the reproductive organs. It also helps to minimize the symptoms of endometriosis by limiting the adhesions caused by endometrial growth and by keeping the scar tissue that does form soft and flexible. The recommended dosage for endometriosis symptoms is 400–800 I.U. daily.

❦ Prostaglandins are a group of compounds produced during times of stress that have a direct influence on regulating levels of inflammation and pain within the body. While some prostaglandins intensify inflammation, others reduce it. Though they are essential to the healing processes in certain situations, in excess they can cause severe menstrual cramps and aggravate endometriosis. Gamma-linolenic acid (GLA) helps to regulate the production of prostaglandins. Found in evening primrose oil, black current seed oil, flaxseed oil, and borage oil, GLA is highly recommended for women suffering from endometriosis. A recommended daily dosage is 500 milligrams twice daily. Omega-3 fatty acids found in fish oils and linseed oil also favor synthesis of inhibitory prostaglandins and should be included in the diet.

❦ Don't underestimate the role that diet plays on the health of the liver. Make a commitment to nourish yourself with wholesome natural organic foods. Avoid refined processed foods, sugar, alcohol, and caffeine-rich foods. All of these deplete the energy of the liver and limit its ability to function properly. Furthermore, sugar and alcohol drain the body of the B vitamins that are essential to the health of the liver. Caffeine not only robs the body of B vitamins but increases the levels of prostaglandins in the system. Make an effort to focus on foods that are rich in B vitamins, protein, and minerals.

❦ Include shitake mushrooms in the diet several times a week. Shitake mushrooms inhibit abnormal tissue growth in the body. They are considered a tasty delicacy as well as a potent medicine. At one time rare and difficult to find, fresh shitakes are now showing up in the produce department of many grocery stores. You can also buy them dry and reconstitute them for cooking. I am a mushroom lover and this is one of those "medicines" I'd gladly take any day.

❦ Avoid foods that tend to raise estrogen levels in the body, such as wheat, citrus, and yams. Herbs that help to elevate estrogens should be avoided also, though most of these herbs have a regulating effect on the hormones, and balance rather than raise levels.

Holistic therapies for endometriosis do not work overnight. Along with the suggestions above, you might wish to explore the herbal treatments for cramps (see pages 117–9) and excess bleeding (see pages 120–2). Make a commitment to work on your health program for four to six months. During that time, you should begin to notice improvement. Your menstrual cycles should become more bearable, your cramping and excess bleeding should diminish, and your overall health should improve. If marked improvement is not noticed, then you might wish to consider more orthodox forms of treatment.

S E V E N T E E N
Vaginal Infections and Genital Herpes

The vagina is the perfect environment for bacteria to grow in. Warm and moist, it is home to many lively microorganisms. Most of these organisms live in symbiotic relationship with one another and are necessary for the overall health of the vaginal area. Some of the bacteria help keep the vagina in its normal state of acidity, which controls the growth of fungus, yeast, and other harmful organisms. (A normal vagina is more than slightly acid, with a pH around 4.0 to 5.0.) When the internal environment of the vagina changes, even slightly, from its normal level of acidity, one or more of the microorganisms can rapidly grow out of control. As they reproduce, they generate metabolic waste material, which in turn causes the inflammation and irritation in the vaginal membranes that we call vaginitis.

There are several kinds of vaginal inflammations, ranging from *candida* and *monilia,* which are caused by a yeastlike fungus, to *trichomonas,* which is caused by a protozoa in the genital/urinary tract, to *gardnerella* and several other vaginal infections which are caused by a variety of microorganisms and are together called *nonspecific vaginitis.* Most of these vaginal inflammations are contagious and tend to be recurrent.

A frequent treatment for vaginitis is antibiotics or sulfa drugs. Both are very effective in killing infection-causing bacteria but both are also very effective in killing the good bacteria needed to maintain a healthy vaginal environment. Though antibiotics quickly destroy microorganisms and miraculously seem to cure the infection, they do not offer long-term relief. With the destruction of the germs, the symptoms of the infection may disappear for a few weeks. However, the problems that created the imbalance in the first place have not been corrected, and the organisms begin to grow again. They often multiply even more quickly now because other organisms that once provided a natural defense against them have also been destroyed by the antibiotics. Seeing her infection returning, a woman may decide to take the medication again, and the circle repeats itself. The only way to treat vaginitis successfully is to correct the underlying causes.

Simple Yeast Infections (Candida and Monilia)

In holistic therapy the major consideration in treating yeast infections is to reestablish the normal vaginal flora, restore the pH level and promote healing from within. When the normal vaginal flora has been reestablished, the bacterial count returns to normal. The yeast bacteria are thus controlled, not by disturbing the natural environment of the vagina or by destroying the yeast bacteria, but by restoring the entire system to balance. It's a beautiful example of holistic therapy and is very effective when followed committedly.

There is a broad spectrum of situations that leads to yeast infections. The vaginal area is very sensitive. It responds not only to the foods we eat and the medicines we take, but also to our feelings. Emotional as well as dietary and other considerations need to be evaluated when considering the cause of a yeast infection. I've known women whose yeast infections would set in right after an intense argument with lovers or husbands. An especially stressful day at work can stimulate the growth of yeast. A change in diet or a few alcoholic drinks can incite one. Even making love can stimulate one; semen, a buffered alkaline solution, raises the vaginal pH level for up to eight hours.

The following conditions are often the cause of yeast infections: emotional stress, general physical weakness, poor diet, hormonal changes (due to menopause, pregnancy), vaginal irritations, excessive douching, birth control pills, hormone pills, stressful sex, and antibiotics, sulfa drugs, and other medications.

The common symptoms of candida and monilia are as follows:

❧ Itching, irritation, and a white cheesy discharge that may smell like baking yeast.
❧ Inflammation of the external vaginal area (the vulva). You may see a discharge, rash, or sores.
❧ Redness, swelling, and discharge from the mucous membranes of the vagina. (This can be seen with the use of a speculum.)

Antibiotics can be used as part of a holistic program to treat yeast infections. They are fast-acting and bring sure relief. However, remember that the continuous use of antibiotics or sulfa drugs will only perpetuate the problem. They will not cure the underlying cause of the infection and are only effective when used as part of a total health program. Frequently, they are unnecessary. Diet, herbs, and rest are often sufficient to correct the problem. My experience has been that unless it is a one-time-only problem, antibiotics will only perpetuate, not cure it.

When using both drug and natural therapy, use the drug medication as the primary medicine for destroying the bacteria and herbal remedies to support the system. Antibiotics are generally strong enough and specific enough to do the job. Do not use herbal remedies for the same purpose. It complicates the body's innate sense and bombards it with too many different kinds of medicine. Use the antibiotics to destroy the bacteria;

use natural/herbal remedies to rebuild the system and restore healthy vaginal flora. In this way the two systems can work harmoniously together.

Natural Remedies for Simple Yeast Infections

Because these yeast infections are so common among women, there are many natural remedies that have been successfully developed to treat them. Natural therapies have as high a success rate as drug therapies in treating yeast infections, and many women choose to use these therapies. The following suggestions are those I have found to be the most valuable and helpful to women. Use them to develop a health program you can reasonably follow.

❦ Wear cotton underpants and avoid panty hose. Panty hose do not permit the vaginal area to "breathe," which further irritates and inflames the yeast infection. There is a reason why manufacturers of women's underwear are required by law to sew cotton crotches into their products. Unfortunately, many of these manufacturers show scant knowledge of the anatomy of the female body; often the amount of cotton used isn't enough to cover a flea's crotch.

❦ Temporarily avoid intercourse. Sexual activity can irritate the already inflamed tissues and force the infecting organisms up into the uterus and fallopian tubes. Semen changes the pH level of the vagina, making it more conducive to the growth of yeast. Also, yeast infections are easily passed back and forth between partners. If you are fighting a yeast infection, it is important that your partner follow a treatment program as well.

During a long-term yeast infection, a restriction on sexual activity may itself contribute a fair amount of stress to a relationship. Though strict adherence may be out of the question, it is important to be careful during lovemaking. Be creative! Find ways to enjoy sex that do not irritate the already inflamed vaginal tissue or pass the infection on to your partner. Or, as one of my students suggested, use condoms. They prevent reinfection without creating serious inconvenience.

❦ Keep the area around the vulva dry. A moist environment encourages the growth of yeast bacteria. Use finely powdered clay as a medicinal talc. (See Yoni Powder below.) And try using a hair dryer after you bathe to dry the vulva. Aside from effectively drying the vulva, it feels quite nice.

YONI POWDER

1 cup fine white clay (available in many health food stores)
½ cup cornstarch
2 tablespoons black walnut hull powder
2 tablespoons myrrh powder
1 tablespoon goldenseal powder
*Optional: a drop or two of tea tree oil

To Make:

Using a wire whisk, mix all the ingredients together. Put some in a spice jar with a shaker top for easy application. The remainder can be stored in a glass jar with a tight-fitting lid. Kept away from moisture, it will last indefinitely.

❦ A good, well-balanced diet is extremely important during a yeast infection. A yeast infection can often be cured by simply eating right. Yeast usually grows in a slightly acidic environment; a healthy vaginal environment is more than slightly acidic. Emphasis should be placed on light, wholesome meals that are healing to the body and help to restore a normal acid/alkaline balance. Meal planning is part of the medicine.

Meals should center around grains (such as brown rice, millet, and buckwheat), soups (such as miso, chicken, and vegetable broths), and steamed vegetables (especially the dark green leafy types). Avoid red meat. Include lots of lemons and grapefruit in the diet, but avoid eating oranges. Unsweetened cranberries and cranberry juice are highly recommended and help to restore acidity to the vagina.

Yogurt and acidophilus should be included daily in the dietary program. If you have allergies to dairy foods, goat yogurt and/or nondairy acidophilus are available. Important components of any problem to cure yeast and yeast-related infection, acidophilus and yogurt help replenish the flora normally found in a healthy vagina.

If you are not getting the desired results from using acidophilus, examine the brand name and the type of culture being used. There are many types and strengths available these days. For medicinal purposes, it is best to use an active strain. These active strains are normally found in the refrigerator department of the natural food store. Many people report better results when using *L. Bifidus* (a type naturally found in humans) rather than the *Lactobacilli* (a type made from animal sources) that is found in yogurt and other fermented milks.

❦ With each meal take a tonic drink made by mixing one teaspoon apple cider vinegar and 1 teaspoon honey in one-fourth cup warm water.

❦ It is important to avoid all alcoholic beverages and sweets (except for your honey/vinegar water). Yeast feeds on sugar and alcohol. A diet high in sweets will promote the growth of yeast bacteria. What do you do when you're baking bread and you want your yeast to grow? You add a little sugar to the warm water and before you know it, the yeast begins to multiply, turns frothy, emits a warm yeasty odor, and smells a wee bit like a vaginal infection! Oftentimes a yeast infection is completely cleared just by eliminating all sweets from the diet. Likewise, a raging infection can be encouraged to grow by continuing to include sugary foods in the diet.

❦ Take two "00" capsules three times daily of the following formula.

ANTI-YEAST CAPSULES

1 part echinacea root powder	1 part myrrh gum powder
1 part pau d'arco powder	2 parts goldenseal root powder
1 part slippery elm bark powder	1 part black walnut hull powder

To Make:

Mix the powders together thoroughly and, following the instructions for encapsulating herbs on page 58, cap the herbs into size "00" capsules.

❧ Each day drink three cups of the following tea between meals or a half hour before eating. For a slightly better flavor and to enhance the medicinal effects, you can mix this tea half and half with unsweetened cranberry juice.

ANTI-YEAST TEA

2 parts sage
2 parts raspberry leaf

2 parts mullein
¼ part goldenseal root

To Make:

Use four to six tablespoons of herb mixture per quart of water. Add herbs to cold water and bring to a simmer over low heat. Keep pot covered. Remove from heat immediately and let steep twenty minutes. Strain. This tea will be quite bitter, so you may wish to mix it with cranberry juice.

❧ Drink eight ounces of unsweetened cranberry juice daily.
❧ Gently douche every few days (or if the infection is severe, each day) with the following formula.

DOUCHE FOR YEAST INFECTIONS

½ ounce Anti-Yeast Tea (above)
2 tablespoons apple cider vinegar
1 tablespoon acidophilus culture or ¼ cup yogurt
Tiny drop of tea tree oil

To Make:

Steep the herb formula in one quart of water for one hour. Strain. Add the rest of the ingredients and mix well. When the mixture has sufficiently cooled (it should be warm, but not hot) place in a douche bag, and very gently, using a slow flow, douche with the mixture.

The above suggestions have worked well for many women. One doesn't need to follow all the suggestions listed, but rather select those suggestions that are most appropriate for you. Definitely more complex than taking prescription pills three times a day, a holistic treatment program requires dedication and work. But considering the results, taking herb teas, douching once a day, swallowing homemade pills, and eating a light nourishing diet are certainly worth the effort.

The preceding suggestions are successful in treating simple yeast infections. But for more persistent yeast infections and those that recur, the following measures may have to be employed. See a holistic doctor if the symptoms persist.

Garlic Suppositories for Yeast Infections

Quick to make, easy to apply, and very effective, garlic suppositories are a favorite remedy of many women. Carefully peel a clove of garlic. (Some women caution against nicking the garlic in the peeling process as they claim the oil burns their vaginas. Most women don't find this a problem, and say that the garlic *should* be nicked or bruised in order for the disinfecting oil to be released. But if you have a particularly sensitive vaginal lining, it is better to be careful when preparing the garlic.) Wrap a piece of thin gauze around the garlic (nicked or not), fold the gauze in half, and twist into a tail. It will look vaguely like a homemade tampax with a tail.

Insert the garlic suppository well inside the vaginal cavity. For easier insertion, a small amount of oil can be rubbed on the end of the suppository. A fresh suppository should be inserted every three to five hours and the old one removed. Repeat for three to five days until the infection is gone. Though this may seem like a rather strange warning, don't forget to remove all garlic suppositories. I've never heard of women leaving a garlic clove in their vaginas, but it has happened with tampons and will cause a raging infection.

Vaginal Bolus for Yeast Infections

Herbal boluses (a type of vaginal suppository) are old-fashioned remedies used for persistent vaginal infections. By changing the herbal formula, you can adapt them for several different problems, including cysts, fibroids, and tumors. The following mixture has had a high success rate for yeast infections. Boluses are easy though messy to make and will take a little time. But they are well worth the trouble because they are very successful in clearing persistent infections. Though I would not necessary recommend their use for a simple yeast infection, they should be tried if the infection persists and is not responsive to other treatments.

VAGINAL BOLUS

1 cup coconut oil	A few drops of tea tree oil
3 parts slippery elm powder	1 part pau d'arco powder
1 part black walnut hull powder	½ part goldenseal powder
1 part myrrh powder (finely ground)	

To Make:

To ensure that the herbs are finely powdered, run them through a nut grinder and a fine sieve. Melt the coconut oil in a saucepan over low heat. When the oil is completely melted, remove it from the heat and stir in the powdered herb mixture. Add enough herbs to make a thick paste. When you have added enough powder so that the oil is thick yet still pliable enough to "work," add the tea tree oil. Quickly roll into boluses the size and shape of your small finger. They will look like herbal tootsie rolls.

Each evening, insert one bolus as far as possible up into the vagina. For easier insertion, you may wish to use a tampon inserter. It will probably be necessary to wear panty liners while doing this treatment. As the coconut oil melts, the bolus may drip.

If you find this formula is too strong for your vaginal membranes, or if your membranes are especially irritated and raw from the infection, use more slippery elm powder. Slippery elm is very soothing and healing to irritated vaginal membranes.

Store the boluses in a glass jar with a tight-fitting lid in the refrigerator. Stored thus, they will last indefinitely. Be sure to label them. (One time, while I was visiting at the herb school, I got very hungry and went searching for a snack. I spotted this unlabeled jar of little tootsie rolls in the refrigerator, decided they must be some sort of new herbal candy, and proceeded to bite into one. Of course, the surprise wasn't too great; much of the herbal medicine I make tastes quite similar!)

Every few days gently douche with the Douche for Yeast Infections. (See page 137) Gentle douching is necessary to wash out any herbal residue. Repeat this process for five days; insert a bolus in the evening, douche every few days, rest for two days. For a persistent yeast infection it may be necessary to repeat the entire process for three to four weeks.

Boric Acid Suppositories for Yeast Infections

When I first heard about the use of boric acid for yeast infections, I was terribly skeptical. Putting boric acid inside the vagina seemed a dubious practice to me. Yet the information was shared with me in a loving and responsible way, and I was curious. Eliana, the young woman who first shared with me the use of boric acid, had had a severe yeast infection for several months. She was currently pregnant and very concerned that she would have an active infection at the time of her child's birth. Complications such as thrush and yeast-related infections could arise for the child. She had tried several herbal remedies and had also tried all the conventional remedies offered by her orthodox doctor. Nothing had worked and she was very despondent over the situation. She learned of the boric acid remedy from her midwife.

Her midwife assured her that there would be no side effects and that the remedy would work. Every day for seven days, Eliana was told to insert two "00" capsules of boric acid deep into her vagina. Her midwife warned her that the boric acid could burn her and be uncomfortable, but that the burning was superficial and would not be problematic. Eliana, having more trust than I would, did as her midwife instructed. The boric acid did burn. She reported that for the first two days, the burning was very uncomfortable, but after that there was no longer any painful sensation. After seven days her long-seated infection was completely gone and did not recur.

The story interested me and I began to share it with my herbalist friends. They reported the same good results as Eliana. I have since recommended it many times, but always with caution. Boric acid can be burning and irritating, though most women don't experience any burning at all. Those who do, say the burning is superficial; no one has ever reported long-term pain. I mention this remedy here because it does seem to eradicate persistent yeast infections when nothing else works. And for many women that is a great blessing.

To use boric acid for yeast infections, fill 14 "00" gelatin capsules with boric acid powder. Both boric acid and gelatin capsules are available in pharmacies. Insert two capsules (600 milligrams of boric acid powder) a day deep into the vagina. The heat of the body will melt the capsules and release the boric acid. Repeat the process for seven days. There may be burning and an uncomfortable feeling for the first couple of days. If the burning persists, discontinue using the boric acid. It is best to insert the capsules in the evening because there is often a lot of vaginal discharge as the boric acid begins to work. A pad may be necessary to absorb the fluid. Note: boric acid is poisonous if ingested. *Do not* ingest the capsules.

C. J.'s Tea Tree Oil Suppositories

This recipe was shared with me by C. J., a woman who was prone to yeast infections for many years. She had literally "tried everything." Both orthodox and nonconventional remedies just didn't work. C. J.'s had been persistent that when she did find a remedy that worked she was delighted to share it. I've found C. J.'s remedy to be a "gold mine remedy" as it has worked for several other friends as well.

To make C. J.'s remedy, mix fifteen drops of tea tree oil in a glass of warm water and drink once a day until all symptoms are gone. C. J. had a rather ingenious method of taking the tea tree oil. Finding the taste of the oil unpleasant, she used an eye dropper to encapsulate the oil in empty gelatin capsules.

A douche can also be made by combining one teaspoon tea tree oil with one teaspoon isopropyl alcohol (rubbing alcohol). Store this solution, which turns milky white, in a dropper bottle. Every day for one week, add ten drops of the solution to one pint of warm water and douche with it. If desired, the treatment can be continued at night by adding five drops of solution to one cup of warm water and saturating a tampon with it. Insert the tampon and leave in place overnight.

Trichomonas and Gardnerella

You may want and need to use both allopathic and herbal remedies to fight these more tenacious infections. While the orthodox drug remedies are killing the bacteria, the herbal remedies will help build, nourish, and heal your system. But remember, if you decide to take antibiotics, to eat yogurt daily and to add acidophilus to your diet. Both yogurt and acidophilus will help restore the proper digestive enzymes and reestablish the intestinal flora that are disrupted by the intake of antibiotics.

Trichomonas

Trichomonas vaginalis, or *trich,* as it is commonly called, is a tiny protozoa, a one-celled organism found in both men and women. At least 50 percent of all women have trich organisms in their vaginas, though often with no symptoms. (Men are usually asymptomatic.) An overabundance of trichomonads within the vagina and urinary tract causes an infection to develop. Trich grows best in a slightly alkaline environment. As blood is alkaline, women are more prone to infection during menstruation. Trich also grows out of control and develops into infections during times of stress, anxiety, and poor health.

Trich usually manifests itself with a yellow or yellowish-green discharge which is thin, foamy, and has a foul odor, often described as "fishy." It can cause a burning sensation during urination, and occasionally, a swelling or bleeding of the vaginal walls. In addition, chronic cervicitis (infection of the endocervical glands that line the cervical canal) can occur. Because trichomonads travel through tiny lymph channels between the vagina and urethra, associated urinary tract infections, such as cystitis, are common.

A simple and effective way of recognizing an early trich infection is by doing a self-examination. Check your discharge. Is it frothy or thin? Yellow, yellowish-green, or gray? Using a speculum (available through clinics and women's health centers), you can look for the discharge that pools just below the cervix. It sometimes appears to have air bubbles in it. There may also be raised, red patches on the vaginal walls and cervix, indicating irritation and inflammation. A diagnosis can also be obtained, of course, at clinics and women's health centers, where a sample of the discharge is examined with a microscope.

Drug Treatments for Trichomonas

Traditionally, Flagyl (metronidazole), an oral drug, is administered for the trich infection. *Women should avoid this drug.* There are indications that it may be carcinogenic. Furthermore, tests have shown that Flagyl can cause birth defects and gene mutations. Flagyl enters the bloodstream and lowers the white blood cell count, decreasing the resistance of the body to infection. *In no case should it be taken by a pregnant woman or by a woman with peptic ulcers.* Nor should it be taken by anyone with an infection elsewhere in the body, by anyone with a history of blood disease, or by anyone with a disease of the central nervous system. *If you do take Flagyl, don't drink alcohol or use vinegar until you have finished the course of treatment.* In combination with Flagyl, alcohol or vinegar can cause nausea, vomiting, sweating, and weakness.

Another drug treatment currently available is the vaginal suppository Betadine. Probably the safest of the conventional drug therapies recommended for trich, Betadine is an antiseptic and can be found in most drugstores.

Natural Remedies for Trichomonas

Because of the harmful side effects that may accompany drug treatments, it is wise to try natural remedies first. Most of the following may be used in conjunction with allopathic drugs:

❦ Abstain from intercourse. Trich is contagious and is easily passed back and forth between partners. Also, intercourse can further agitate the already inflamed vaginal lining.
❦ Use garlic suppositories daily. Take garlic oil capsules internally. Garlic has proven to be especially beneficial for trichomonas. (See page 138.)
❦ Try boric acid capsules inserted in the vagina each day. (See instructions and cautions for using boric acid, pages 139–40.)

❧ Vinegar douches are very helpful when treating trich. Since trich grows best in a slightly alkaline environment, douching with acidic solutions like vinegar can eliminate the infection. Gently douche every couple of days with the Douche for Yeast Infections.

❧ Oat straw herb (not oatmeal) is a specific for trichomonas and should be used in conjunction with other teas. Drink oatstraw tea both as a curative and a preventative.

❧ Take two capsules of Chaparral Combo (below) three times a day until symptoms disappear.

CHAPARRAL COMBO CAPSULES

2 parts chaparral powder   2 parts pau d'arco powder
1 part osha root powder   ½ part black walnut hull powder

To Make:
Follow directions for encapsulating herbs on page 58.

Gardnerella

Gardnerella is a yellow, white or mucusy discharge which may or may not have blood in it. It is usually accompanied by itching or vaginal irritation and sometimes cystitislike symptoms. The walls of the vagina may be cloudy, puffy, and coated with pus. Gardnerella may also be accompanied by lower back pain, cramps, and swollen glands in the abdomen and thighs. The symptoms are similar to those of trichomonas, though the discharge tends to be creamy white or grayish rather than green and frothy. The odor can be especially strong-smelling and rather fishy. Some cases of gardnerella are symptomatic and are only found by a pap smear. In much the same way as other yeast infections, gardnerella often begins when a woman's natural resistance is lowered by anxiety, tension, lack of sleep, poor diet, sexual activity with an infected partner, birth control pills and other medications, and/or an imbalanced diet.

To combat bacterial infections, eat plenty of garlic—a safe natural antibiotic—and eat a diet rich in high-quality protein (antibodies are made of protein). Though raw garlic is best, there are several brands of garlic capsules available today that contain the active ingredients. Be sure to eat a diet rich in a full spectrum of vitamins and minerals. Concentrate on B vitamin complex and on vitamins C, E, and A. Comfrey/oatstraw tea is highly recommended, both as a preventative and a remedy. An excellent tonic high in protein, vitamins, and minerals and rich in chlorophyll, comfrey/oatstraw tea is a natural cleanser of the system.

Natural Remedies for Gardnerella and Nonspecific Vaginitis
❧ For the itching and irritation caused by gardnerella, apply a comfrey/St. John's Wort salve (see page 55 for directions how to make) directly on the lips and inside the vagina. Medicinal Yoni Powder (see page 135) should be sprinkled over the area several times

daily. This will not only help with the odor but, more important, help heal the infection. Cultured buttermilk or yogurt applied directly to the area of irritation is very soothing and healing. Insert the yogurt inside the vagina, using your fingers or a tampax applicator. At first the yogurt and/or buttermilk may burn slightly, but the burning sensation will quickly pass.

❦ Take two capsules of Chaparral Combo three times a day.

❦ Use a garlic suppository daily. (See page 138.)

❦ Gently douche with the following formula every two days until the infection clears.

APPLE CIDER VINEGAR DOUCHE

1 quart warm water
2 tablespoons apple cider vinegar
1–2 teaspoons garlic oil (to make see page 50)

❦ Abstain from intercourse. Gardnerella is easily spread from one partner to another. It is also important to avoid further agitation of the vaginal lining.

❦ Use boric acid suppositories. (See directions for use and cautions on pages 139–40.)

❦ Help acidify your system by drinking eight ounces of unsweetened cranberry juice every day. The cranberry juice can be mixed half and half with comfrey/oatstraw tea.

Allergies as a Cause of Vaginal Infections

If a woman has tried both natural remedies and drug therapies to no avail, her vaginal infection may be the result of allergies—either to various foods or to some other environmental factor. Though the culprit can be any food, it is most often dairy food: milk, yogurt, cream, butter, cheese, etc. Sometimes citrus fruit is the cause of the problem. Sugar, honey, and other sweeteners, though certainly detrimental once the infection sets in, do not seem to *create* an allergic response.

Specific allergens are often difficult to determine. If you suspect a certain food, try eliminating it entirely from your diet for two weeks. (It must be eliminated entirely because even a small amount is enough to trigger or sustain a reaction.) Begin by eliminating all dairy foods, since they are most often the problem food item in vaginal infections. Take note of any improvement in the status of your infection after two weeks. Even the slightest improvement can be a confirmation. After the two-week trial period, introduce dairy foods back into the diet in a big way. Do you notice any yeast-like symptoms returning?

After you test dairy foods, try the same procedure on citrus and any other food group you might be suspicious of. Though this is not an "official" allergy test, it is quite effective if done correctly and often indicates which food(s) are possible troublemakers. I've found it almost as effective as clinical food-allergy tests in determining offending foods—and certainly far less expensive.

If you have any concern at all that certain foods may be the underlying cause of a chronic vaginal infection, quickly eliminate those food groups from your diet. Correcting the infection may be that simple.

Hot tubs, though wonderfully relaxing, can also be the cause of severe vaginal infection. Two factors seem to be precipitate infections. One, there may be an allergic reaction to the variety of strong chemicals used in the tubs. Second, the warm, moist, and not always perfectly clean environment of the hot tub can foster the infection. Infections set off by hot-tub immersion are especially persistent and extremely irritating. Symptoms are often felt within hours and begin with an achy, sore sensation in the vagina. The vaginal wall will appear irritated and raw and a cheesy white discharge will begin to flow. Symptoms will progressively get worse, so act quickly and be persistent with your treatment. The outer labia will need special attention also, as they will often be raw and inflamed. A good herbal salve, such as comfrey/St. John's Wort Salve (see page 56) and Vitamin E oil are often soothing and healing.

Genital Herpes

I remember the days when I used to work in my old herb shop, Rosemary's Garden. It was a small nook of a place lined with hundreds of jars filled with herbs. When anyone walked into that tiny store, they were instantly noticeable. There were no corners in which to hide. I could always spot the people who came to talk about herpes. They would check to be sure no one else was in the shop before coming in. Once in, they would stall, first looking over the herb books, then move to the card section before slowly making their way to the counter where I sat. They would usually begin their conversation by asking me general questions, possibly about herbs or remedies, or life on the river or the time of day. Eventually there would come a long pause and then the painful admission that they had herpes. I would always recognize these customers because they would be so shy and embarrassed to talk about the "horrors of herpes." This was back in the days when time moved more slowly and my customers and I had the leisure just to wait until the time was right to share. It was also the time when herpes was the "new" venereal disease and people didn't know much about it or what to do for it. They were usually very fearful and discouraged. Often they came to see me shortly after a visit to the doctor. The prognosis at that time was pretty depressing. "Herpes was incurable; once contacted, you would always have it. It was highly contagious, and it was necessary to abstain from sex." If I had received a diagnosis of herpes, I would have been depressed, too. The truth of the matter is, the prognosis hasn't gotten much more enlightened. But there is a lot more information to share about herpes and there are certainly successful treatments for it.

Herpes is caused by a tiny organism, the herpes simplex virus. Little is known about this organism except that it is antagonistic to the human body. It enters the body via the skin and mucous membranes, and makes its way along the nerve endings, where it settles in and makes itself at home. Once established in the system, it becomes permanently incorporated into the DNA of the cells. There are basically two types of herpes. The first is herpes simplex virus I (HSV I), which is usually found above the waist and is characterized by raw sores called fever blisters or cold sores. The second is herpes simplex virus II (HSV II), or genital herpes, which is usually found below the waist, predominately around the genitals.

The Symptoms of Genital Herpes

The first sign of genital herpes is an inflamed sensitive area which is often accompanied by swollen glands in the groin. Within a few days this sensitized area erupts into sores that quickly become small red blisters. These can be quite painful. As the blisters rupture, they often bleed or weep a clear fluid. Usually after five to seven days a crust forms on the blisters. Then they heal and disappear until the next outbreak. For a small minority of women, the first outbreak is the only one they ever experience. But most women (upwards to 75 percent) experience recurrent episodes within the next few months and years. Many women report that symptoms get milder with each ensuing outbreak, possibly due to herpetic antibodies being produced as a natural line of defense by the system.

A Three-Step Program for Treating Genital Herpes

Over the years I have seen several cases of HSV II respond remarkably well to natural treatment. At any rate, since Western medicine has nothing to offer in the way of treatment except symptomatic relief from the blisters, trying alternative treatments seems a wise and sensible thing to do.

Step 1 in an alternative treatment program is to build and strengthen the nervous system with nervine adaptogenic herbs and foods. Herpes virus resides in the nerve endings located at the base of the spine. Not surprisingly, they are activated by stress and nervous conditions. Adaptogenic herbs and foods increase the body's ability to respond to the stresses of the environment while calming and relaxing the nervous system. The following nervine adaptgens strengthen, nourish, and maintain the homeostatic mechanisms of the nervous system, enabling it to deal more effectively with stress:

❦ Include B vitamin-rich foods in the diet such as whole grains, nutritional yeast, bee pollen, wheat germ, spirulina, blue green algae, seaweeds, cereal, nuts, seeds, and peas.
❦ Add a vitamin B supplement to your daily diet.
❦ Drink Stress-Less Tea (see below) every day for several weeks and whenever there are high levels of stress in your life thereafter.

STRESS-LESS TEA

4 parts nettle	1 part St. John's wort
3 parts oat straw	1 part skullcap
3 parts chamomile	1 part passionflower
1 part comfrey leaf	

St. John's wort

To Make:

Use four to six tablespoons of herb mixture per each quart of water. Add herbs to cold water and bring to a simmer slowly, over low heat. Keep pot covered tightly. Immediately remove from the heat and let it sit for twenty minutes. Strain.

❦ For chronic cases of nervous tension take one-fourth teaspoon of the following tincture three times a day.

TENSION TINCTURE

2 parts valerian   1 part skullcap
1 part hops

To Make:

For instructions on how to make tinctures, see page 66.

Step 2 in a holistic therapy for herpes is to strengthen your immune system so that viruses, bacteria, and other infectious agents are less able to attack your body, and that when they do, they can be warded off better. A healthy immune system and strong nervous system support the foundation of a program to reduce or eliminate herpes outbreaks.

❦ Echinacea is highly recommended as a preventive measure for women prone to herpes. Take it daily for a period of three months, and thereafter, whenever there are periods of susceptibility in your life. To take full advantage of echinacea's immune-enhancing effects, take it for five days, then stop for two days and repeat the cycle. If you are taking echinacea tincture, the recommended dosage is one-fourth teaspoon, three times daily. If you are taking it in tea form, the recommended dosage is three to four cups daily. If you are taking echinacea capsules, the recommended dosage is two capsules, three times daily.

❦ Include pau d'arco every day in the diet for three to six months. It may be used in tincture, tablet or tea form. Use the same dosages as recommended for echinacea (see above). The following formula contains pau d'arco and is a good preventative tea.

IMMUNE SUPPORT TEA

4 parts pau d'arco
2 parts echinacea
1 part burdock root
Optional: cinnamon, orange peel, licorice root, or other tasty root herbs to taste.

To Make:

Use four to six tablespoons of the herb mixture per quart of water. Add herbs to cold water and bring to a simmer over low heat. Keep pot tightly covered. Simmer gently for twenty minutes. Remove from heat and let infuse twenty minutes. Strain. Drink three to four cups daily.

❧ Include daily dosages of chlorophyll, wheat grass, and/or blue-green algae in your diet. Each of these substances strengthens the immune system and provides antiviral activity. The ultimate green herbs, they are also extremely cleansing and nourishing to the system. These nutritional substances are found in natural food and herb stores.

Step 3 in the herpes treatment program is to thoroughly evaluate your diet to see what foods might be agitating the condition. Sweets, both natural and otherwise, arginine-rich foods such as peanuts, chocolate, and soft drinks (especially those with cola), and stimulants can all activate the outbreak of herpes. Likewise, the lack of certain elements in the diet can exacerbate the situation. People prone to herpes need to include foods high in B vitamins, calcium, iron, Vitamin C, and lysine.

A dear friend of mine had a severe case of herpes. Though hers was nongenital herpes—it appeared as large red crusted welts on her face—dietary considerations for genital and nongenital herpes are the same. A beautiful woman concerned with her appearance, these unsightly, as well as painful, sores caused enormous stress in her life. When she asked me for suggestions, the first thing I did, to her chagrin, was review her diet. Knowing her well, I knew that her diet consisted of rich foods, sweets, coffee, and chocolate. She was reluctant to give them up. So I made a friendly bet with her.

I challenged her to give up totally all foods that might be aggravating her condition. Just for one month. Just as an experiment. And to include a simple tea (Adapto-Tea) in her diet each day. She agreed rather reluctantly. The horrible case of herpes she had been hosting for some time cleared up. Hoping it might be coincidental, she began heartily eating the suspected foods again. The results were immediate. Herpes sores began surfacing again. After several aborted attempts to "prove" that her herpes was not related to diet, she finally became convinced. At that point she had a very clear choice: either continue eating the foods she so much enjoyed and suffer the consequences, or make some changes in her diet. Below is the program that I recommended for her and which she has faithfully followed ever since.

Dietary Suggestions for Treating Herpes
❧ Obviously, my first suggestion is to eliminate the known offenders: chocolate, sugars (including honey, jam, and so on), alcohol, caffeine and other stimulants. A pretty strict order, but the results are well worth it. Also high on the list of offenders to be eliminated are arginine-rich foods like peanut butter, chocolate, cola. There seems to be a connection between high levels of arginine and herpes attacks.
❧ If you are prone to herpes, include zinc (a supplement available in natural food stores) in the diet during periods of vulnerability, such as emotional stress, menstruation, menopause, illness, when traveling, and so forth. The recommended daily dosage ranges considerably. High doses of zinc can depress immunity, so I generally never recommend more than twenty to thirty milligrams daily during periods of susceptibility.
❧ Though lysine, an amino acid, is not a cure, it has been found to be effective in suppressing the early symptoms of herpes. It is most effective for herpes simplex I, but I also suggest using it for genital herpes. Dosages tend to be high, ranging from 700 to 1,000 milligrams daily during the active stages. Many women use lysine on a daily basis to prevent herpes

outbreaks, but I have not found it to be especially effective as a preventive. Lysine primarily counteracts and balances the effects of arginine in the system. It's more effective to avoid arginine-rich foods than to supplement your diet with lysine on a daily basis.

❧ Include lots of garlic (in salad dressing and added to food at the end of cooking) and/or garlic oil capsules in the diet. Garlic has eighteen known antiviral and antibacterial substances in it and definitely helps control herpes. At the very first signs of a herpes flare-up, take a large amount of fresh garlic and/or garlic oil capsules immediately. A standard dosage would be twelve capsules at the onset, then three every four hours until all symptoms have vanished. That's a lot of garlic, but it works! You may feel confused by the variety of garlic oil capsules available in the health food stores these days. Even pharmacies have begun to carry them. It's important to get good-quality garlic oil capsules. If uncertain of which ones to purchase, I recommend the Kyolic and Kwai brands.

❧ The following tea contains adaptogen herbs that help raise the level of immunity and strengthen the system. Drink about a quart daily. Adjust the flavors so that you enjoy the taste of it and look forward to drinking it each day.

ADAPTO-TEA

3 parts pau d'arco	1 part astragalus
2 parts echinacea	½ part yellow dock
1 part dandelion root	

Optional: sassafras, cinnamon, and orange peel to taste.

To Make:

Use four to six tablespoons of herb mixture per quart of water. Add herbs to cold water and bring to a simmer over low heat. Keep pot tightly covered. Simmer for twenty minutes. Remove from heat and let infuse for twenty minutes longer. Strain. Drink three to four cups daily.

The fourth and final step of a holistic program for herpes is to give yourself symptomatic relief from the pain by treating the herpes externally. Below are the suggestions I've found bring the most relief to the greatest number of people. Obviously, you don't need to, and shouldn't, use all of these suggestions! You may need to do a little experimenting to find the one(s) that work the best for you.

❧ Aloe vera gel soothes, dries, and effectively helps to heal herpes sores. Apply the aloe vera gel directly to the sores. You can use the gel pressed fresh from the leaf of a plant, or purchase the gel directly from a health food store.

❧ Though some women feel that keeping the sores moist only prolongs the healing process, others find the comfort of salves and ointments very healing. It all depends on the individual. Try both methods and see which works best for you. The best healing salve I know of for herpes is St. Johns Wort Salve. (See the recipe on page 56). You can also make St. Johns wort/calendula oil for herpes.

❧ If you find that your particular case responds better to an astringent, drying type medication than to a salve, make a St. Johns wort/calendula tincture. (See pages 66–67 for directions on making tinctures.) Apply this topically to the open sores. But be careful; it will sting! Dilute it with water before applying.

❦ My dear friend and fellow herbalist, Jane Bothwell, has found essential oil of myrrh to be very effective when applied directly to the lesions. She has also had success mixing powdered myrrh into a paste with water and applying this as a poultice for herpes sores.

❦ The Anti-Herpes Paste below makes an excellent poultice when applied directly to the sores.

ANTI-HERPES PASTE

1 part goldenseal powder
1 part black walnut hull powder
1 part echinacea root powder

To Make:

Mix the powdered herbs together, then moisten the mixture with a bit of St. Johns wort/calendula tincture.

❦ Warm herbal baths are soothing and healing. I've found two types of baths that seem to bring relief and aid in healing the herpes outbreak. You might wish to alternate both types or find the one that works best for you. The first is a soothing, relaxing bath that relieves the itching. It also strengthens one's spirit, gives a deep sense of cleanliness, and promotes a feeling of inner strength and support. The second bath is an astringent cleanser. After bathing, gently but completely dry the groin area. I recommend using a hair dryer set on warm. You might wish to sprinkle a dusting of Yoni Powder over the sores. (See page 135.)

RELAX AND SOOTHING BATH

3 parts chamomile
1 part hops
2 parts calendula

1 part instant oatmeal (dry)
1 part comfrey leaf
1 part comfrey root

To Make:

Mix these ingredients together and place a big handful or two in a large handkerchief or cotton bath bag. Tie it onto the nozzle of the tub and let hot water stream through it for several minutes. Adjust the temperature of the water, untie the bag, and let it float with you in the tub.

ASTRINGENT CLEANSER BATH

1 ounce dry chaparral leaves
4 tablespoons baking soda

1–2 drops tea tree oil

To Make:

Mix dry ingredients thoroughly, then mix in oil. Place mixture in a large cotton handkerchief or bath bag. Tie it onto the nozzle of the tub and let hot water stream through it for several minutes. Adjust the water temperature, untie the bag, and let it float with you in the tub.

Herpes and Pregnancy

Most of us have heard of the problems associated with herpes and pregnancy. There is a slight increase in the risk of miscarriage and premature delivery among women who are first exposed to herpes while pregnant. These women need to take extra precautions and follow the dietary guidelines listed above as well as the general guidelines listed for pregnancy in Part V. There is also a slight possibility that the herpes virus may infect the child while it is in the womb, but the greatest threat is having active sores while giving birth. If there are open sores present at the time of birth, there is a high possibility (60 to 70 percent) that the child will be born with birth defects. The thought itself is enough to create stress in the pregnant mother and trigger a herpes outbreak! Generally, women with active sores present at their birth will opt to have a cesarean birth. There are some hospitals and practitioners using a special bandage to cover the sores if they are on the labia, allowing for a safe vaginal birth.

Prevention, then, is the key here. Follow all the guidelines listed above. Though there are certainly risks, the actual incidence of babies being born brain-damaged, blind, or in any way impaired is extremely rare. Choose as your midwife and/or doctor a holistic practitioner who has an openminded attitude about the situation and an unbiased understanding of your concerns.

Fibrocystic and Related Breast Conditions

There is an overwhelming amount of information available these days about breast lumps. Practically every woman's magazine contains a monthly feature on breast exams, how to look for lumps, and what to do about them if you find them. There is a wonderful range of high-tech hospital tests available for diagnosing breast tissue. As women living in a cancer-plagued world we are acutely aware of what lumps can mean and have been well educated to check for them on a regular basis.

It is often difficult to tell the difference between fibrocystic benign breast condition and cancer. For safety's sake and for peace of mind, you should always consult a medical doctor or a qualified holistic practitioner at the first signs of unfamiliar breast lumps and/or if there are any noticeable changes in your breast tissue.

In my work as an herbalist, I have known several women who have had fibrocystic breasts and/or cancer. These women have been teachers to me as each chose the healing modalities that felt right to them, once they had obtained a diagnosis. The best system of healing is the one that both empowers the individual and is eclectic enough to include the most appropriate and effective techniques from different systems.

One woman I knew quite well over the years was a feminist, a wonderful artist, and a goat herder. Grace lived by herself on the top of a mountain overlooking the sea. She used to come to town once every few weeks and always stopped by the herb shop. That's how I got to know her. When she first showed me the lumps in her breast, I felt immediately that she should seek medical advice. The lumps were quite large, hard, and did not change with her monthly cycle. But Grace had developed a fanatical mistrust of the medical profession and was adamant about not seeking medical help. She'd just buy her herbs, go home, and do her home treatments. Grace was an older woman, well-informed about health matters, and definitely very opinionated about them. Though I have always felt that each person has the right to chose the healing path she wishes to walk, and that the prime role of a healer is to support each person on her individual path, I was truly very worried about Grace. After many months, I finally talked her into seeing a wonderful healer/doctor whom she quickly came to trust.

Eventually Grace did go to the hospital, a route she deeply feared. Her breast had become quite enlarged, and open sores had formed. Seeking medical help was the first step in Grace's healing. She developed close relationships with many of the nurses and doctors and slowly grew out of her deep-seated mistrust of the medical profession.

Unfortunately, Grace had to have a complete mastectomy, but her decision seemed only to free and empower her. After her incision had healed and she was up and about again, full of spunk and energy, she accompanied us on several of the herb school's backpacking trips into the mountains. I always admired the way she would throw her clothes off and, like a proud one-breasted goddess, jump into the mountain rivers and streams, unabashed, full of womanly joy and charm.

A number of years went by. I hadn't seen Grace since I moved from California, though I'd heard she was doing fine—tending her goats, weaving and spinning, and painting fantastic pictures. Just a few weeks ago I received a letter from a mutual friend who told me that Grace had died peacefully and comfortably in her home. Though the success of a healing modality for cancer is often judged on the basis of how long a person lives, Grace's success, though she did live for quite a number of years, was not based on the length, but on the quality, of her life. Her particular story is one of healing, growth and self-empowerment.

My own experience of breast lumps was very different from Grace's, because mine were cyclic: they came and went each month in association with my menstrual cycle. Nonetheless, they often worried me and made me feel helpless. Fortunately, they also empowered me by forcing me to take control of my life. Through the use of diet, herbs, and self-guided meditation, I eventually learned to regulate and control these cyclic lumps.

I was in my midtwenties when I first noticed small, hard lumps in my breast. I was unworried at first, probably more because I was so naive than for any other reason. For several years I was vaguely aware of them, noting that they regularly fluctuated in size, depending on where I was in my menstrual cycle. I accepted that fact as a good sign and went on ignoring them.

When I was in my late thirties I went through a major life crisis. I was very successful at what I did, loved my work and my community, but had exhausted myself with projects, work, and family. I owned a lovely little herb store and a mail-order herb business, ran a large herb school, gardened, raised horses, and had a family. It was really more than I could handle, even in "superwoman mode," and my family life suffered both from my lack of time and from the fact that I was worn out a good deal of the time. Nonetheless, caught up in the busyness of it all, I prided myself on the fact that I was holding everything together—until it all began to unravel! Just when I was thinking I was on top of the world, the Great Cosmic Mother laughed at me and turned my world upside down.

It seemed as though it happened overnight, though in truth, I knew that this crisis had been building for several years. I woke up one morning feeling as if I didn't know who I was anymore. Though I loved my work, I found I was sick of working. My marriage was falling apart. I felt an inner longing to leave Sonoma County where I had spent most of my adult life, but I had no idea where to go. Moving would mean leaving the friends I had known all my life, the herb school that I had founded and deeply loved, my herb shop and the community I felt such an integral part of. Of course, these great changes were preceded and heightened by wearing myself out with work until I was utterly exhausted. I was emotionally and physically wrung out, a typical result of "the superwoman syndrome" and a poor example of a healthy herbalist.

At about this time, the lumps in my breast began to grow. One lump in particular began to grow at an alarming rate. It felt like a hard walnut turning into a golf ball in the soft fleshy tissue of my right breast. Though I was conscious of it, the last thing in the world I wanted right then was to focus on myself or on my breasts, the feminine symbol of nourishment. So, like many good women in similar situations, I continued to ignore my problem.

It was the night voices, the strong voice of Artemis, and the power of the moon shining down on my vulnerable, dreaming self, that finally awakened me to the potential seriousness of my situation. I woke up one night from a dream in a panic, sweating profusely, my hand grasping my right breast. Deeply alarmed, I knew it was long past time and I needed to do something right away. The next morning I worked out a schedule for myself, following suggestions from several of my herbalist friends and a very supportive woman doctor. I began a very rigorous program that included herbs, vitamins, and dietary changes. Just as important, I undertook a reevaluation of my life and reorganized it in a manner that worked better for me. I made the move and the other changes I needed to. I rested, slept a lot, and ate the foods and herbs I knew were helpful. Within a few months the lumps completely disappeared. (The program I followed is outlined on pages 154–6.)

These two stories certainly do not convey the full range of symptoms or problems associated with breast lumps. There are many types of growths that can develop in our breasts. Most of them are not cancerous. More than seventy percent of women are reported to have a fibrocystic breast condition; fewer than 10 percent of women develop breast cancer. Yet, our immediate response to any growth is, "Maybe it's cancer." Consequently we experience the panic that particular word strikes in our hearts each time we feel a lump. We are trained to look *for* cancer, not the lack of it, when we examine our breasts. Maybe that's why so many women unconsciously choose *not* to do breast exams. Even though it's a simple process that can save lives, each time a women searches her breasts she feels, albeit unconsciously, that she is looking for cancer. It's a very negative concept. Perhaps we really do believe the old adage, "What we seek, we shall surely find."

I do not underestimate the present threat of breast cancer, and I encourage women to do self-examinations of their breast on a regular basis. But I also advocate doing these examinations in a positive and empowering manner. Breast exams should be a life-affirming experience, geared toward training us to recognize normal breast tissue and teaching us to appreciate and honor our breasts and the rhythms and cycles they go through. I recently saw a pictorial in a magazine showing how to do a breast exam. I had to stop to appreciate it because it was so beautifully done. The woman was slowly and sensuously enjoying her own body. We seldom slow down enough to acknowledge our bodies. The need for breast exams allows us to touch, feel, and appreciate the beauty of our own unique breasts and what they represent.

Breast tissue is composed of fat- and milk-producing glands that are controlled by a monthly cycle of changing estrogen, progesterone, and prolactin levels. During the month, hormonal changes often cause the milk glands to swell and retain fluid. Small cysts may form and are especially prevalent in the lymph nodes under the armpits. Fibrocystic lumps feel like small balloons filled with fluid and seem to "float" when pressed. They've often been compared to feeling like an eyeball under a closed eyelid. The swollen enlarged tissue is often painful. When menstruation begins, hormonal stimulation ceases and the breasts return to normal.

Not a disease but a condition, fibrocystic breast lumps are benign breast tissue. They are as normal in some women as menstruation, pregnancy and menopause. They are a typical characteristic of the hormonal changes we experience each month. It is common, not uncommon, for women to experience them. They are generally easy to detect because they change with our monthly cycles, usually becoming more painful and inflamed a few days before menstruation begins, and disappearing shortly after menstruation is over.

Though neither cancerous nor malignant, fibrocystic breast tissue is painful and worrisome to many women. It makes detecting cancerous lumps more difficult. It can be a signal that our hormones are out of balance. Too much free circulating estrogen in the system causes the tissue to swell and hold water. A deficiency of essential fatty acids (EFA) is also indicated. Essential fatty acids are needed to regulate prolactin and prostaglandins in the system. This cyclic condition can be regulated by diet and herbs.

It is also important for women to take a serious look at their breasts and how they feel about them. A symbol of nourishment, breasts are often misrepresented as sexual objects. Our culture, so lacking in self-nourishment and love, has become totally preoccupied with the size and shape of breasts, and out of touch with the marvelous nurturing energy they represent.

Our challenge comes in learning to distinguish normal breast changes from abnormal growths that can indicate cancer. Unfortunately, we are not taught to recognize these normal changes. We live with the fear that every change in our breast tissue is a symptom of cancer. However, it's not the scope nor purpose of this book to distinguish between the different types of breast tissue nor how to distinguish benign growths from potentially cancerous ones. For additional information I highly recommend *The New Our Bodies, Ourselves* by the Boston Women's Health Collective.

The following program is the one I followed faithfully for several months and the one I recommend to other women experiencing similar benign breast growths. Many of the following suggestions can also be used as an adjunct therapy for a woman undergoing orthodox treatment for breast cancer. Always consult with your doctor on these matters. However, if he or she is not favorably disposed toward holistic treatment, you may find that the doctor is not supportive.

My Personal Program for Treating Fibrocystic Breasts

IMMUNE CLEANSER

1 part yellow dock root	1 part ginger
3 parts dandelion root	1 part dong quai
2 parts burdock root	1 part astragalus

1 part licorice root   4 parts pau d'arco
1 part vitex (chaste berry)
Optional: cinnamon, orange peel, sassafras, and stevia to taste.

To Make:

Use four to six tablespoons of herb mixture per quart of water. Add herbs to cold water and simmer over low heat for twenty minutes. Keep pot tightly covered. Remove from heat and allow to infuse twenty minutes longer. Strain. Drink three to four cups a day.

❦ Take two tablespoons of spirulina daily.
❦ Take two capsules of 500 milliliters black current seed oil, evening primrose oil, or borage oil three times a day.
❦ Take two capsules of dong quai three times a day, except during menstruation.
❦ Take Floradix+Iron, NatureWorks, or other liquid mineral/vitamin formula, following the dosage recommendations on the container.
❦ Take 600 I.U. vitamin E capsule daily (see caution on page 212).
❦ Eat shitake mushrooms several times a week. These can be sauteed, steamed, and/or eaten raw. I love the rich woody flavor of these mushrooms. They are available dried in natural food stores, and sometimes found fresh in supermarkets.
❦ I found the following drink to be an excellent source of nourishment. I made it in bulk and stored it in the freezer. I always had a glass in the morning for breakfast and sometimes again later in the day. Though you can mix it with any fruit juice, I found it tasted best mixed with pineapple and/or orange juice. The recipe makes about one and a half pounds of dry mix. Use one to two tablespoons per cup of juice. It is difficult to mix, so use a blender or beater.

SPIRULINA GREEN DRINK

1 pound spirulina   6 ounces powdered apple pectin
½ pound bee pollen   6 ounces granulated lecithin

In addition to the above suggestions, it is important to follow a diet that reduces exogenous estrogen while supporting the endocrine glands. The following dietary suggestions are designed to achieve these goals.

❦ Eliminate sugar, white flour, and refined foods.
❦ Eliminate all methyl-xanthines, such as caffeine, theophylline, theobromine (coffee, chocolate, cola, and black/green teas).
❦ Eliminate red meat, which is a source of exogenous estrogen. If you wish to include red meat in your diet, do so on a limited basis, and be certain it is organically raised.
❦ Decrease fats, especially animal fats. Replace with unsaturated vegetable oils which are high in unsaturated fatty acids.

❧ Decrease milk and dairy products which are sources of exogenous estrogen. Yogurt and cultured milks are acceptable.

❧ Increase foods that are high in vitamins C, E, and selenium. These are antioxidants and help increase the detoxification of estrogen.

❧ Include complex carbohydrates, which are found in vegetables and whole grains. Also, include foods high in sulfur-containing amino acids such as garlic, onions, beans, and eggs.

External Treatments of Fibrocystic Breasts

It is sometimes helpful, in cases of large or generalized fibrocystic breast tissue, to apply external poultices directly to the mass. The following three poultices are the ones I've found to be the most effective.

Green Clay

Various types of clay will work as a poultice for cysts and tumors, but volcanic green clay is so rich in minerals and has such exceptionally fine drawing abilities that it is the one I always recommend. Mix it into a paste with water and spread it directly over the desired area. Cover with plastic wrap. Leave on until completely dry. You may leave it on overnight (though it will dry and crumble, making a mess in your bed) and rinse off in the morning.

Castor Oil Pack

Use a large, soft, cotton cloth. Heat the castor oil until it is very hot. Soak the cloth in the castor oil until it is thoroughly saturated. Place the cloth directly over the lumps. Cover the cloth completely with plastic wrap and leave it on overnight. This will help keep the heat in and also keep the oil from getting on everything. Repeat this five nights in a row and rest for two nights. Then repeat the cycle again. It is best to do this treatment in three-week cycles. Castor oil is very messy and will require some commitment on your part, but the packs are very effective.

Poke Root

Poke root is an old remedy for treating breast inflammation. I am always cautious recommending remedies I've only heard about and have not seen work for myself. In the case of poke root, I actually have seen it in action, but am still hesitant to recommend it!

Janice, the wife of one of the residential herb school teachers, was having mastitis (breast inflammation). She had recently given birth to their second child and shortly after had developed the inflammation. One of the visiting herb teachers, Michael, who is quite a remarkable herbalist and healer in his own right, suggested poke root poultices. We had a lot of fresh poke growing in the garden, and since Michael was adept at using this strong root, it seemed like a good idea. One of the students was sent to gather the fresh poke.

Now, fresh poke root, though a powerful medicine, is very irritating. The juice from the root can cause an ugly and very irritating skin rash. The berries are quite toxic, and the stalks and leaves, once they are past their youthful prime, are also poisonous. This isn't a plant to mess around with. (Yet thousands of people, including myself, enjoy the young leaves, properly prepared, as an early spring green and employ the root for medicine.)

So in came the student, fresh from the garden with a bag of fresh root. His arms were already itching and a red streaked rash was developing. Janice's eyes opened wide and I could see her getting a little nervous in her already feverish state. Michael quickly and very professionally mixed up a mash of the fresh root and applied it to her aching breast. We watched with a mixture of compassion and curiosity.

A red swelling quickly developed beneath the poke poultice. Janice reported a throbbing in that area and said it was getting increasingly painful. The blood and infection seemed to be concentrating there. Michael said that this was a good sign; the infection was coming to a head. But just about then, Janice decided that, good sign or not, she had had enough. The poke root was unceremoniously composted in the garden, and our first experiment with fresh poke root was over. We went back to nursing Janice with cool vinegar packs and sage poultices. Though slower-acting, they were soothing to her soul and effective in eliminating the infection.

I have since used poke root tincture on my own breasts as well as on other women's and can report excellent results. However, that first experience taught me to be cautious when using poke. I generally recommend using poke root tincture, not the fresh root, when making poultices.

Use fresh poke root tincture. Apply fifteen to thirty drops to a piece of cotton cloth and apply the cloth directly to the lump in the breast area. Secure in place with plastic wrap. Leave on overnight. Remove in the morning. Repeat for five nights, rest for two. Repeat this cycle for three weeks. Rest a week, then repeat if necessary.

For especially tenacious lumps, you can also take fifteen drops of tincture diluted in one-fourth cup warm water once a day. *Warning: poke root should be taken only in the recommended dosages!* Do not decide that, since a little is good for you, more may be better. It is not.

When You Have Breast Cancer

If you have breast cancer you may wish to try some of the herbal and nutritional remedies recommended in this section *in addition to, not in place of,* your allopathic orthodox treatment. I would suggest the dietary suggestions mentioned above, and the poultices, and the following:

❦ Chaparral tincture: one teaspoon three times a day
❦ Chaparral tablets: two tablets three times a day
❦ Chlorophyll and/or wheat grass juice: one teaspoon three times a day
❦ Blue-green algae: one teaspoon three times a day
❦ Pau d'arco/echinacea tea: one cup three times a day
❦ Reishi mushroom: three capsules three times a day

NINETEEN
Uterine Fibroids, Ovarian Cysts, Cervical Dysplasia, and Hysterectomies

Like benign breast lumps that develop with changing hormones, stress, and/or periods of ill health, ovarian cysts and uterine fibroids fluctuate and grow with the changing conditions of our lives. They do not automatically signal cancer, nor does a routine response to them have to be surgical removal, chemotherapy, or radiation. Often these therapies only perpetuate the problem. Radical medical techniques add additional stress to an already stressed system. Stress will perpetuate any health problem and appears to be an underlying cause of abnormal growths. Avoid it whenever possible. Though surgery and chemo/radiation therapy may be necessary, I would hardly recommend them as a first line of defense.

It is estimated between 40 and 50 percent of American women will have their uteruses removed by the time they are sixty-five. What a frightening statistic! For a while, hysterectomies became almost as common as tonsilectomies. Women were routinely persuaded to have what were sometimes unnecessary operations. The medical professional seemed to be saying to women that if they didn't want to have children, why carry around a useless piece of baggage? The uterus was easy to remove and, of course, the operation had a hefty price tag attached to it which, because of insurance coverage, didn't serve to deter women from the operation.

Like all operations, hysterectomies may at times be necessary, but this should be the exception, not the norm. Examine all other options before having this operation. The uterus is an integral and vitally important part of our inner ecology. It is almost as essential to life as our heart and liver and blood. Maybe even more so, since it is from this uniquely feminine organ that our creativity and fertility rises. Not only the organ of biological fertility, our uterus also houses the essence of our inner creativity and vital juices. We may be able to live and even function without one, but it is like removing a jewel— the hearthstone—of the center of the earth and replacing it with nothing. This is not something that should be done without careful consideration.

If your health care professional recommends a hysterectomy, be sure to get a second, and even a third, opinion. If you find it necessary for your long-term health to have a hysterectomy, do not despair. Surgical menopause is easily supported by good eating habits, a healthy life-style, and a good herbal program. For suggestions see the last two chapters of this book.

Most often when a woman discovers she has a benign growth in her vagina or womb, there is still time to attempt to eradicate it with natural, noninvasive therapies like nutrition and herbs. If these remedies do not have the desired effect and the cyst or benign growth continues to grow, there is always the second choice of surgery or other orthodox treatments. A third choice—one that is seldom considered and that I would be reluctant to recommend—is to just leave it alone. Nonetheless, it is not uncommon for these growths to disappear of their own accord.

Uterine Fibroids

Fibroids are benign tumors, generally solid in nature, that grow on the uterus. Small fibroids can be totally symptom-free. As they grow larger and/or more numerous, they may cause some pain, bleeding between periods, and excessive bleeding during periods. Large fibroids can also prevent pregnancy and/or cause miscarriages, but this is rare and occurs only if the fibroid has grown quite large. Though their cause is not fully known, we do know that they are dependent on estrogen for their growth. Estrogen treatments, oral contraceptives, and pregnancy stimulate their growth. Lowering estrogen levels in the body slows the growth of fibroids. Uterine fibroids will often shrink considerably or disappear completely during and after menopause, when estrogen levels naturally decrease.

Ovarian Cysts

An ovarian cyst is a sac containing fluid or semisolid material that develops in the ovarian tissue. Like fibroids, ovarian cysts are often symptom-free in the early stages. If they continue to grow, excessive bleeding, painful menstruation cycles, and pain in the pelvic area may be experienced. The most common symptoms are lower abdominal discomfort, together with distention of the abdomen. As the cyst enlarges, the abdomen begins to extend and will begin to mirror the early stages of pregnancy. Cysts seem to develop when a follicle fails to rupture or release an egg during its normal development. These follicles fill with clear fluid or become semisolid and develop into little sacs. Cysts seldom require surgical removal and most disappear by themselves with a little added help.

Usually, ovarian cysts and uterine fibroids are discovered during routine pelvic exams or testing done for other problems. They may also be detected when they've grown quite large or numerous and are causing physical problems such as excessive bleeding, painful menstrual cycles, or distention of the abdominal wall. Once the discovery is made, you will usually have time to try natural remedies. If your doctor recommends immediate surgical removal or other radical treatments, consider your second and third options. And get at least one second opinion.

According to the work of Dr. Catherine Kousimine, who has treated degenerative illnesses such as cancer for over forty years, cysts and fibroids are a part of the body's normal defense system. When the liver isn't able to detoxify the system, she believes, a "second liver" is created in the form of a cyst or fibroid. This second liver performs the role of storing toxins and maintaining the organism's equilibrium.

Medical science doesn't know the exact reasons or what causes growths to form on the ovarian and uterine walls, nor are they able to provide answers for preventing them. New Age "science" has all kinds of suggestions for why we might develop these extra growths in our wombs. I heard one explanation recently that made me smile, though I'm sure there is some validity in it: "A cyst/fibroid is a replacement or a mourning for what one wishes she were growing in her uterus." I'm sure the answers are as complex as the internal structure of our organisms and as mysterious as the great universe we live in. We don't have to know all of the causes just now; but it is certainly helpful to have some sense of how to correct the imbalances.

Natural Therapies for Uterine Fibroids and Ovarian Cysts

Below are some suggestions designed to help the body rid itself naturally of abnormal growths like fibroids and cysts. It generally takes three full menstrual cycles for most growths to either disappear or shrink in size. If they are large, it may take longer. If the growth(s) are already dangerously large when discovered, you may wish to consider orthodox therapies. But be sure to follow up with a good natural cleansing/building program that will both heal your womb area and prevent further growths from occurring.

❧ Follow the program outlined for fibrocystic breast condition. (See pages 154–6.) The focus should be a diet that helps lower estrogen levels and slows the growth of benign tumors. Avoid estrogenic foods such as dairy, eggs, red meat, and fat. (For a more complete list of these foods see page 155.) Emphasize a diet rich in dark green leafy vegetables, whole grains, and fresh fruit. Diet is essential in any cleansing/building program and should be carefully considered when developing a natural program for cyst or fibroid conditions.

❧ Take two Chaparral Capsules, below, three times a day for three months.

CHAPARRAL CAPSULES

1 part chaparral powder	1 part yellow dock root powder
1 part pau d'arco powder	1 part vitex (chaste berry) powder

To Make:
See page 58 for instructions on encapsulating herbs.

❧ Drink Liver Cleanse Tea, below, to cleanse and strengthen the liver so that it can effectively balance hormonal levels in the body.

LIVER CLEANSE TEA

1 part yellow dock root   1 part oregon grape root

2 parts wild yam root   2 parts burdock root

1 part dandelion root   1 part vitex (chaste berry)

Cinnamon, ginger, sassafras, and orange peel to taste.

To Make:

Use four to six tablespoons of herb mixture per quart of water. Add herbs to cold water and bring to a simmer over low heat. Keep pot tightly covered. Gently simmer for twenty minutes. Remove from heat and infuse twenty minutes longer. Strain. Drink three to four cups daily.

❦ Drink Spirulina Green Drink daily. (See page 155.)

❦ Use the formula below to make a vaginal bolus. Apply it five nights in a row, then rest from the application for two nights. Repeat this cycle for several weeks. Be sure to gently douche every few days to rinse out the herbs that accumulate in the vagina. Use a mild cleansing douche such as the Douche for Yeast Infections. (See page 137.)

VAGINAL BOLUS II

1 part yellow dock root powder   1 part witch hazel bark powder

1 part chaparral leaf powder   ½ part black walnut hull powder

1 part goldenseal root powder   1 to 2 drops of essential oil of myrrh

3 parts slippery elm bark powder   and/or tea tree oil

To Make:

See page 138 for directions on preparing a bolus. Note: If this particular formula irritates your vagina, add more slippery elm powder and/or some comfrey root powder.

❦ Make use of castor oil packs. This is a remedy that has proved extremely beneficial for women with cysts and fibroids. Edgar Cayce made these packs well known, and they continue to be helpful to many people. For complete instructions on applying a castor oil pack, see page 156. These packs should be applied three to four times a week, more often if your schedule allows.

❦ Make use of green clay packs. Clay is the essence of the mountains, ground down over the ages into a smooth powder. It is the rich substance of the earth, blessed by thousands of sunrises, sunsets, wind, and rainstorms. When we take the minerals that we call clay, mix them with water, and place the resulting paste over our wounds, we are using a powerful, age-old medicine.

The French and other Europeans have used clay as a remedy for hundreds of years. Here in this country Native Americans have long been acquainted with its healing power. Clay has strong drawing properties and will help draw blood to the area of the cyst or fibroid and concentrate it there. The strong flow of blood to an area disperses energy and helps break up the congestion and stagnation that often contribute to growths and blockages in the body.

There are many different types of clay. The colors are determined by the different concentrations of minerals found in it. For instance, red clay is very high in iron; yellow clay is rich in sulphur; green clay, my favorite medicinal clay, is rich in volcanic matter, minerals, and decomposed plant material. You can use local deposits of clay, but be sure it is smooth and free of pebbles and gravel. It needs to come from "clean" natural areas. Don't collect it from stagnant ponds or near areas that have been heavily fertilized or sprayed. Just as it is important to work with high-quality grown herbs, it is important to work with high-quality chemical-free clay. You can also purchase good-quality clay at health food and herb stores.

To make a green clay poultice for a cyst or fibroid, take one-half to one cup of clay and mix it into a paste with warm water. Spread a little vegetable oil directly over the area of the fibroid or cyst. Next, spread the clay thickly over the area. Cover it with a thick piece of gauze or cotton cloth and leave it on until the poultice is completely dry. The longer you leave it on the better. I generally suggest leaving a clay poultice on for one to two hours or overnight. Rinse off with warm water. For the clay poultice to be most effective, it is necessary to apply it three to four times a week for several weeks.

❦ Make use of sitz baths. An old European hydrotherapy treatment, sitz baths are probably the single most effective method, next to diet and herbs, for shrinking abnormal growths in the reproductive organs. They are easily done, but are a bit awkward at first. You will have to get used to them to fully appreciate the benefits! See page 113 for instructions on how to do them.

Sample Treatment Program for Uterine Fibroids and Ovarian Cysts
The following program should be adhered to for at least three full months.

❦ Concentrate on a diet low in estrogenic foods—low in fat, meat, eggs, cheese, and dairy. Limit your sugar, alcohol, and coffee intake. Eat foods rich in whole grains; dark green leafy vegetables; protein, such as tofu, tempeh, fish, organically raised chicken; fresh fruits; and herbal teas.
❦ Take two Chaparral Capsules (see page 160) three times a day.
❦ Drink three to four cups of Immune Cleanser Tea (see page 154) or Liver Cleanse Tea (see page 161) every day.
❦ Take a sitz bath (see page 113), followed by a castor oil pack (see page 156) and Vaginal Bolus II (see page 161) five nights a week.

Cervical Dysplasia

As is so often the case in many reproductive problems, no one really knows what causes cervical dysplasia—nor what "cures" it. In medical terms, it is termed an idiopathic disease, a disease of unknown origins, though there does seem to be some indication that women exposed to synthetic hormones (like daughters of women who took DES during pregnancy) are more susceptible to dysplasia. Also, exposure to sexually transmitted diseases, such as vaginal warts, herpes, chlamydia, and trichomoniasis, may make one more susceptible. Many of the reports I have read about cervical dysplasia link it to multiple sexual partners.

I'm sure there is no simple answer to a problem so complex as cervical dysplasia. We find it much easier to understand and accept a disease if there is a germ or a virus it can be pinned on rather than having to look to the world as a whole and our relationship with it as the "holistic" cause of the problem. Many of the illnesses we experience are a result of our environment, of our mental and emotional states, and are but reflections of the times we live in.

Cervical dysplasia has only been recognized as a condition since the advent of the pap smear, because without a pap smear it is not detectable. Dysplasia means abnormal cell growth in the cervix. Because cervical dysplasia is often considered a precancerous condition, being diagnosed with CD can create great anxiety in women. But dysplasia is not cancer and generally does not develop into cancer. In its most advanced stages it indicates a tendency toward cancer, but in its early stages the cells often return to normal of their own accord.

The abnormal cervical cells are generally classified according to the degree of their abnormality and are rated on a scale of I to V. Class I is considered a normal or "negative" pap smear. Class II is considered atypical and indicates that there are some abnormalities. Class III is considered "suspicious." About 30–50 percent of the women with a Class III pap smear may develop cervical cancer. If cancerous cells have already established themselves in the cervix, the pap smear tests will be classified as "positive" and labeled Class IV and V, depending on the severity of the condition.

When getting a pap smear, it is important to be aware that there can be some variation in the test results. There has been so much publicity about these errors recently that pathology labs are making a concerted effort to correct the problem. I have had several friends who have had pap smears done within a few days of each other and each test shows a different class of dysplasia. One close friend was diagnosed as having a Class III dysplasia after a routine pap smear. Needless to say, she was very concerned. On the recommendation of her doctor, she returned a few days later to the same lab and had another test. The diagnosis this time was a Class I. The reason for a discrepancy of this kind may lie in the quality of the lab work, in the quality of the tests themselves, or in changes in the cervix itself. Because of the potential for error, you should have more than one pap smear. You should even have a third one at a different lab if your pap smear registers abnormal cell growth or if the results of the first two tests are markedly different.

If a pap smear continues to register Class III or above, it is important to consult your physician and/or a qualified holistic health practitioner immediately. They will want to monitor any cervical changes with more frequent pap smears and will probably suggest laser surgery or other procedures to destroy or remove the abnormal cells. Though it is always automatically assumed this is what a woman should do, I am not so quick to make this recommendation. I think it is a personal choice that a woman makes after consultation with her doctor (preferably a holistically oriented one). Allopathic treatments address only the symptoms, not the cause of dysplasia. These invasive procedures often irritate the cervix, aggravating the underlying cause. If a woman does decide to have the cells removed, she should be informed of the different procedures available and the advantages and disadvantages of each of them. (See Appendix I, General Books on Women's Health, for a list of references that cover this material.)

If you have dysplasia cells that register Class I or Class II, doctors will often recommend a wait-and-see period. This creates a perfect opportunity to try to correct the problem by natural means. You can, if you choose, work with diet, herbs, guided meditation, and other natural therapies during this period to promote cervical well-being. Below is the program that several women I know have used successfully. The objective of a holistic approach to dysplasia is to balance hormonal activity, strengthen and support the immune system, and normalize and restore the cellular integrity of the vagina. If possible, work with a holistically minded practitioner who can provide guidance and support. If the wait-and-see period is used wisely as a period of grace and healing and as a time to reevaluate your life, making necessary life-style changes, then this period can be an empowering and healing time.

Internal Therapies for Cervical Dysplasia

❦ Take two Chaparral Capsules (see page 160) or one-fourth teaspoon chaparral tincture (see page 66) three times a day. Chaparral is excellent for inhibiting cancerous cells.

❦ Take one-fourth teaspoon pau d'arco tincture (see page 66) four to six times a day.

❦ Take two tablespoons of wheat grass juice three times a day. Wheat Grass juice is frequently used in precancerous and cancerous conditions. It is made by juicing the stalks of fresh young wheat. Wheat grass juice is available in most natural food stores in the freezer section.

❦ Take two Anti-Yeast Capsules (see page 136) every day.

❦ Drink three to four cups of Hormonal Regulator Tea (see page 117) or Endo-Liver Tea (see page 127) every day to cleanse the system and build the health of the liver.

❦ Follow general diet recommendations given on page 113.

If it is difficult to make dramatic dietary changes, as it often is for many people, then at least cut back on or eliminate foods that are known irritants: caffeine, alcohol, fried, fatty foods, and sugar.

External and Vaginal Therapies for Cervical Dysplasia

❦ Take a sitz bath two to three times a week. (See page 113 for directions.)

❦ Use vaginal boluses. They are a bit messy and time-consuming, but produce good results. Use the Vaginal Bolus II formula on page 161 and follow the instructions for making boluses on page 138. Be sure to douche every few days when using the bolus to clear out any residual herb build-up, using Douche for Yeast Infections (see page 137).

❦ Some women have reported good results using wheat grass juice as a douche. Dilute six tablespoons of wheat grass juice in one quart warm water and douche gently three to four times weekly.

❦ Vaginal Depletion Pack is made and distributed by the Eclectic Institute (14385 S.E. Lusted Road, Sandy, Oregon 97055). This rather dubious-sounding bolus was developed by Eclectic physicians in the early 1900s and is still used today for cervical erosions, abnormal pap smears, and pelvic inflammatory conditions. It has been used successfully to normalize dysplasia cells.

T W E N T Y
Fertility/Infertility

CHILD-
BEARING
YEARS

•

165

Infertility, or the inability to conceive, has become a major problem for women—and men—in recent times. Not too long ago, the big problem for women was preventing fertility. Women conceived more often than they wanted to and ended up spending most of their adult years either pregnant or nursing. But for an increasing number of modern-day couples the problem is infertility, and the cause is not always known. Physical problems, including infected, scarred, or abnormally formed reproductive organs, are often a major factor in infertility. Uterine fibroids or ovarian cysts are sometimes the cause of infertility. Endometriosis is considered to be a leading cause of infertility. These problems can be detected by modern medical tests and are often, though not always, correctable. But causes of infertility are often termed "idiopathic," which means that no one knows the cause for sure. When this is the case, a woman must be creative and determined in reestablishing her fertility.

I've frequently found that infertility is due to imbalances in the energy levels of the reproductive system. The reproductive organs are often "weak" in women—excessively "yin." That is, they hold many deep inward emotions and are, in a sense, "weeping" with these held-back feelings. This condition may manifest itself in an infection of a yeast or mucus nature. There is frequently a continuous, though slight, discharge, as if the vagina is weeping. Often, too, there are menstrual difficulties. The organs feel cool or even cold; there is no heat generated in them. When you visualize your reproductive organs, think of them as being warm and alive, pulsing with life and creative potential.

Stress and tension are often the root of infertility. A person may dream and wish for a child, a family, but be exhausted from her work and the stress of modern-day living. It is hard to nurture another soul if your own body is exhausted. You may be strong enough to function adequately; your menstrual cycles may be normal and nothing may seem to be wrong. But there may be a deep sense of exhaustion, an absence of reserve energy. I think one of the reasons that young women conceive so easily is that even though they may not desire children, their energy is still strong and vital. As women grow older and take on the burdens of life, they exhaust themselves, often without replenishing their inner reserves of energy. So their bodies get very tired. It is not aging that exhausts us of our fertile potency, but unhealthy aging. Dona Josefa, a powerful and beautiful shaman healer from the Huichel tribe in Mexico with whom I had the pleasure of studying, had her last child when she was well into her sixties. Her husband, Don Jose, was over eighty.

A poor flow of energy circulating through the reproductive organs will also weaken fertility in women—and men. This is often due to imbalances in hormones caused by improper diet and life style. If a women frequently experiences irregular or painful menstrual cycles, it may be an indication that energy is not circulating strongly or smoothly through the pelvis. Herbal teas, sitz baths, a healthy diet rich in vitamins and minerals, and outdoor exercise that stimulates the spirit as well as the body, are all helpful in removing energy blockages in the reproductive organs.

The reproductive organs of women are extremely responsive organs. Often problems of infertility are due to blocked emotion and feelings stored in our memories. By coming to terms with the deep feelings that may have scarred our innermost beings, we can often unleash our creative powers and awaken our fertility.

Though I've known many women who have conceived after long periods of infertility, it is hard to say how much the herbs I've suggested have helped. There are so many factors involved. I do know that herbs help heal the reproductive organs and balance hormonal levels. They aid in restoring overall vitality and health. All these factors are important when one is considering pregnancy or lack of it. If one were attempting to restore or increase fertility, it would certainly be safer, less invasive, and less expensive to first try herbs and diet before attempting the standard medical route. (At least one never has to worry about the possibility of quadruplets when trying herbal fertility therapies!)

Herbs are most helpful when infertility is due to endocrine imbalances. However, even if the cause is structural problems or scarring due to endometriosis, pelvic inflammatory disease, sexually transmitted diseases, and so forth, herbs can play a vital role in correcting the problem by restoring the body to an overall state of health, and thus increasing fertility. Herbal therapies should be tried for at least three months and possibly longer before results are looked for.

Laurie, a close friend and a student at the herb school, had tried for several years to conceive. As she approached her late thirties, her biological clock was ticking away and her urge to conceive was growing strong. Having experienced a lot of previous reproductive problems, including an ectopic pregnancy, a miscarriage, severe monthly cramps, and cervical dysplasia, both her reproductive system and her emotional being were deeply scarred.

Still, she yearned to conceive and have a family. Over the years her persistence, her belief in herself and her love of herbs continued to grow. As her knowledge of herbs blossomed, she improved her diet and her life-style. Even her love life blossomed. She and John had met at the herb school and were married a few years later. Though acutely aware of the possible effects of Laurie's reproductive history, they were intent on having children and raising a family.

Meanwhile, many of Laurie's reproductive problems were clearing up. Her menstrual cycles had become regular and seldom painful. Her cervical dysplasia had responded to diet and herbs. Much of the emotional scarring had healed, too. But after four years of marriage, the longed-for baby had still not arrived. John wanted her to begin fertility testing. Fertility drugs were even discussed. But Laurie was reluctant; it just wasn't her way.

Her tenacious belief in herself amazed me. Over a period of several years Laurie had regained the health of her reproductive system. Her own body had become a powerful teacher to her, and in many ways, was the most valuable teaching she had to offer her students. "Walking her talk," she lived what she believed. She had changed her life-style to support a radiantly healthy body. Her diet, her use of herbs, her life work were all conducive to fertility. And at last it happened: Laurie became the mother of a baby daughter. Born on the spring equinox, she is a baby conceived in love and made possible by self-renewal and empowerment.

Herbs to Increase Fertility

The following herbal formulas are recommended to increase fertility. Most of these suggestions are applicable to the man in the family, also.

❦ Take two capsules of dong quai three times a day except during menstruation. (Men should take two capsules of ginseng every day.)

❦ Take Liquid Floradix Iron with Herbs regularly, following the dosage recommendations on the bottle. Or take a vitamin/mineral formula you make yourself. (See page 62 for directions.)

❦ Take Fertility Tonic, in capsule or tonic form, daily. (See page 58 for directions on making capsules, page 66 for directions on making tinctures.) If taking Fertility Tonic in capsule form, take two, three times a day. If taking it in tincture form, take one-fourth teaspoon three times a day.

FERTILITY TONIC

4 parts rehmania
1 part astragalus root
1 part dong quai root
   (for men, substitute ginseng)

2 parts false unicorn root
3 parts wild yam root
1 part vitex berries

FEMALE FERTILITY TEA

3 parts wild yam root
2 parts licorice root
4 parts sassafras bark of root
1 part vitex (chaste berry)
½ part dong quai root
   for men, substitute ginseng)

a pinch of stevia
1 part ginger root
1 part cinnamon bark
½ part false unicorn root
¼ part orange peel

To Make:

Use four to six tablespoons of the herb mixture per quart of water. Add the herbs to cold water and bring to a slow simmer over low heat. Keep pot tightly covered. Simmer gently for twenty minutes. Remove from heat and allow to infuse for another twenty minutes. Strain. Drink three to four cups daily.

CASCADE'S FERTILITY FORMULA

1 dram dong quai tincture
2 drams squaw vine tincture
2 drams wild yam tincture
1 dram ginseng tincture
1 dram ho-shou-wu (polyganum multiforum) tincture
1 dram dandelion leaf/root tincture

To Make:

See pages 66–67 for directions on making tinctures. Mix tinctures together well. Take thirty drops of the mixture twice daily, before meals, immediately following cessation of menstrual flow, and continuing until next period. Discontinue during menses and repeat cycle for up to four months. If pregnancy occurs, discontinue. (Cascade says that this formula works best while on a romantic outing!)

❦ Drink ginseng tea or take ginseng capsules regularly. Ginseng is often helpful for women who have fertility problems, especially if the infertility is related to weak or cool sexual organs. Ginseng increases heat to the pelvic region and helps remove blockages.
❦ Take sitz baths several times a week for several months. (See page 113 for directions.)
❦ Make use of acupuncture. It is very effective for removing stagnation and energy blocks and has been used successfully for problems of infertility.
❦ Try homeopathic remedies. They have often proved helpful in increasing fertility. Consult a homeopathic physician for an appropriate remedy.

A CLOSING NOTE

I have heard so many stories of couples who have tried to conceive for years, but with no luck. They finally decide to adopt, and shortly after signing the adoption papers they ended up pregnant. I certainly would not suggest this as a fertility "cure," but it's a wonderful way to satisfy your parenting needs while caring for and loving a child. And, who knows, you may just conceive. It's certainly not uncommon.

Pregnancy and
CHILDBIRTH

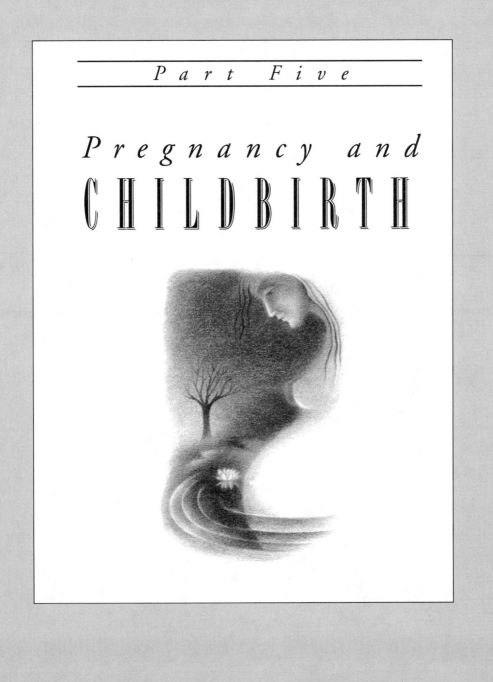

A Healthy Pregnancy

Nothing is so beautiful as a ship at full sail, or a woman great with child.

—Author unknown

Ideally, of course, each and every woman should have an herb garden—perhaps tucked amongst the vegetables and flowers, or a separate space, to wander in and dream of a babe's sweet face.

—Rosemary Sutton

Pregnancy and childbirth provide the opportunity to become active participants in the grand fertility plan of the Great Mother. What greater wonder is there than seeing the belly stretched taut with the fullness of creation? What more profound task than creating life with all of its hopes and dreams and possibilities? Though indisputably one of life's great miracles, pregnancy and childbirth bring with them a unique set of challenges. Caught up in the dramatic changes our bodies undergo, we sometimes lose sight of the great wonder of this time. Miraculously, for a few short months of our lives, we become the cocreators of life. The food we eat, the processes of our bodies, the air we breathe, and the water we drink become the building blocks for a soul unfolding. Perhaps more than at any other time, it is wise to have a knowledge of the healing herbs and a trust in the rhythmic nature of the universe.

Most early herbalists were trained in the skills of midwifery, and most midwives were also trained in the use of herbs. The two trades went hand in hand, each intimately linked with the flow of life. The herbs used today for pregnancy and childbirth are the same herbs used for centuries. Passed down from mother to daughter for generation upon generation, the age-old lore of herbs has been distilled into the wealth of information available to us today.

The effectiveness of herbal remedies is often traced to their high concentrations of vitamins, minerals, and other chemical constituents. An even greater source of their power is the life force inherent in them. Steeped in ancient genetic strength, born of the earth and nourished by what is essential in life, herbs possess powers not measurable in terms of chemical components only. Impregnated with life energy and an inherent will to reproduce, they provide a living source of nourishment for the pregnant mother and unborn child. The life force found so strongly in the plants infuses the mother's very blood and is carried to the seed within.

One of the great joys I've experienced as an herbalist is participating in the ritual of birth with several of my friends. Most recently, I had the great honor of assisting at the birth of my first grandchild. What a monumental experience it was to welcome that beautiful little boy into the world. I've had the privilege of guiding women in herbal ways throughout their pregnancies, helping them with herbs at the time of birth, and comforting them with herbal teas and sitz baths afterwards. Some of these women were children themselves when they first came to the herb shop with their mothers. It was wonderful to watch the fullness of the circle and the traditions passed on. We called these babies "herbal babies," and their pictures fill the pages of my photo albums.

Though most of these births flowed easily enough, it would be presumptuous to say that complications and problems never arose. As I have said before, herbs are not always the appropriate choice of medicine. They do not provide the cure or solution for many health problems; it is sometimes modern medicine that renders the necessary miracle. One birth in particular stands out as an example of this.

Joanne was an excellent herbalist. She ran an herbal center in the Midwest, and we were very good friends and coworkers. Even more so than I, she was a devout herbalist; she practiced herbalism as a way of life. When she became pregnant, a joyous moment in both her own and her husband's life, she decided that this was going to be a totally natural pregnancy and childbirth. She and her husband were respected members of their community, and the joy of Joanne's pregnancy, coming late in life, was shared by all her friends and family.

Nine months later, after gallons of raspberry leaf tea, all the other "right" herbs, and the best diet, Joanne and Stephen awaited the moment, with their house in order and several midwives to assist. When labor began, there were early signs of a potentially difficult birth. But Joanne was very determined to have a natural birth, at home, with her midwives and herbs. After two days of continuous labor, however, Joanne was exhausted and her energy was running out. Labor continued to be painfully intense but there were no signs of delivery in sight, and both Stephen and the midwives were strongly suggesting that Joanne go to the local hospital, where a doctor had been called and was waiting.

For Joanne, I think, it was almost a humiliation, a surrender of her ideals. Here she was, the outstanding herbalist of her community, the "natural" woman, having to turn to mainstream medicine and go to the hospital! Yet what more wise and natural thing to do? Her baby's life and perhaps her own were at stake. When in trouble it is wise to choose the form of medicine that works best. That is medicine at its most truly holistic. Afterward, when Joanne called and told me, almost apologetically, what had happened, I congratulated her enthusiastically on the birth of their son and the wise choice she and her husband had made. I smiled, knowing what a great teacher her son was going to be for her and that this was just the first of many lessons he would teach her. The whole experience was also an excellent lesson for her students and would broaden their ideas of holistic living.

Though generally a healthy and joyous time for most women, problems and complications do occur during pregnancy and childbirth. A knowledge of herbs, though certainly not the answer for all problems that arise, is invaluable to women during this time. Knowing which herbs to use as well as which herbs *not* to use can prove helpful time and again.

Most herbs are remarkably safe to use during pregnancy and provide a gentle alternative to orthodox medical treatments that are often not recommended at this time because of their possible side effects. During pregnancy, herbs provide an excellent source of concentrated nutrition. Because they are naturally biochelated, their high vitamin/mineral content is easily assimilated. During labor, they can be helpful in promoting contractions, easing pain, and assisting in the childbirth process. And following childbirth, herbs can once again rise to the occasion by helping restore the vitality and strength of the mother.

Perhaps it's not just the herbs themselves that heal, but the ritual of using them. While pregnant and after giving birth, a woman needs time to reflect, to nourish her inner self, and to form a bond with her newborn. But time is an element missing from most people's lives. During pregnancy, the expectant mother often feels driven to get things done before the "deadline" of her child's birth. And after the baby arrives, she may feel driven again to get "back on her feet" so that she may return to work. Using herbs on a daily basis can help her reconnect with the deeper rhythms of life—her own, her baby's, and the natural world's. Making herbal teas, enjoying the beauty of an herb bath, massaging her baby with the herbal oils she's made herself—each of these moments can gently remind her of time's sweet timelessness and deepen her experience of creating life.

Which Herbs Can One Use Safely During Pregnancy?

Many modern herb books provide a long inventory of herbs to avoid during pregnancy. Though I certainly believe it's important to exercise caution in this area, I also feel that many herbs end up on this "herbal blacklist" and there they stay, inadvertently passed from one list to another.

Though there is little information to support the bad press some herbs receive in this matter, I do emphasize caution. "Better to be safe than sorry," as the old saying goes, I have, however, established some guidelines that may be useful to the pregnant woman in helping to decide which herbs can be safely used.

❦ During pregnancy, use herbs that are considered food, or tonic, herbs. These herbs are used like food and can be eaten every day with no residual buildup. Examples of such herbs are: alfalfa, nettle, dandelion, raspberry leaf, oat straw, melissa, and chamomile. (See the "Favorite Herbs for Pregnancy" list beginning on page 174.)

❦ Avoid all herbs that can be toxic to the system. Among these herbs are tansy, rue, cotton root bark, pennyroyal *oil,* and goldenseal (which may be potentially harmful only when taken in large quantities).

❦ Avoid herbs used during menstruation to stimulate the menstrual cycle. Some of these herbs are considered abortifacient because they can cause premature contractions of the uterus and thus a possible miscarriage. Herbs in this group are in fact sometimes used during the first trimester of pregnancy to precipitate abortions, though to do so they must be taken in large quantities and even then, are often not successful. Though non-toxic to the system as a whole, they work through the action of their high concentrations of oxytocins to cause uterine contractions. These herbs are also used during the last few days of pregnancy to help open the womb and ensure an easier childbirth. Herbs in this group include angelica, black cohosh, blue cohosh, motherwort, pennyroyal leaf, parsley leaf (when used vaginally), and yarrow. Dong quai, though a strong uterine tonic, is also not recommended during pregnancy because it is used to regulate and/or stimulate the menstrual cycle. (See pages 178–79 for a fuller discussion of the uterine-stimulating herbs that should be avoided during most of the nine months of pregnancy.)

❦ Avoid herbs that are high in alkaloids and/or have a strong medicinal action on the body. These herbs may be perfectly safe to use and are often highly recommended as herbal medication at other times, but during pregnancy a woman should use milder tonic herbs.

❦ Herbs used for specific illness are often too strong to be used on a regular basis by a pregnant woman. However, if you are sick during pregnancy and would benefit from taking small amounts of these herbal medicines, you can assess the situation and evaluate the herb individually. Herbs for specific illnesses should be avoided or used with caution not because they are toxic or because they are abortifacient, but because they have very powerful physiological actions and may irritate the system. Examples of such herbs are goldenseal, coffee, cascara sagrada, senna, and angelica.

❦ When using an herb that you're unfamiliar with, especially during pregnancy, research it in one of several good herb books. (See Appendix I.) Never use herbs during pregnancy whose safety is questionable. Comfrey is a good example. Though I have used comfrey leaf and root successfully for many years, the herb is currently being scrutinized for potentially hazardous side effects. Until this controversy is settled, it is best to avoid it during pregnancy.

The following are my favorite herbs for pregnancy and childbirth. All of them are remarkably safe and easily obtainable in natural food and herb stores. Most of them are also listed in the Materia Medica at the back of this book.

Favorite Herbs for Pregnancy

Black haw (Viburnum prunifolium) Black haw is used in much the same way as its cousin, cramp bark. It has proven a useful preventative of miscarriage through a long history of folk medicine. It "quiets" the uterine muscles and eases the tension that often precipitates uterine contractions.

Blessed thistle leaf (Cnicus benedictus) Blessed thistle, like its cousin, milk thistle (Cardus marianus), is highly regarded as a liver tonic and builder. But it's most valued by pregnant women because it stimulates blood flow to the mammary glands and increases and enriches the flow of mother's milk. It is often combined with fennel and raspberry leaf to make an effective and tasty tea. Blessed thistle's hemostatic properties also reduce the chances of hemorrhaging during childbirth.

Burdock root (Arctium lappa) Often sold as a vegetable in Oriental markets under the name "Gobo," burdock root is a delicious and very nourishing herb. It was used by ancient herbalists for weak uteruses and as an aid during childbirth. Though these days it is not generally considered a pregnancy herb, I always recommend it because of its high concentrations of vitamins, minerals, and trace minerals. It is also a mild diuretic and an excellent herb for the liver. It is a pleasant-tasting tea and can be used to camouflage the bitter taste of dandelion root. (Add a bit of ginger and cinnamon bark for flavor.)

Chamomile flowers (Matricaria chamomilla, and related species) This delicate, gentle flower is a must for pregnant women. Its sunny disposition is helpful for lifting the spirits and its calming relaxing attributes are very soothing to the soul. Chamomile is recommended for the daily stresses of life and can be enjoyed as a relaxing tea. Better yet, it can be used as an infusion for the whole body. Fill the bathtub with warm water and add a large cloth bag full of chamomile and lavender blossoms. Then immerse yourself in this giant cup of tea. A nice massage with chamomile oil can follow, soothing away any tired, achy muscles or bothersome thoughts.

Because of its mild, bitter constituents, chamomile is a specific for digestive disorders and, combined with ginger, is recommended for morning sickness. Its high calcium content makes it an excellent tonic herb for the nervous system. The beautiful colored essential oil of chamomile, called azulene, is an antiinflammatory substance and helps explain chamomile's effectiveness in healing swellings, achy joints, and other inflammatory conditions.

Cramp bark (Viburnum opulus) Though this herb is not absolutely necessary as a tonic herb during pregnancy, it is an excellent remedy to have on hand in case of a threatened miscarriage or spot bleeding. It is possibly one of the best herbs known for preventing miscarriage due to stress and anxiety and is specifically used for relaxing the uterine muscles. If miscarriage is a potential problem during pregnancy, cramp bark can be used over an extended period of time with no harmful side effects.

Dandelion greens and root (Taraxacum officinale) For centuries the greens of dandelion, that brightly flowered common pest of garden and field, have been relished as a potent source of vitamins and minerals. You'll not find many food sources that have a higher percentage or quality of vitamin A, calcium, and iron. The bitter compounds so readily found in dandelion greens aid digestion and stimulate bile flow. Not only are the greens nourishing and toning to the system, they also have gentle remedial properties that are helpful to pregnant women. Dandelion leaf tea

dandelion

is a mild diuretic and helps eliminate excess water from the system. Because the leaf is high in natural potassium, it does not deplete potassium in the system as do synthetic diuretics. If a pregnant woman is experiencing high blood pressure during pregnancy, she might want to try a combination of dandelion leaf tea, garlic oil capsules, and stress release techniques before resorting to medical drugs. Many women have had success in lowering high blood pressure with this combination of natural remedies.

While the leaf is fairly well known as a salad green and herb tea, dandelion root is often neglected. But it too is a wonderful tonic herb and a gentle remedial for pregnant women. The root is used primarily for digestive disturbances and for cleansing and toning the liver. It is especially useful for fatigue and that exhausted feeling many pregnant women experience. The bitter principles found in such high concentrations in dandelion root nourish and activate the liver so that it can function at its optimum.

Ginger root (Zingiber officinale) A warming tonic herb for the entire reproductive system, ginger is specifically recommended during pregnancy for morning sickness and digestive problems. It is also a safe herb during pregnancy for colds, sore throats, and congestion. And ginger tastes so good! Freshly grated and combined with honey and lemon, it's a delicious, effective remedy. During prolonged labor, ginger oil can be massaged over the lower back to restore energy. (To make ginger oil, see instructions for making herbal oils on page 50).

Lady's mantle leaves (Alchemilla vulgaris) Though little used in this country, lady's mantle is highly regarded as a "woman's herb" throughout Europe. It is a lovely, easily cultivated plant. Though used for many women's problems, it is especially valued during pregnancy for toning the uterus. Because of its astringent qualities, it's helpful in reducing the chances of hemorrhaging during childbirth. Lady's mantle also helps settle the stomach and is useful in treating morning sickness.

Peter and Barbara Theiss write, in *The Family Herbal,* "Lady's mantle is associated with the qualities of gentleness, elegance, and grace in combination with powerful authority. If a woman finds difficulty in accepting a maternal role, is troubled by thoughts of abortion, and suffers from morning sickness and other disorders during the first months of pregnancy, depression after birth, and so on, Lady's mantle is her herb."

Lemon balm leaves (Melissa officinalis) Though not generally considered a specific herb for pregnant women, lemon balm has so many excellent properties and is so safe, effective, and tasty that I often suggest it during pregnancy. It is primarily used to calm and relax the nervous system. A cup of warm lemon balm tea, sweetened with a touch of honey, is a wonderful remedy for headache, depression, and insomnia. Combined with chamomile flowers, it helps take the edge off a stressful day.

Lemon balm can also be used by pregnant women for digestive purposes. Possessing a high concentration of essential oils, it has antispasmodic powers and helps relieve gas pains. Because of its antihistaminic properties, it is also used to reduce the effects of allergies. Combined with nettle, lemon balm provides an effective, nontoxic tea for women who suffer from allergies during pregnancy. But the best thing about lemon balm is its delightful flavor. Fresh and invigorating, lemon balm makes a delicious tea and is a wonderful addition to salads and soups.

Nettle leaf (Urtica dioica) Rich in calcium, iron, and many other vitamins and minerals, nettle is an excellent nourishing herb for the pregnant woman. It is also tasty as freshly steamed greens and makes a pleasant-tasting tea. Nettle is highly recommended for pregnant women who suffer from chronic fatigue and low energy due to insufficient iron. The tea is also a mild diuretic and aids in the elimination of excess water from body tissues. Nettle's reputation as a specific herb for general female problems and as a tonic during pregnancy stems from its use by Native American women as a tonic throughout pregnancy and as a remedy for hemorrhaging during childbirth. It is still used by Native American women to enrich and increase the flow of milk and to aid in restoring and rebuilding the mother's energy following childbirth.

Oat straw stalk and unripe fruit (Avena sativa) Rich in calcium and magnesium, oat straw tea is highly recommended during pregnancy for calming nervous stress and tension. It is a safe natural tonic herb for the nervous system and is very relaxing and tasty when combined with chamomile flowers. It is also a safe remedy for the yeast infections that may occur during pregnancy. People often confuse oat straw with oatmeal. I've had several people write to ask me if their oat straw tea was supposed to look and taste like a breakfast cereal! Though both are great food, the tea is made from the young stalks and slightly unripe grain; oatmeal is made from the rolled pressed grain.

Oat straw is readily available in natural food and herb stores. I always found it amusing that as a child growing up on a farm I played in barns full of oat straw. My father bought it by the ton. As an adult working in the herb store, I sold it by the ounce!

Red raspberry leaf (Rubus idaeus and related species) Considered the "herb supreme" for pregnancy, raspberry leaf tones and nourishes the uterine muscles, is rich in vitamins and minerals, and is especially high in naturally chelated iron, which the body can readily assimilate. It enriches and increases the flow of milk, helps restore the system following childbirth, and is a good all-purpose, pleasant-tasting herb to drink during the entire nine months.

Slippery elm bark (Ulmus rubra and U. fulva) Though this is a favorite medicinal herb of mine and one I've used for years, I've cut back on my use of it due to the Dutch Elm disease that has destroyed so many of these grand old trees. But when necessary, I still recommend it in small amounts, for it is the herb of choice in many health situations. Rich in mucilage, slippery elm is both nourishing and medicinal. It is excellent for any type of mucous membrane inflammation and/or irritation. During pregnancy, it can be safely used for colds, infections, vaginal irritations, and as a nourishing, soothing gruel for morning sickness.

If you read in some books that slippery elm is dangerous and not to be used, consider the source of that myth. Historically, Native American women used long sticks of the soft inner bark of slippery elm inserted into their wombs to induce abortion. State legislatures passed laws forbidding the sale of slippery elm sticks. This particular use of slippery elm continues to taint its reputation. It has absolutely no toxic properties when taken as tea or food.

Squaw vine (Mitchella repens) Indigenous to the North American continent, squaw vine was first used by Native American women as an aid in pregnancy and childbirth. Considered one of the best of the herbs used for toning and nourishing the uterus, it is often combined with raspberry leaf for a perfect pregnancy tonic.

Strawberry leaf (Fragaria vesica and related species) Well known for its delicious red fruit, strawberry's leaves are also used by herbalists. It has qualities similar to those of its cousin, raspberry. Though it is not as famous, it, too, is used as a tonic during pregnancy. The leaves are slightly acidic and cooling to the system. I've found strawberry leaf tea especially pleasant in the hot humid days of summer for women in the later stages of pregnancy. A pleasant-tasting tea, strawberry can be combined with raspberry leaf and squaw vine for an exceptional tonic blend to drink during the entire pregnancy. Jeannine Parvati, in her excellent women's herbal, *Hygia*, recommends strawberry leaf to prevent miscarriage. It is also used for fevers and diarrhea.

The following herbs are useful during pregnancy and childbirth but must be used with caution and only for specific remedial situations. DO NOT USE THESE HERBS CARELESSLY. See cautions on each herb in the Materia Media at the back of the book.
Angelica (Angelica archangelica, A. sylvestris) A strong, stately herb often used to correct menstrual irregularity and delayed menstruation, angelica promotes blood flow to the pelvis and causes uterine contractions. Therefore, *it is not recommended for use during pregnancy,* though it is sometimes employed by midwives during childbirth when labor is prolonged or delayed. Angelica is the herb of choice of most midwives to help expel the placenta following childbirth.

Black cohosh (Cimicifuga racemosa) Considered a marvelous woman's tonic herb, black cohosh is both a uterine stimulant and a uterine relaxant. Possessing estrogenlike qualities, it is used to promote menstruation and regulate hormonal action. Eclectic physicians believed black cohosh to be one of the most useful and powerful uterine tonics; some of the early patent medicines contained high concentrations of the herb. However, because of its stimulating effects on the uterus, *it is not recommended for pregnant women except during the last week of pregnancy.* It is often combined with blue cohosh and used during the last week to prepare the uterus for childbirth. Its unique properties enable it to stimulate contractions while relaxing the tension and stress that concentrates in the uterine muscles.

Blue Cohosh (Caulophyllum thalictroides) Blue cohosh is considered one of the best uterine stimulants and menstruation-promoting herbs available. It is often combined with black cohosh and used as a tea and/or tincture during the last week of pregnancy to prepare the uterus for an easy birth and to stimulate uterine contractions.

Caulopsaponin, a chemical component of blue cohosh, actively stimulates uterine contractions and promotes blood flow to the pelvic region. *Because of its strong uterine stimulant properties, blue cohosh should not be used at any time during pregnancy, except in the last week.* It is very beneficial when labor is long and drawn out.

Motherwort (Leonurus cardiaca) Though motherwort is used during the last few days of pregnancy to prepare the uterus for childbirth, *its menstruation-promoting properties make its use undesirable throughout pregnancy.* Concentrations of leonurine and stachydrine, two chemical constituents that promote uterine contractions, are found in motherwort, substantiating its traditional use to promote menstruation and hasten childbirth.

Pennyroyal leaf (Hedeoma pulegioides and Mentha pulegium) Pennyroyal is one of the best-known herbs for stimulating blood flow to the pelvis and activating uterine contractions. *Because of its ability to stimulate uterine contractions, it should never be used by pregnant women except during the last few days of pregnancy.* Though pennyroyal herb is often listed as toxic, it is not poisonous and has, in fact, proven quite useful as a birthing aid. *However, the essential oil of pennyroyal, if taken internally, is extremely toxic and has killed women who have tried to take it to stimulate abortions.* While the herb can be used safely during the last few days of pregnancy, the oil should not be used by pregnant women at any time.

Shepherd's purse (Capsella bursa-pastoris) This plant is listed here not because it should be used with such great caution, but because it has a specific remedial action for pregnant women. Shepherd's purse is the herb par excellence for hemorrhaging during childbirth. Its high concentrations of tannin, tyramine, and other amines are very helpful in arresting the flow of excessive bleeding. The herb should be used *fresh* or tinctured from fresh plant material for maximum effectiveness. Tinctures made of the fresh herb are almost always effective in curbing excessive bleeding and are included in the birthing kits of most midwives I know. Because shepherd's purse is high in oxytocin, a uterine contractor, it may also help stimulate contractions at the end of labor, though I have never seen it used for this purpose.

Yarrow (Achillea millefolium) Yarrow, an excellent hemostatic, is used in combination with shepherd's purse to arrest hemorrhaging during childbirth. Yarrow is generally considered a safe, nontoxic herb and is commonly used for colds, flus, and fevers. However, *because of its stimulating action on the uterus, it is one of the herbs that should not be used during the early stages of pregnancy.*

General Formulas for a Healthy Pregnancy

The following are some of my favorite herb tonics to use during pregnancy. The formulas can be adjusted to make the flavors more appealing to individual tastes. In general, you should make a quart of tea at a time, store it in a thermos or quart jar, and drink it throughout the day.

PREGNANCY TEA

3 parts red raspberry leaf
2 parts nettle
1 part alfalfa leaf
4 parts peppermint and/or spearmint

3 parts lemon balm
2 parts squaw vine
A pinch of stevia for sweetness

To Make:

Use four to six tablespoons of herb mixture per quart of water. Place herbs in cold water and bring to a simmer over low heat. Immediately remove from the heat. Keeping the pot covered, let mixture infuse for twenty minutes or longer and strain.

CALCIUM-PLUS TEA

2 parts oat straw
1 part alfalfa

2 parts nettle
½ part shave grass (horsetail)

To Make:

Use four to six tablespoons of herb mixture per quart of water. Place herbs in cold water and bring to a simmer over low heat. Remove from stove immediately. Keeping pot covered, let mixture infuse for twenty minutes or longer and strain.

IRON-PLUS-CALCIUM TINCTURE

3 parts nettle
2 parts yellow dock root
1 part watercress

2 parts spirulina
1 part kelp
1 part lamb's quarter

For instructions on making tinctures, see page 66.

GENTLE RELAXATION TEA

3 parts lemon balm
1 part passion flower
2 parts oat straw

3 parts chamomile
¼ part valerian

To Make:

Use four to six tablespoons of herb mixture per quart of water. Place herbs in cold water. Bring to a simmer over low heat. Remove from stove immediately. Keeping pot covered, let mixture infuse for twenty minutes or longer and strain.

3 parts peppermint
1 part squaw vine
1 part ginkgo

1 part gota kola
1 part raspberry leaf
½ part ginger

To Make:

Use four to six tablespoons of herb mixture per quart of water. Place herbs in cold water. Bring herbs to a simmer over low heat, keeping pot covered. Remove from stove immediately. Let mixture infuse for twenty minutes or longer and strain.

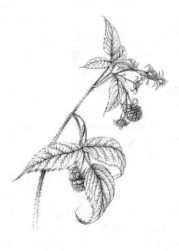

raspberry

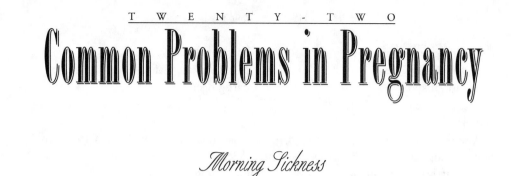

T W E N T Y - T W O

Common Problems in Pregnancy

Morning Sickness

Morning sickness is the most common and irritating problem encountered in the first trimester of pregnancy. About half of all pregnant women experience it to one degree or another. For some women, it is an all-day problem, not just something that afflicts them in the morning. Generally the unpleasant symptoms of morning sickness are over after the first three months, but unfortunately, some women experience them well past the first three months of pregnancy. In severe cases they can make this otherwise happy period quite miserable, and the memory of pregnancy downright unpleasant.

A combination of factors, including sudden hormonal changes, shifting dietary needs, an insufficient amount of B vitamins, and/or low blood sugar, give rise to morning sickness. In particular, a rapid increase in the hormone chorionic gonadotrophin (CG) during the first few months of pregnancy is thought to be a cause of the complaint.

Formerly, morning-sickness medication offered by the orthodox medical community contained antihistamines, which caused possible problems with the immune system and immunological disorders. Antihistamines have also been linked with birth defects in animals. Thankfully, these days most doctors offer nothing more than fluids and encouragement if things get out of hand.

Wild yam root, which balances hormonal production and tones and nourishes the liver, is one of the best remedies for morning sickness. Some women have found that just sipping wild yam tea during the day alleviates the nausea. A combination of two parts wild yam, one part dandelion root, and one part chaste berry also makes an excellent remedy for morning sickness. Because wild yam is a tonic herb, its effects may not be felt immediately. I've found it works best if taken in small amounts (one-fourth cup every hour or two) over a period of several days.

Since morning sickness often occurs first thing in the morning and during prolonged stretches without food, low blood sugar levels may be implicated. A long-standing remedy for morning sickness is to eat small meals frequently, avoid large meals, and snack on wholesome nourishing protein foods between meals. Some women have found that popcorn sprinkled with nutritional yeast is a satisfying between-meal snack. Yogurt is also excellent. Whole grain crackers with nut butter (almond, hazelnut, or peanut) or another high-protein spread make a good between-meal snack. High-mineral vegetable broths are also satisfying to sip between meals, particularly in cold weather, and provide good nutrition in an easily assimilated form.

Most experts agree that insufficient B vitamins, especially B_6, can contribute to the symptoms of morning sickness. Pregnant women are often deficient in Vitamin B$_6$. The increased stress on the body as it adapts to pregnancy depletes the B vitamins quickly. Because they are water-soluble, the B vitamins do not store readily in the system, and sufficient supplies must continuously be made available. A pregnant woman's diet should contain foods rich in B vitamins. Nutritional yeast, yogurt, bee pollen, spirulina, wheat germ, whole grains, egg yolk, cabbage, and organ meats are particularly valuable at this time. (Use only organically raised meat to eliminate the possibility of consuming synthetic hormones.) A B-vitamin supplement may also be necessary during the first trimester of pregnancy to avoid or lessen morning sickness.

Pregnant women are also frequently deficient in hydrochloric acid, especially in the early stages of pregnancy. Some women have found relief from morning sickness by taking a supplement called Betaine HCl, which is hydrochloric acid in tablet form. If you experience bloating and/or queasiness after eating, especially after eating protein foods, and experience a craving for sour foods (pickles) it may indicate a deficiency of hydrochloric acid. Later in pregnancy (the last trimester), digestive discomfort is generally not caused by a lack of digestive acids, but by an overproduction of them, leading to heartburn. (See suggestions for dealing with heartburn on page 185.) A suggested dose is one to four tablets of HCl with each meal. Begin with one tablet. If you experience any discomfort, discontinue taking it.

For those days when nothing seems to stay down, make a broth containing equal parts barley and whole oats. When the broth has cooked sufficiently, strain out the grains and add a little slippery elm powder. Slippery elm is difficult to mix, so blend it in the blender for a smooth consistency. Though bland, this mixture is both soothing and nourishing. The flavor can be enhanced by adding miso, tamari (a high-quality soy sauce) or other soup-seasoning mix. The mucilaginous nature of this mixture is also soothing to the intestines and will reduce any inflammation or irritation caused by digestive disturbances. You may also try eating yogurt or oatmeal and kefir, easily digested and highly nourishing foods that are soothing to the intestinal tract.

A hot water bottle can be a comforting remedy during bouts of extreme nausea. Cuddle up in bed with a hot water bottle on your agitated tummy, a cup of Ginger/Peppermint Tea (see page 184), a box of crackers, and a good book. Two great books to read while you're pregnant are *Nature's Children* by Juliette de Bairacli Levy, and *The Wise Women's Herbal for the Childbearing Years* by Susun Weed.

Herbal Remedies for Morning Sickness

WILD YAM COMPOUND FOR MORNING SICKNESS

2 parts wild yam root   ¼ part ginger root
1 part dandelion root   ½ part vitex (chaste berry)

To Make:
Prepare a tincture (see page 66 for instructions) and take one-fourth teaspoon three times daily. During acute episodes of morning sickness, this formula may be taken frequently throughout the day.

Ginger root has been an old-time favorite for nausea, morning sickness, and motion sickness. It is delicious made with honey and fresh lemon juice.

GINGER ROOT TEA

1–2 teaspoons fresh ginger root
Honey and lemon

To Make:
Grate from a fresh root and simmer for a few minutes. Add honey and lemon to taste. If the weather is hot, ginger root tea can be served at room temperature. Do not serve it cold, as cold liquids are irritating to the system and will further agitate nausea. For extreme cases of nausea, ginger root powder can be encapsulated and taken throughout the day.

GINGER/PEPPERMINT TEA

1–2 teaspoons fresh ginger root
1 teaspoon peppermint

To Make:
Follow instructions for making Ginger Root Tea. After the ginger root has simmered for a few minutes, remove from the heat and add one teaspoon of peppermint per cup of tea. Cover and let mixture infuse for ten minutes. Strain. Sweeten with honey if desired.

PEACH LEAF TEA

1 part red raspberry leaf
1 part peach leaf

2 parts peppermint leaf
¼ part ginger root (grated)

To Make:
Use four to six tablespoons of the herb mixture per quart of water. Add herbs to cold water and over a low heat, bring to a simmer. Remove from heat immediately and infuse for twenty minutes, keeping pot covered. Strain.

The following formula was shared by a student of mine who had several months of intense morning sickness. She said this was the only preparation that brought relief.

BANCHA COMBO

1–2 teaspoons Bancha tea
¼ teaspoon umboshi plum paste

1 teaspoon tamari (a high-quality soy sauce)
A pinch of fresh ginger

To Make:

Simmer one minute, let cool, and sip slowly. Umboshi plum paste is specific for nausea and upset stomach. All of these ingredients are found in natural food stores.

Heartburn

Heartburn is another side effect of pregnancy. For the majority of pregnant women, it is not a big problem, though it may make eating unpleasant. For some, it is a major cause of distress. Heartburn usually occurs in the later weeks of pregnancy and is caused by overproduction of digestive acids, by relaxed or stressed stomach muscles, or by nervous tension. The remedies are simple. Eat small, frequent meals. Avoid acid-forming foods. Among these are foods high in sugar (all sugars, including natural sugars, are acidic to the system), cheese, citrus fruits (except for lemons and grapefruit, which are alkalizing to the system), and processed wheat. Eat slowly and chew foods well. Avoid liquids with meals. Yogurt, kefir, and warm milk with cinnamon are helpful, tasty remedies for heartburn when it is caused by overproduction of digestive acids.

Herbal Remedies for Heartburn

Papaya tablets and papaya leaf tea have proven very helpful. But the most effective way to take this remedy—and the best tasting—is to eat fresh papaya. (That may entail a trip to Hawaii or another tropical paradise, which is highly recommended for morning sickness as well as any other of the maladies of pregnancy.) Mucilaginous herbs such as slippery elm and marshmallow root are also very soothing to the intestines and help pacify heartburn. Mix one tablespoon of slippery elm powder in a cup of warm milk and flavor with honey and cinnamon for a soothing, tasty remedy.

Other digestive herbs that help with heartburn are fennel seeds, anise seeds, cumin seeds, and dill seeds. An old-fashioned remedy for digestive disturbances like heartburn was to combine these seeds in a tasty combination and chew them before and after meals.

TEA FOR HEARTBURN

2 parts anise seed
2 parts fennel seed
3 parts peppermint

1 part cinnamon
⅛ part lavender

To Make:

Use four to six tablespoons of herb mixture per quart of water. Add herbs to cold water and slowly bring to the simmering point over low heat, keeping pot covered. Immediately remove from heat and infuse for twenty minutes. Strain. Drink in small amounts throughout the day.

Fatigue

Many expectant mothers experience a sudden and overwhelming need to go into hibernation around the second month of pregnancy. While it's true that the body may need more rest now and added time for contemplation and introspection, there are things one can do to lessen the feelings of fatigue. Often the exhausted feeling originates in poor dietary habits. The growing baby has a tremendous need for nourishment. If mom's diet doesn't supply the nourishment the baby demands, then the mother's own body will, leaving her feeling drained and tired. A lack of B vitamins and/or a lack of iron (which can lead to anemia) may also cause fatigue.

Include a tonic tea like Pregnancy Tea (see page 180) or Iron-Plus-Calcium Tincture (see page 180) in your daily diet. The herbs in these teas provide a rich supply of vitamins and minerals. Alfalfa is loaded with vitamins A, D, E, and K, eight digestive enzymes, and numerous trace minerals. Nettle is so rich in biochelated iron, calcium, and protein—as well as a host of other important nutrients—that it is virtually a pregnancy tonic by itself. Red raspberry leaf, considered "the herb supreme for pregnancy," is the all-time favorite herb for pregnant women. First mentioned in Pliny's herbal of the 1500s, it has been used almost universally for centuries to soothe nausea, prevent miscarriage, ease labor pains, and build up a healthy milk supply. Its impressive array of vitamins and minerals make it a great all-round pregnancy tea.

A lack of iron is often a contributing factor in fatigue during pregnancy. Include a good daily iron tonic, such as liquid Floradix Herbs with Iron or NatureWorks Herbal iron, or make your own, using the recipe on page 62. Liquid iron, made from organic plants, is the best form in which to take this supplement. Iron from organic sources and from biochelated plants is more easily transformed into a usable form in the human body than is iron from tablets. Be certain your diet is high in such naturally iron-rich foods as molasses, egg yolk, dark-green leafy vegetables, beets, beet greens, and iron-rich herbs. (Organ meats also are high in iron. But use only organically raised meat. Nonorganically raised animals contain high concentrations of chemicals, growth hormones, and pesticides, and are not recommended.)

Herbal Remedies for Fatigue

❦ Take one to two tablespoons of spirulina daily.

❦ Take Floradix or a similar organic iron/mineral formula daily. (See instructions for making your own on page 62). If you prefer iron tablets, be certain they are biochelated so that your body can utilize them efficiently. The container will clearly state if they are biochelated.

❦ Take one to two teaspoons of bee pollen daily. (Some people may be allergic to bee pollen. See caution on page 213.)

❦ If it's the season of wild greens and fresh garden vegetables, make a daily green drink by blending fresh wild greens in the blender with tomato or pineapple juice. Add spirulina and nutritional yeast.

❦ Eat seaweeds daily in soups, salads, or as a between-meal snack. Powdered seaweeds like kelp can also be added to juice or other food.

❦ Take the time to rest and relax. Don't ignore the need for extra sleep. Your psyche may need some extra time to prepare for this life-changing event.

❦ Take the following tea formula daily. It provides many of the vitamins and minerals needed during pregnancy and will help reduce or eliminate the feelings of fatigue.

UPLIFTING TEA

2 parts raspberry leaf
2 parts nettle leaf
4 parts peppermint

1 part alfalfa
1 part squaw vine
¼ part ginger root, grated

To Make:

Use four to six tablespoons of herb mixture per quart of water. Add herbs to cold water and bring to a simmer over low heat, keeping pot covered. Immediately remove from the stove and allow to infuse for twenty minutes. Strain. Drink three to four cups daily.

❦ Take the following tea formula frequently throughout the day. It will taste bitter, but it is very effective in restoring energy.

HIGH-IRON TEA

1 part yellow dock root
1 part nettle leaf

1 part raspberry leaf

To Make:

Brew this mixture extra strong by infusing two tablespoons of the mixture per cup of water and allowing it to steep overnight. Take by the tablespoon every hour or two throughout the day.

Anemia and Iron Deficiency

Anemia has long been a concern of obstetricians and has often been blamed as the primary cause of fatigue and low energy during pregnancy. (I often wonder whether the tremendous physiological and hormonal changes going on during pregnancy are the root of our need to rest and contemplate and if, perhaps, the correct thing to do would be to follow those impulses.) It used to be routine for pregnant women to be prescribed iron tablets for iron-poor blood. Though constipation and upset stomachs often resulted and the blood count often didn't rise very much, iron tablets were routinely prescribed throughout pregnancy. I myself remember having iron tablets prescribed when I was pregnant with my son. Fortunately, after a few days of constipation and upset stomach, I decided that this wasn't the way I wanted to get iron into my body and discontinued the iron tablets.

Amazingly, there is startling new evidence that indicates that iron deficiencies are not quite what they were thought to be and that iron supplementation may not be as necessary as previously believed. In fact, inorganic iron supplements are coming under severe attack as the potential cause of many health problems. Nutritional research journals are full of interesting new facts and studies about the side effects of iron tablets. Though iron is a main component of hemoglobin and is essential to the health of the fetus and mother, a moderately low iron count may be part of the natural physiological changes the body undergoes during pregnancy and not a cause for alarm at all. During pregnancy, blood volume increases dramatically; lower hemoglobin levels may be a reflection of increased blood volume.

Dr. Andrew Weil states in his book *Natural Health, Natural Medicine,* "Unless you are a menstruating woman or have had a significant blood loss, you should *never* [his emphasis] take supplemental iron except on orders from a physician after appropriate blood tests have documented iron deficiency anemia. Not only can excess iron accumulate in the body to toxic levels, it may also interfere with immunity and promote cancer." On the same subject, Susun Weed writes in her book *Wise Woman Herbal for the Childbearing Years,* "It is possible that many diagnoses of iron deficiency anemia during pregnancy are a result of misinterpretation of the body's natural physiological changes while pregnant, and that lower hemoglobin levels, especially during the second trimester when the blood volume increases sharply, are normal."

No one questions that iron is an important mineral and is necessary during pregnancy. However, the "how much" and "in what form" are in question. A major constituent of hemoglobin, iron is indispensable in the oxygenation of cells. During pregnancy, extra iron must be available for both the mother and infant. The mother needs extra reserves of iron during childbirth, while the child must store sufficient quantities in its liver to be used during its first months of life after the womb.

Iron is readily found in dark-green leafy vegetables and in dark-red vegetables such as red chard, beets, and red cabbage. It is found abundantly in molasses, dried fruit (primarily black mission figs), cherries, prunes, and apricots. Sea vegetables are high in iron and should be included often in the diet; try mild-tasting seaweeds like dulse and hiziki. Wheat germ, brewer's yeast and fresh seeds and nuts are excellent sources of iron. Egg yolks also are high in iron, as are all organ meats (which are safe as long as they come from organically fed animals). There are many herbs rich in organic iron: nettle, rose hips, watercress, yellow dock root, burdock root, parsley, and horsetail.

Without the presence of calcium, protein, copper, cobalt, and other trace minerals, iron cannot be absorbed. Iron is fairly useless in tablet form. For the most efficient absorption of iron, it should be taken in a naturally biochelated form, the form that nature provides. If assimilation of iron is poor, and iron deficiency results, use a good herbal liver tonic to stimulate digestion and absorption. If necessary, supplement the diet with natural iron supplements such as Iron-Plus-Calcium Tincture (page 180) or spirulina. You can also take Floradix Herbs with Iron or NatureWorks Herbal Iron, liquid iron supplements made from wildcrafted and organic herbs and available in natural food stores. Finally, try to cook in cast-iron pots as much as possible. Though an old fashioned remedy, cooking foods in cast-iron pots provide the system with an extra boost of iron.

Symptoms of iron deficiency are very obvious; they are probably better signals of anemia during pregnancy than hemoglobin tests are. Shortness of breath, fatigue, weakness, heart palpitations, pallor, and breathlessness are all common signals and alert one that reserves of iron are low.

Water Retention

Water retention (edema) is another commonly experienced discomfort associated with pregnancy and usually begins to occur during the second and third trimesters. Some water retention is normal and is to be expected. Pregnancy hormones, mainly estrogens, cause connective tissue throughout the body to swell and retain extra fluid which serves as a protective device for the mother and child. However, excess edema, aside from being very uncomfortable, is a sign of stressed, overburdened kidneys. This can be due as much to emotional stress as to physical imbalance. It is essential during pregnancy and while nursing to drink sufficient water. My midwife friends recommended up to twelve cups daily! This large quantity of water does not cause the kidneys to overwork. Quite the contrary; it enables the kidneys to function better.

If you are suffering from edema, it's helpful to drink mild herbal diuretics that gently stimulate the kidneys to perform more proficiently. Dandelion greens, chickweed, cleaver, and nettle are very beneficial as mild, nonirritating diuretics. If a stronger diuretic is needed, add uva ursi to the formula. Herbal diuretics are amazingly effective and will correct most cases of edema.

Herbal Remedies for Water Retention

❧ Dandelion greens alone will often create the proper water balance the body needs. They are high in potassium and won't (unlike synthetic diuretics) cause a deficiency of that mineral. Drink several cups a day of dandelion green leaf tea and/or mix it with other herbs. For instructions on making dandelion leaf tea, follow instruction for making tea on page 47.

❧ Eat plenty of steamed burdock root and/or drink it as tea. The roots of burdock and dandelion blend well together and an effective tea can be made by combining them.

❧ Eliminate the intake of salt. Do not use table salt at all during pregnancy and eliminate snack foods such as chips, pretzels, crackers, nuts, and salted popcorn.

❧ Either of the following two formulas can be drunk daily to tone the kidneys and eliminate excess water.

DANDY LION TEA

2 parts dandelion leaf   1 part uva ursi
2 parts chickweed   3 parts nettle

To Make:

Use four to six tablespoons of herb mixture per quart of water. Add herbs to cold water and bring to a simmer over low heat. Keeping pot covered, remove from stove and infuse for twenty minutes. Strain.

DANDY ROOT TEA

2 parts dandelion root   1 part marshmallow root
2 parts burdock root

To Make:

Use three to four tablespoons of herb mixture per quart of water. Add herbs to cold water and bring to a low boil. Simmer fifteen minutes. Remove from heat and strain immediately.

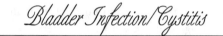

Bladder Infection/Cystitis

Many women experience cystitis at least once during pregnancy. The blood volume increases up to 50 percent during pregnancy, causing the kidneys to work double time. In addition, pressure placed on the kidneys by an ever-expanding womb causes further stress. The result is often a raging bladder infection.

Bladder infections are easy to detect. A frequent need to urinate, painful and/or incomplete urination, and a burning sensation during urination are the obvious signs. Antibiotics, the usual medication for cystitis, are not recommended during pregnancy. Most bladder infections are easily correctable with natural remedies if treatment is begun early.

Herbal Remedies for Cystitis

❧ The most widely known and accepted treatment is cranberry juice. It is best to use unsweetened cranberry juice, which is easily obtained at natural food stores. If unsweetened cranberry juice is not available, you can make your own juice by blending frozen cranberries with fresh water. Though unsweetened cranberry juice is the remedy of choice, I have found that even commercial brands will work. In order to be effective, several glasses of cranberry juice must be consumed daily.

❧ Avoid sugar. Sugar will feed the bacteria in the bladder that causes the infection and contributes to the continuing growth of the infection.

❧ The following herbal formula is a very effective treatment for cystitis.

TEA FOR CYSTITIS

1 part nettle   2 parts corn silk (the golden tassel from
1 part dandelion greens   garden corn)
1 part pipsissewa   2 parts uva ursi

To Make:

Prepare an infusion, following directions on page 47. Drink one fourth cup every half hour throughout the day.

❦ Some women find it helpful to take a double dose of acidophilus (double the amount recommended on the container) to help cure cystitis. Also, large doses of vitamin C— up to 2000 milligrams twice daily—help eliminate infection by restoring the proper acidity of the bladder.

Constipation

Constipation is often a problem during the later months of pregnancy. In part this is due to the relaxing effect of hormones on the smooth muscles. Women also tend to move and exercise less as they continue to grow. A woman's system seems to slow down as the process of forming and developing a new life is accelerated. Simple measures are often all that are needed to correct constipation. It is important to drink plenty of water, to continue to exercise, and to eat a diet rich in fiber and nutrients.

If constipation occurs, avoid synthetic laxatives. They are harsh and irritating to the colon and, though they may cause successful elimination of the bowels, they will not correct the underlying problem. In addition to avoiding synthetic laxatives, do not use harsh herbal laxatives. Their purgative effect will leave the body quite exhausted and cause further stress to the colon. Also, many laxatives are not recommended during pregnancy because they can cause premature labor.

Herbal Remedies for Constipation

❦ Eliminate starch and refined foods from the diet and replace with foods high in fiber and bulk. Eat salads two or three times a day. Fresh and dried fruits, such as apricots, prunes and grapes, should be included daily. These foods, aside from being good for the colon, are excellent during pregnancy in general. Include foods that are high in mucilaginous material, such as oats, barley, slippery elm, psyllium seeds, and marshmallow root. These herbs are soothing to the mucus membrane lining of the lower intestines and colon. They also swell up with water, providing a lubricating bulk that aids in elimination.

❦ Nonstressful exercise, especially toward the end of pregnancy, is one of the most important remedies for constipation. It also helps the expectant mother avoid many other problems associated with pregnancy and childbirth. The peristaltic action of the lower bowel is stimulated by movement. A good bowel movement often follows a long walk, yoga exercises, or other forms of exercise. You may find that a few simple changes, such as eating a more wholesome diet and exercising more frequently, are all that is necessary to get those lazy, resistent bowels moving.

❦ Herbs to add to the diet on a daily basis for constipation include: carob powder, slippery elm, flax seed, psyllium seeds, licorice root, and aloe vera. These herbs can be incorporated into cereals and blender drinks, mixed in with different foods, or rolled into candy balls. Sometimes a pinch of cayenne added to food and/or warm lemon water also proves helpful in treating constipation.

MILD LAXATIVE JUICE

1 cup pineapple juice

¼ cup aloe vera juice

½ cup grape juice

To Make:

Blend ingredients in a blender.

MILD LAXATIVE BLENDER DRINK

2 cups pineapple juice

¼ cup aloe vera juice

½ cup yogurt

1 tablespoon slippery elm powder

½ banana

1 tablespoon psyllium seed husks

To Make:

Place all ingredients in a blender and blend until smooth.

LIVER CLEANSING TEA FOR CONSTIPATION

3 parts dandelion root

1 part licorice root

1 part yellow dock root

1 part flax seed

2 parts burdock root

⅛ part senna pods

2 parts slippery elm bark

⅛ part turkey rhubarb root

To Make:

Use two teaspoons of herb mixture to two cups of water. Add herbs to cold water and bring to a low simmer over low heat. Simmer gently for ten minutes. Remove from heat and infuse for twenty minutes. Drink one cup in the morning and one cup in the evening.

LAXATIVE TEA WHEN NOTHING ELSE WORKS

1 part slippery elm

⅛ part cinnamon bark

1 part flax seed

⅛ part senna pod (increase senna

4 parts fennel seed

   if necessary)

2 parts licorice root

To Make:

Add two teaspoons of herb mixture to two cups of cold water and bring to a slow simmer over low heat. Simmer gently for ten minutes. Remove from heat and infuse, keeping pot covered, for twenty minutes. Strain. Drink one cup in the morning and one cup in the evening. Senna is the active laxative herb in this formula; increase it if necessary.

During the last months of pregnancy, the circulatory system is doing double duty and the veins often suffer because of it. The added pressure of weight gain and an increase in blood volume put tremendous pressure on the veins, especially those that carry blood from the legs to the heart. The high levels of progesterone produced during pregnancy can further complicate the situation by causing relaxation of the smooth muscles and a decrease in muscle activity. Since contracting muscle activity is the primary force used to pump blood through the veins and back to the heart, decreased activity can cause stagnation and a pooling of blood in the lower extremities. Surface veins and capillaries, with their relatively weak walls, may become swollen, twisted, and enlarged.

A lack of nutritional elements in the diet, especially vitamin C, rutin, and other bioflavonoids, combined with the extra stress on the circulatory system, can cause the fragile capillaries to break. A tendency toward varicose veins and hemorrhoids may also be inherited. If you bruise easily or have had trouble with varicose veins and/or hemorrhoids in the past, practice preventative medicine at the onset of pregnancy. Wear support hose, avoid standing for long periods of time, and include those foods that aid in building and repairing the blood veins in your diet.

I have seen cases of serious varicose veins in pregnant women that could have been completely avoided if only the proper precautions had been followed. A lovely young friend of mine named Ann was a case in point. When Ann got pregnant, she was already suffering from an advanced case of "superwoman syndrome." Married to a loving but not particularly warm man, she was very thin and starving for warmth and affection. One had the sense that she carried the weight of the world on her shoulders. She was delighted by her pregnancy, but it only seemed to increase her burdens.

Early in her pregnancy the veins in Ann's legs began to distend. I believe that even then, had she followed the advice offered by her friends, she would not have had to suffer as she did. As it was, her aching legs did not slow her down; she remained thin, anxious, and overworked throughout most of her pregnancy. But the veins began to protrude in purple highways up and down her legs, making even walking difficult. Finally, during the last trimester of her pregnancy, there was no recourse but to retire to bed. I think in many ways it was the best thing that could have happened to her. At last she could rest, be waited on, and cared for.

Ann consulted a holistic physician, who recommended many of the suggestions that follow. In her two ensuing pregnancies, she followed the preventive measures advised by her doctor, and, though her legs troubled her somewhat, the problem with her veins was never as severe again.

Herbal Remedies for Varicose Veins

❦ Diet is essential in the prevention and treatment of varicose veins. Vitamin C and related bioflavonoids strengthen the capillaries and are especially beneficial for healing them if they are injured. Foods high in vitamin C and bioflavonoids include buckwheat, nettles, rose hips, oranges, lemons, grapefruit, peppers, whole grains, hibiscus flowers, and the white rinds of organically grown citrus fruits.

❧ The allium family, which includes garlic, onion, chives, and leeks, helps maintain elasticity in the veins and capillaries. These foods are very helpful during pregnancy to prevent varicose veins.

❧ Lecithin, vitamin E, and rutin supplements are also recommended during pregnancy to prevent and repair varicose veins.

❧ The following astringent liniment is very helpful for varicose veins. Rub the liniment up the legs toward the heart two to three times a day, using a soft cotton cloth. This is invigorating and healing for the injured veins. Always rub toward the heart.

ASTRINGENT LINIMENT

1 part yarrow
1 part shepherd's purse
1 part calendula
¼ part cayenne

To Make:

Cover the herbs with warmed vinegar and/or witch hazel extract (available at pharmacies) and let the mixture sit for two to three weeks. Strain and rebottle. This liniment will last indefinitely and may also be used as an astringent for muscular pains and aches.

❧ To ease the pressure on the veins, spend some time every day with your legs slightly elevated. While sleeping and whenever sitting, elevate your legs with pillows. This allows the blood to flow smoothly and freely to the heart and relieves pressure on the veins.

❧ It may be necessary to wear support hose and/or Ace bandages to lend support to the veins during pregnancy. Don't neglect to do so if necessary, and don't wait until the veins become congested and swollen. Prevention is the key. Once the delicate capillaries and surface veins become distended, their elasticity is very difficult to restore.

❧ Deep breathing as well as muscular contractions can help ensure a healthy return of blood to the heart. Breathe deeply. You can feel the blood surging into the chest region. If circulation is a problem and varicosities result, do regular deep breathing exercises.

❧ Butcher's broom *(Ruscus acluteatus)* has a great reputation as an antiinflammatory for the vascular system. It promotes circulation from the lower extremities and has been used successfully as both a preventive and a curative for varicose veins. Butcher's broom may be difficult to locate; you may have to get a natural food or herb store to order it for you. Butcher's broom comes in the form of capsules, tea, and tincture.

Hemorrhoids

Many of the suggestions listed above are also effective in treating hemorrhoids. Hemorrhoids, after all, are just another form of varicose veins. In addition to the suggestions above and below, do Kegel exercises daily. These not only help prevent hemorrhoids, but also help heal them once they've formed. (See page 221 for instructions on how to do Kegels.)

Herbal Remedies for Hemorrhoids

❦ One of the most effective salves I know of for hemorrhoids is the comfrey/St. John's wort salve listed on page 56. Keep it in the refrigerator (the cold temperature helps constrict the veins) and apply it two or three times daily.

❦ Cold compresses also constrict the blood vessels and will aid in disengorging the hemorrhoidal veins. The witch hazel extract available in most pharmacies makes an excellent compress for constricting and shrinking the veins. It is best if kept in the refrigerator. Moisten cotton cloths with the extract and apply as a compress. It may feel a bit shocking to apply a cold compress to the highly sensitive anal area, but cold compresses constrict enlarged and engorged blood vessels and are effective in healing hemorrhoids.

❦ If the hemorrhoids are quite enlarged and painful, apply a comfrey/St. John's wort poultice to the area and leave on for one hour. Use fresh or dried herbs and make into a paste with cold water. Wrap the herbs in cheesecloth or muslin and apply directly to the hemorrhoids. Sit in a comfortable chair and read a good book while the poultice does it work.

❦ Another poultice I've found to be quite helpful for hemorrhoids is green clay. Mix the clay with water and/or witch hazel extract into a paste and apply directly to the hemorrhoids. Leave the poultice on until it is completely dry. Though a bit messy, it works. After all, dealing with a bit of flaky green clay is a whole lot better than having sore and swollen veins. To remove the clay poultice, soak in the tub or take a shower.

Stretch Marks

Stretch marks are the maps of our children's womb life etched permanently in the soft folds of our skin. Nevertheless, no one really wants to get stretch marks, and the best way to avoid them is by taking steps to prevent them. As with any scar tissue, once the stretch marks are formed, they are a permanent part of the landscape of our body. Time may erase the depths of the lines, but however faint, they will remain a part of our living history.

To prevent stretch marks it is necessary to keep the skin elastic. During pregnancy the skin has to do a tremendous amount of stretching. If it has natural elasticity and is kept well lubricated and cared for throughout pregnancy, it can often make that stretch with no signs of wear. The best time to begin "belly care" is at the very beginning of pregnancy or, even better, prior to conception.

Herbal Remedies for Stretch Marks

❦ Massage a rich lubricating oil over the belly and breasts daily. Take time to enjoy the blossoming of the life within and to feel the fullness of your belly unfolding. Drinking lots of water and other liquids is essential to the skin's elasticity and will contribute to its pliability. Take 200 to 400 I.U. of Vitamin E daily. (If suffering from high blood pressure, heart disease, or diabetes, take only 50 I.U.). Also, mix vitamin E oil into your massage oil or cream base and massage in daily.

❦ Any good rich natural oil can be used for massage, but my favorites for pregnant bellies are cocoa butter and coconut oil mixed with sweet-scented essential oils. Vitamin E oil should be mixed in, using 20,000 units per cup of oil. The following massage oil is excellent and an all-time favorite of mine. Thick, rich, and luxurious, it is a pleasure to massage it daily over the miraculously expanding womb.

BELLY OIL

½ cup cocoa butter	20,000 I.U. vitamin E oil
½ cup coconut oil	2 teaspoons grated beeswax
¼ cup apricot, almond, or grape seed oil	1 teaspoon lanolin

To Make:

Melt all ingredients together. You may wish to scent the mixture with your favorite essential oil, but I love the rich chocolaty smell as is. Rub this rich oil over the belly and breasts two or three times daily to keep the skin supple and help eliminate stretch marks. This is the richest, most emollient oil I know to use as a lubricant for the expanding belly.

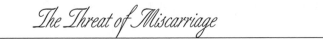

The Threat of Miscarriage

The threat of miscarriage is a very serious matter. You will want to consult your midwife and/or physician right away if you experience any unusual symptoms. Occasionally miscarriage is the body's natural response to certain conditions and no intervention, whether herbal or medical, can or should oppose the body's purpose. However, when miscarriage is threatened because of stress, inadequate diet, hormonal imbalance, trauma, or weak uterine muscles, herbs can provide the extra nourishment and strength needed to correct the imbalanced flow of energy. *Bed rest and removal of the stress factors supersede everything.* Follow with herb teas and gentle strengthening meals. Call a friend to help out with meals and housework. One of the worst things you can do is to try to get back on your feet and take control. Rest and relax. Let others do for you.

If possible, your home room should be light and airy, with fresh air circulating. Open the curtains and windows if the weather permits. Have sprigs of fresh herbs such as lavender and lemon balm, if available, to hold and press, and don't overlook a bouquet of fresh flowers placed by your bedside. The aroma from the fresh plants gives courage to the soul. This is generally a time of emotional crisis, and friends should make it as comfortable and life-sustaining as possible for the expectant mother, father, and infant.

Many women have early miscarriages and never suspect it. It is estimated that upwards to forty percent of all pregnancies are terminated in the very early stages and are mistaken for heavy or late menstrual cycles. Excess bleeding, cramps, and clotting associated with irregular or heavy menstrual cycles are frequently spontaneous miscarriages. If you are trying to conceive but having difficulty and at the same time experiencing symptoms of early pregnancy—swollen breasts and delayed menstruation, followed by a heavy period—it may be that you are pregnant. If the miscarriage happens within the early weeks, low progesterone levels may be at fault. Progesterone is the hormone necessary for maintenance of pregnancy. Check with your doctor, who can give you tests to determine if a low progesterone level is the problem. However, it is *not* recommended to take synthetic progesterone. Long-term results have not been adequately studied and the tests that have been done indicate that synthetic progesterone therapy may cause birth defects in children. We do not want to repeat the mistake of the infamous synthetic estrogen (DES) that was used to prevent miscarriages and produced daughters and sons with DES-related abnormalities.

Wild yam root is specifically recommended as a progesterone-stimulating herb. Many other herbs, such as chaste berry, help regulate and normalize hormones and can be safely used.

Herbal Remedies to Prevent Miscarriage

Vitamin E, in doses up to 600 I.U. per day (50 I.U. if you have high blood pressure, heart disease, or diabetes) can help prevent miscarriage. The following herbal formulas have also proved helpful in preventing miscarriage.

TINCTURE FOR PREVENTION OF MISCARRIAGE

3 parts cramp bark
1 part black haw
1 part false unicorn root

To Make:

It is wise to make this formula into a tincture at the beginning of pregnancy. (See page 66 for directions for making tinctures.) If for some reason miscarriage does threaten, you will have an excellent remedy prepared. Add one-half teaspoon of the tincture to one-fourth cup warm water or tea and drink every half hour. It may be taken as a tea also.

TEA FOR PREVENTION OF MISCARRIAGE

2 parts wild yam root
1 part black haw
1 part cramp bark

To Make:

Use four to six tablespoons of herb mixture per quart of water. Add herbs to cold water and bring to a slow simmer over low heat. Simmer gently for twenty minutes, keeping pot tightly covered. Take one-fourth cup every half hour until symptoms cease. Use the tea in conjunction with the tincture above. Decrease the dosage of tea as symptoms subside.

TEA TO ARREST SPOT BLEEDING

2 parts shepherd's purse
1 part raspberry leaf
2 parts nettle leaf

To Make:

See instructions on making infusions on page 47. If you start to bleed during pregnancy, immediately begin to drink the tea, one-fourth cup at a time, every half hour until bleeding subsides. *Notify your midwife and/or physician.*

TINCTURE TO STOP BLEEDING

1 part fresh shepherd's purse
1 part fresh yarrow flowers and leaves

To Make:

See page 66 for instructions on making tinctures. Take one-fourth teaspoon of the tincture every half hour. Use in conjunction with Laxative Tea When Nothing Else Works. The tincture may be diluted in the tea. *Notify your midwife and/or physician.*

TEA FOR NERVOUS STRESS

2 parts chamomile
3 parts lemon balm
1 part squaw vine
1 part skullcap
⅛ part valerian

To Make:

Use four to six tablespoons of herb mixture per quart of tea. Add herbs to cold water and bring to a slow simmer over low heat. Immediately remove from stove. Keeping pot tightly covered, infuse for twenty minutes. Strain. Drink one-fourth cup every hour. Use in conjunction with Belly Oil.

The Final Countdown and Postpartum

The last few weeks before your due date are an excellent time to prepare your body for the actual birthing process. Do an inventory of your herbs and herbal remedies and stock anything you may need for birthing and immediately afterward. Along with herbal remedies and teas, it's nice to include in your "birthing kit" some of the herbs women have traditionally used in the birthing room. Sprigs of lavender, lemon balm, and rosemary have historically been used to bring courage to laboring women. Especially in a hospital birthing room, fresh herbs and bouquets of flowers add light and vitality. I used to make mobiles of natural things—beautiful pieces of driftwood, shells, sprigs of dried herbs and flowers—to hang in the birthing room. It brought a touch of nature, beauty, and serenity to the sacred space of birth.

The herbs I recommend for labor and postnatal care are as follows:

Blue cohash is used in prolonged labor to help bring on and/or stimulate contractions.

Chamomile calms and relaxes a laboring woman.

Comfrey heals tears and injuries caused during birthing. It also strengthens muscles and tissue, and provides nutrients to rebuild the body. (For information on the comfrey controversy, see the entry for this herb in the Materia Medica.)

Fennel seed enriches and increases the flow of milk.

Lady's mantle (the herb of the alchemist—and what greater alchemy has just been performed?) restores life force and vitality following childbirth.

Nettle enriches the flow of milk and restores energy and vitality.

Pennyroyal leaf is used in prolonged labor to help bring on and/or stimulate contractions.

Raspberry leaf enriches milk flow, builds energy, restores muscle tone, and serves as an excellent overall strengthener.

Sage decreases the flow of milk (necessary if infection or complications arise).

Shepherd's purse arrests internal and external bleeding during childbirth.

Squaw vine restores vitality and strength following childbirth.

Yarrow arrests internal and external bleeding during childbirth.

When Labor Is Prolonged

Do not use teas to hasten labor simply because you are impatient. Each child has its own birthing rhythm and it should not be disturbed. Frequently, that rhythm does not correspond to the designated calendar birthing time (or the doctor's schedule), but unless the birth is very overdue there is generally no need to worry. The tea formulas are used only when a prolonged labor has become debilitating to the mother and/or child and when it is necessary, for health reasons, to manipulate the timing. Sometimes a warm bath made with chamomile and/or valerian is relaxing and soothing enough to hasten delivery. Herbal tinctures and teas can be used in conjunction with warm herbal baths to facilitate labor.

A special massage oil made of fresh grated ginger combined with valerian and lavender has proven useful when massaged over the back and stomach muscles. Make the oil ahead of time. Follow the directions for making herbal oils on page 50.

TINCTURE TO FACILITATE LABOR

1 part blue cohosh   3 parts pennyroyal leaf (not oil)
1 part black cohosh

For instructions on making tinctures, see page 66. Dilute one-half teaspoon of the tincture in one-fourth cup of warm water every thirty minutes, or as often as needed. The taste is somewhat unpleasant. You may wish to dilute the tincture in peppermint tea to camouflage the flavor.

Sometimes a shift in energy is all that's needed to encourage the birth. Years ago, on the land where the herb school was located, a friend wished to have her child in our tepee. Circular, white, and sacred, it was located next to the pond and seemed like a lovely place to give birth. Several weeks before her due date, she and her family settled in. Life in the tepee was good. But the weather in coastal California in the middle of the summer can get really hot. And in that tepee in the open sun-drenched meadow, with a belly stretching to give birth, my friend found it hot indeed.

When her birthing time came, the breeze stopped, the sun beat down hotter than ever, and it seemed as if everything—including her contractions—had come to a standstill. She'd start and then she'd stop. This went on for several days. Her frustration began to reflect the hot, still days of that California summer.

One afternoon when I stopped in to check on my friend, I was appalled at how thick and heavy the energy was in the tepee. Something needed to happen. The wind needed to blow, the trees to dance, the energy in the tepee to move. Instinctively, I began to sing to my friend. And then I began to dance. Luckily, there were a couple of other women in the tepee who joined in the singing, for my own voice is notoriously out of tune. The midwife present happened to be an accomplished belly dancer (the dance of birth) and she began to sway in a beautiful rhythm. It was really lovely and exotic. And, of course, very soon thereafter the wind began to blow and the energy to undulate in the tepee. Within hours, my friend gave birth to her fifth child. Today, on the small knoll beside the tepee, there's a lovely tall eucalyptus tree growing where the placenta was planted.

To Stabilize Blood Pressure

Low blood pressure can be due to dehydration and/or low blood sugar as well as to a loss of blood. Black cohash, linden flowers, hawthorne berries, and shepherd's purse will help stabilize blood pressure during labor. Be certain to drink sufficient fluids. It is good to have a birth attendant who watches and regulates the amount of fluid you are drinking. During the intensity and excitement of labor pains, one is often not aware of how much liquid one is consuming.

TEA FOR STABILIZING BLOOD PRESSURE

1 part black cohosh
1 part linden flowers
3 parts hawthorne berries

2 parts squaw vine
1 part shepherd's purse

How to Make:
Use four to six tablespoons of herb mixture per quart of water. Place herbs in cold water and bring to a slow simmer over low heat. Immediately remove from the stove and infuse for twenty minutes. Keep pot tightly covered. Strain. Drink one-fourth cup every half hour or as often as needed throughout labor.

In Cases of Heavy Bleeding or Hemorrhage

A doctor and/or midwife should always be consulted in cases of heavy bleeding or hemorrhage. The following suggestions are emergency measures only, and should be used when further medical assistance is being sought. Occasionally they succeed in slowing or stopping the bleeding, making more heroic measures unnecessary, but it is always wise to consult a health professional when heavy bleeding begins.

The following formula is a favorite of many midwives and is an integral part of their birth kits.

SHEPHERD'S PURSE/YARROW COMPOUND

1 part yarrow
1 part shepherd's purse

To Make:

Prepare a tincture (see page 66 for instructions) and drink at least one-half teaspoon diluted in warm water every half hour. If you make the recipe in tea form, drink one-half cup of it every half hour. For ease in administering, the tincture may be diluted in the tea.

Another excellent remedy for heavy bleeding is Raspberry/Nettle Tea (below). Both herbs are mild astringents and effective tonics.

RASPBERRY/NETTLE TEA

1 part raspberry leaf
1 part nettle

To Make:

Use four to six tablespoons of herb mixture per quart of water. Add herbs to cold water and bring to a simmer over low heat. Remove from the stove immediately. Infuse for twenty minutes. Strain and drink one-fourth cup of tea every half hour.

In cases of severe heavy bleeding, when nothing else seems to work, try taking one-fourth teaspoon cayenne powder every fifteen to twenty minutes. Dilute the cayenne in warm water to facilitate its going down. It will be hot, but it often works wonders. Because cayenne doesn't contract the uterus sufficiently to halt postpartum bleeding permenently, I recommend taking it with a tea made of a combination of raspberry, lady's mantle, and shepherd's purse.

To Heal Tears and Stitches

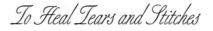

To help heal tears to the perineum, take comfrey sitz baths (see instructions, page 113) several times a day for at least five days. Drink a tea made of equal parts of comfrey and nettle for a week or two to help repair any internal damage. (See the Materia Medica for cautions regarding comfrey. If you do not wish to use comfrey, oat straw can be substituted.)

You may find it helpful to keep an atomizer containing comfrey tea with a little aloe vera gel in it next to the toilet. Before urinating, squirt a little of the tea over the stitches to keep the urine from stinging. (The tea should be made fresh every couple of days.) Comfrey salve is helpful too, though you should not apply it for the first day or two, as the stitches need time to dry.

To Encourage and Enrich Milk Flow

To ensure a healthy, rich flow of milk, drink at least three cups of the following formula every day.

3 parts fennel seed

½ part fenugreek seed

½ part blessed thistle leaf

¼ part hops

To Make:

Use four to six tablespoons of herb mixture per quart of water. Add herbs to cold water and bring to a simmer over low heat. Remove from the stove immediately and infuse for twenty minutes. Strain. Drink three to four cups daily. You may wish to adjust the amount of blessed thistle and hops you add to this tea. Both are *very bitter* herbs. This formula can also be made into a tincture. (See page 66 for directions on making a tincture.)

Another tea that helps increase the flow of milk is the following.

BLESSED THISTLE TEA

1 part blessed thistle

(also called our mother's milk thistle)

4 parts fennel seeds

2 parts nettle

2 parts raspberry leaf

To Make:

Use four to six tablespoons of herb mixture per quart of water. Add herbs to cold water and bring to a slow boil over low heat. Remove from heat and infuse for twenty minutes. Strain. Drink three to four cups daily.

To Decrease the Flow of Milk

A vibrant young mother came to visit me one day while I was working at the herb shop. She was having a very difficult time producing a sufficient flow of milk for her infant child. She was quite willing to try the herbal teas I suggested. After a few days she returned to say that in spite of regular use of the teas, her milk flow remained scanty. I was puzzled, as the herbs were generally quite helpful to women in her situation. Upon further questioning, she revealed to me that as part of a very conscious attempt to eat well, she was eating quantities of dark-green leafy vegetables. I asked her if she was including parsley in her diet. I had guessed correctly. She had read that parsley was an outstanding source of vitamins and minerals. Since it was plentiful, inexpensive, and tasty, she was eating fairly large amounts of it. At any other time, this would have been great, but parsley is one of the main herbs used to halt the flow of mother's milk. As soon as the young woman stopped eating parsley, her milk flow increased substantially.

Sage is the other herb used with excellent results to decrease or stop milk production. These herbs are especially useful when weaning your child, and during breast infections such as mastitis. However, you should avoid both sage and parsley if you do *not* wish to decrease your milk flow.

One of the best times to use your knowledge of herbs is the season immediately after pregnancy and childbirth. Herbs will aid in restoring your vitality and fill the depleted reservoir of strength that sometimes follows birth.

Drink plenty of mild herbal nervines. They will encourage nursing, help you adjust to the demands of the newborn, and generally calm and renew your system. Skullcap, lemon balm, valerian, lavender, motherwort, and chamomile are all excellent for calming the nervous system and inducing a state of peace in the hectic days following childbirth. For a good herbal nervine, see Gentle Relaxation Tea on page 180.

In your daily teas be sure to include herbs that provide concentrated nourishment, such as raspberry leaf, nettle, oat straw, alfalfa, seaweed, peppermint, and dandelion greens. Create several herb tea blends that satisfy your need for a beverage while providing food and nourishment for your miraculous body, which has just delivered a miracle. See Pregnancy Tea on page 180 for a good all-round tonic formula.

Don't neglect to drink herbs that lift the spirits. Herbs such as borage flowers, hawthorne berries and flowers, rose blossoms, chamomile, and lavender blossoms have long been used to celebrate life. You can formulate your own tasty and uplifting blends, mixing and blending the herbs into delicious, personalized formulas, or use the following formula.

JOY TEA

2 parts chamomile
3 parts lemon balm
1 part hawthorne berries and blossoms
2 parts hibiscus flowers
2 parts rose petals (from unsprayed bushes)
⅛ part lavender flowers
⅛ part cardamon pods, chopped

To Make:

Use four to six tablespoons of herbs per quart of water. Add herbs to cold water and place in direct sunshine. If winter, place in a south-facing sunny window. Let sit for several hours or overnight. Strain and enjoy. This lovely, exhilarating tea is best made with fresh herbs and flowers.

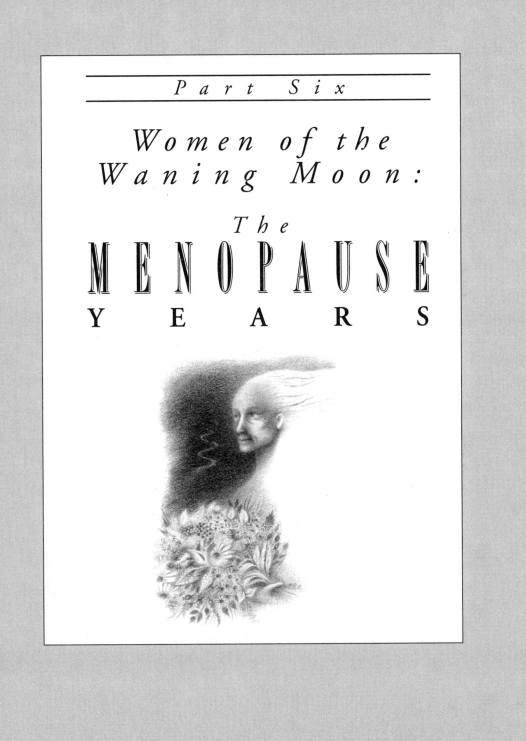

Part Six

Women of the Waning Moon:

The MENOPAUSE YEARS

A New Cycle of Life

There is no more creative force in the world than the menopausal woman with zest.

—Margaret Mead

As long as they think we're crazy, we're safe.
—Adele Dawson

Just as puberty awakened the creative flow and power of our menstrual cycle and marked our emergence as young women, so menopause marks the completion of that cycle and our entrance into the third major cycle of womanhood. Even though menopause may be a positive or neutral experience for many women, in our culture these powerful cyclic changes do not occur in a supportive or nourishing environment. Without the support and understanding of the society in which we live, much of what we experience becomes confusing, stressful, and painful.

In traditional cultures, the older woman was respected as the village elder. Trusted as the care-person or guide for the children of the tribe, she also served as teacher and wise woman. She was respected as an elder, and she held an honored place in her community. Even as recently as two generations ago, the older woman held a firmly rooted place in society. Our great-grandmothers were honored as useful members of society, and accorded special respect as their years advanced.

Though my grandmother's dying was long, a slow surrender to the tides of time, she occupied a revered and respected place at the family hearth until the day she died. And she was little affected by society's changing attitudes toward the older generation. My mother, now also a great-grandmother, has been little affected by society's attitudes toward the elderly. With her rounded body, silver-streaked hair, and skin etched with the tales of time, aging has brought her peace, a larger garden of wild flowers, and many lovely grandchildren. To her Taurean being, that spells ultimate contentment. Having just become a grandmother myself—to a beautiful baby boy—and having had the good influence of these two powerful elderly women in my life, I, too, am experiencing the grace and strength of this cycle of life.

Unfortunately, however, fewer and fewer women escape the contemptuous attitudes toward the elderly now common in our society. Our model of the older woman leaves much to be desired. In a culture where extreme emphasis is placed on youth, beauty, and sex, the older woman's place of honor has been usurped. The stereotype of the menopausal and postmenopausal woman is of someone "past her prime," someone who is unsexy, unproductive, and hard to live with. Fortunately, *none* of these stereotypes is true. It is time for us to stop supporting these myths and create a new mythology that speaks of the inner power of this stage of womanhood.

Even when physical "symptoms" are minimal, menopause is often still viewed as a negative time in a woman's life. In part this is because of lack of information or blatant misinformation. Even now, too few books deal with the subject in a positive or creative manner. What information is available is often neither enlightening nor particularly informative. Many of us are still entering this stage of our lives just as ignorant and ill-informed as when we entered puberty twenty-five years earlier. Remembering the awkward, often embarrassing introduction we had to our first moon cycles and the negative associations that still surround menstruation, it is hardly surprising that menopause, too, is surrounded with negative images and mystery. Given that menopause is more often associated with loss—of fertility, youth, and vitality—than with gain—of wisdom, contentment, and respect—is it any wonder few of us look forward to it? In our society, a man's getting older, grayer, and more wrinkly only makes him seem wiser and more distinguished. This is not so for the women in our society, who have allowed themselves to be valued for youthfulness, beauty, and sexuality only. It is hard to envision a way to age gracefully in the cultural atmosphere we have created for ourselves. Unlike the respect that men command as they age, our own transformation occurs in an entirely negative framework and continues crippling us with the biases of our culture. If we can change our self-image and attitudes, this moment in our lives can be an empowering, celebratory rite of passage as indeed it should be.

Many of the unpleasant aspects of menopause are not physical problems at all, but the emotional results of the transitional nature of these particular years of a woman's life. Life changes abruptly. The children have grown and are leaving home. Parents are reaching their later years and may be becoming more dependent. This is a time when relationships undergo major changes and often end abruptly. Careers may suddenly shift and change. We often find our innermost belief systems questioned and examined. Any one of these situations is enough to create emotional and physical havoc. Just when we thought we had all the answers and life was neatly tied in a package, it turns itself upside down. We are once again faced with the ongoing challenge of life and the great mystery that leads us into the exploration of self. Though these can all be positive changes, transition is, by its very nature difficult.

In the arrogance of my youth, I believed I would be unaffected by such changes. I looked forward to getting older and possessing the "wisdom of the old." I thought that people would take me more seriously, and be respectful of the great wisdom and experience I would have to offer. (My image of myself as an older, wiser woman was probably based, I now think, on my continuing to look and feel twenty years old!) But when I actually began to approach menopause, I realized how deeply affected I was by my culture's perception of youth and aging. Surprisingly, I found myself experiencing my society's images and feelings about menopause. Aware that my hair was silver-streaked, perplexed by energy that was clearly not as boundless as it used to be, feeling my body shape change, I was acutely conscious that there was a metamorphosis occurring in the deep inner recesses of my being. Life was slowing down for me on the outer levels of activity while accelerating on the inner, a gift, to be sure, if I chose to view it as such. The wise older woman, the "Crone" of ancient cultures, was visiting and instructing me. I could feel those powerful hormonal changes beginning to take place in my body as I prepared for menopause.

As I felt my energies shifting and menopause approaching, I experienced a great yearning to understand these cyclic changes. What better place to learn than from the women who were already experiencing the changes of menopause? Invited to speak at conferences, I suddenly shifted my focus to subjects aimed at the older women. Often I included workshops specifically for menopausal women. All this was designed, of course, to deepen and expand my own awareness. I could offer herbal formulas and remedies easily, for I had already developed a clientele of older women and knew the problems associated with menopause and the herbal therapies that were helpful. But what I wanted to understand was the inner workings of the heart, how the body accommodated the changes it was undergoing, how the mind influenced the rhythms of the physical self.

These workshops were conducted in the safety of a circle. The speaking stick was passed around. It always amazed me, placed in a circle of trust, how much we women could open and share. For many women this was their first opportunity to speak of their fears and anxieties about menopause. For others, it was the opportunity to share the power and excitement they felt. A theme I heard often in the circles I sat within was the sense of loss, of sadness about the passing of the menstrual cycle and the end of the fertile years. Interestingly, but not surprisingly, many women reported having had long, painful years of menstruation and/or having harbored resentment toward their menstrual cycles. After years of growth gained through the therapeutic process of living life, they had recently come to terms with their monthly cycles, and now, with hardly time to take a breath, it was time to change again.

The "symptoms" so many women my age begin to experience have been successfully reduced or eliminated by understanding this process called menopause. Though menopause does have physiological symptoms, these are not always uncomfortable or inevitable. In fact, the majority of women do not experience much discomfort at all. It is estimated that 10 percent of women experience no disagreeable symptoms and 80 percent experience symptoms but find them tolerable. Only 10 percent find them so disagreeable that they seek medication.

As a woman approaches menopause there is a period of great hormonal change that may last for several years. This change begins some years before menstruation ceases and menopause begins. The hormonal changes are marked by a gradual decrease in the cyclic release of estrogen and progesterone. Eventually, the ovaries stop producing a monthly egg and secrete a smaller supply of estrogen. At the same time there is a decline in the production of the hormone progesterone, which each month has been building up the lining of the uterus in preparation for a fertilized egg. This is a tremendous amount of physiological change to adjust to. It is only normal that its effects are felt not only physically but emotionally as well.

Many of the symptoms associated with menopause are similar to those of adrenal stress. It is interesting to note that the adrenal glands take over the biological function of the ovaries by continuing to produce small amounts of estrogen once menopause begins and continues to do so until about age seventy. But often, due to stressful living and poor eating habits, the adrenals are prematurely worn out in many women by the time they reach the age of menopause. Exhausted and depleted, the adrenals are unable to function in optimum capacity in their new job. The symptoms of adrenal stress are similar to those of menopause: nervous disorders, severe depression, irritability, fatigue, and unpredictable mood swings.

Most women go through menopause sometime between the age of forty and fifty-five and experience some type of noticeable change over a period lasting six months to two years. Some of the signs of menopause can be attributed to the dramatic hormonal changes occurring during this time. But general physical health and attitudes are primary factors in our well-being and contribute to our ability to adjust to the changes. Many of the disagreeable "symptoms" associated with menopause are a reflection of "ungraceful aging," a direct result of poor eating habits, stressful living, and lack of exercise. Men experience many of these symptoms in this age frame also. These "symptoms" in both men and women can often be corrected with good nutrition, exercise, and life-style changes.

The three most predominant and unpleasant symptoms of menopause are hot flashes, vaginal dryness, and emotional instability. Other uncomfortable symptoms associated with menopause include insomnia, depression, stiffening joints, sore breasts, osteoporosis, dry skin, and abdominal congestion (constipation, gas, and bloating). Fortunately, many women do not experience any of these and no one experiences all of them at once. All the symptoms are transient and all are correctable.

Nutritional Therapies

Dietary imbalances and unhealthy eating patterns can cause many of the supposed "symptoms" of menopause; likewise, a well-balanced diet will support a harmonious transition. The following are suggestions for foods that provide the essential vitamins and minerals specifically needed during the menopausal years. Because these are foods and not vitamin/mineral pills, they contain all the necessary nutrients needed by your body. Do a checklist of these foods and see how many are included on a regular basis in your diet. If any are lacking, you may wish to begin to include them daily.

Calcium
Calcium-rich foods are essential during the menopause. Calcium helps prevent osteoporosis and other bone problems. It also helps prevent hot flashes. Calcium in easily di-

gestible form is found in seaweeds, yogurt, and other milk products, almonds, sesame seeds and sesame products, and in most dark-green leafy vegetables such as spinach, chard, broccoli, turnip greens, and kale. There are many herbs that provide high amounts of calcium to the diet: comfrey, oat straw, nettle, dandelion greens, mustard greens, horsetail, chickweed, amaranth, and watercress.

Seaweeds are particularly high in calcium. Though they are a major food source in many parts of the world, they are often neglected in American diets. Three and a half ounces of cow's milk contains 118 milligrams of calcium. The same amount of hizike (a mild-flavored seaweed) contains 1400 milligrams; kelp, 1093 milligrams; and wakame, 1300 milligrams.

Along with foods high in calcium, you may wish to add a calcium supplement to your diet. If using pills, be certain the calcium is from an organic source and is biochelated for easy assimilation. An excellent calcium/mineral supplement made from herbs and organic sources of minerals is liquid Floradix Iron with Herbs and Nature-Works Herbal Iron. Both products are widely available in natural food and herb stores. You can also make your own high-iron formula. See page 62 for instructions.

HIGH-CALCIUM CANDY

1 cup sesame butter
½ to 1 cup honey
Powdered milk (enough to thicken the candy)
¼ cup ground or chopped almonds
¼ cup ground apricots
2–4 tablespoons powdered calcium
¼ cup toasted sesame seeds and/or coconut flakes

To Make:
Mix honey and sesame butter together. Add remainder of ingredients. Adjust flavors. Thicken with powdered milk to form into balls. Roll in toasted sesame seeds or coconut flakes.

HIGH-CALCIUM SHAKE

2 cups fresh orange juice and/or pineapple juice
½ cup yogurt
1 frozen banana
2–4 tablespoons calcium powder
2 tablespoons sesame seeds
1 teaspoon bee pollen (Some people are allergic to bee pollen. See caution on
  page 212.)
½ teaspoon spirulina
½ teaspoon dong quai powder

To Make:

Place all ingredients in blender and blend on high speed until creamy. A frozen banana gives the shake a nice creamy consistency.

Iron

An adequate intake of iron is essential for robust health and high energy. Its major role is keeping the blood oxygen-rich and it is found in every cell in the body. Even though it is found abundantly in food sources, the average diet is low in iron. Iron-deficient cells cannot get enough oxygen and exhaustion, fatigue, and stress result.

Iron is found in spinach, beets and beet greens, seaweeds, apricots, whole grains, wheat germ, bran, cereal (especially oats), raisins, tofu, molasses, sunflower seeds, and eggs. It is highly concentrated in many herbs: parsley, watercress, nettle, comfrey, alfalfa, yellow dock root, and horsetail. Along with iron-rich foods, you may wish to add additional iron in the form of liquid Floradix Iron with Herbs or NatureWorks Herbal Iron. Both these formulas are available at natural food and herb stores.

Vitamin E

Vitamin E is both a wonderful nutrient for the reproductive system and a specific remedy for hot flashes, muscle cramps, and vaginal dryness. It provides energy to the system by oxygenating the cells. Vitamin E is found in whole grains, cold pressed oils, dark-green leafy vegetables, bee pollen and some nuts.

Along with a diet containing many foods rich in vitamin E, a vitamin E supplement is often recommended during menopause. A suggested dose is 400–600 I.U. daily. But please note: For women with diabetes, a rheumatic heart, or high blood pressure, the recommended dose is no more than 50–150 I.U. daily. Purchase d-alpha and mixed tocopherol vitamin E (from natural sources) rather than the synthetic dl-alpha variety. Though more expensive, d-alpha and mixed tocopherol vitamin E is of much better quality and more effective.

Bee Pollen

This potent food source is a concentration of nearly all known nutrients. It is a complete protein containing all twenty-two amino acids. It has a higher concentration of the eight essential amino acids (those not produced in our bodies) than most other forms of protein. In addition to its protein content, bee pollen contains high levels of twenty-seven different minerals, enzymes, and coenzymes, vitamins B_1, B_2, and B_6, niacin, pantothenic acid, folic acid, vitamin C, and the fat soluble vitamins A and E.

A combined miracle of flowers and bees, the tiny grains of pollen provide some of nature's finest nutrition. A wonderfully uplifting food, bee pollen captures the essence of flowers and the energy of bees. Pollen is highly recommended for women during menopause; it seems to definitely lift the spirits and create greater energy levels. Interestingly, pollen is the male germ plasm of the flowering plant and is essential to life. Use only small amounts of bee pollen out of respect for the energy that the bees put into collecting it. It is recommended that you eat no more than one to two teaspoonsful a day (each teaspoon contains 4.8 billion grains of pollen!). For the best quality pollen, use it fresh, not in tablet form. Always eat it raw, sprinkled over salads, in yogurt, by itself, or in blender drinks.

Some people suffer allergic reactions to bee pollen, though others claim it helps clear their allergies. The first time you try some, take just a few grains to test for allergic reactions.

Spirulina

A tiny aquatic plant, spirulina is a blue-green algae that grows on freshwater ponds. It has been traced to the first forms of plant life on earth. Respected as an excellent source of nutrition in many cultures for centuries, it has only recently been introduced in America.

Spirulina is 60–70 percent protein by weight. It is considered the plant with the highest proportion of usable protein and is second only to dried whole eggs when compared with animal forms of protein. It is included here as a wonder food for women of menopause years not only because of its high-quality protein, but because of its concentration of B vitamins and gamma-linolenic acid (GLA). The B vitamins help build a strong nervous system and help with the balancing of mood swings and depression. GLA is excellent for preventing degenerative diseases such as osteoporosis and arthritis.

Spirulina is available in tablets and powder form. I recommend the powder for quality and economy. However, most people find the "green" taste and look overpowering and opt for the tablets. A recommended amount would be two tablespoons of the powder or six tablets daily. An added benefit of spirulina is that it gives one a feeling of fullness and lessens the desire to eat.

Dong Quai

This is one of the most wonderful herbs known for the female system and is used for the treatment of almost every gynecological ailment. As well as being an effective medicine when needed, it is a powerful uterine tonic and hormonal regulator and is used as a food supplement for these purposes. During menopause, dong quai helps tone and feed the reproductive organs and make for an easier hormonal transition. It is excellent for the circulatory system, is a blood tonic, and is also high in minerals, especially iron.

Dong quai is available at herb stores, natural food stores, and in Chinese pharmacies. It comes in many forms: tinctures, powder, tablets, whole root, and whole, pressed root. My personal favorite is the whole pressed root. They are beautiful to look at and easy to eat. The suggested daily dose is two tablets two times daily or one-eighth inch of the whole root eaten twice a day. If using dong quai in tincture form, the recommended dose is one-fourth teaspoon of tincture mixed in tea or water and drunk twice daily. A taste for dong quai is easy to acquire; it is rather bittersweet and exotic, but pleasant.

Ginseng (Panax Ginseng and Related Species)

Though many people relate ginseng to the male system, I find it an excellent tonic herb for some women, especially those who need the "yang" or grounding energy it is famous for. Considered the "king of all tonics," ginseng builds life force slowly and surely. It helps the body overcome fatigue and stress and is excellent for long-term deficiencies and imbalances. For women going through menopause it serves as a rejuvenator of the entire system and as a hormonal balancer. It will restore and build energy if used over a period of time. One of its great values during menopause is its ability to produce a steady flow of grounded, well-balanced energy and to aid in the elimination of mood swings and depression.

There are many varieties and grades of ginseng. The better the quality, the more effective the herb will be, of course. Do not use "instant" ginseng; it is of poor quality and ineffective at best. Buy your ginseng from a reputable source, i.e., a good herb store or natural food store. The herbalist there should be able to help you select a good-quality root. Chinese pharmacies have excellent selections but you have to know what you're looking for or be able to speak Chinese. Ginseng comes in many forms: tinctures, extracts, whole root, and powder. I prefer American ginseng and/or white or red ginseng roots from China. (Do not buy wild American ginseng; it is a highly endangered plant.) The suggested dose is two tablets twice daily; or one-fourth teaspoon in warm water (or in tea) twice daily; or a one-eighth-inch piece of the whole root chewed each day.

One of my favorite ways to prepare ginseng is this: Take a root four to six inches long and slice it. Put the slices in a small glass jar (or ceramic ginseng cooker), cover with three to four cups of water, and seal with a tight-fitting lid. Place the jar in a large pot with enough water to cover the jar about three-quarters of the way up. Put a lid on the large pot and slowly simmer for about six to eight hours. Keep an eye on the water level and add more water if it gets too low. This is a concentrated, powerful ginseng tonic and will help restore vital energy if taken once a month. Fast or eat very lightly of grains and steamed vegetables when you drink this. Have one cup of this ginseng broth in the evening, and one in the morning. Repeat until the liquid is gone.

Foods to Avoid

The above dietary suggestions, though general, will enhance your health greatly. But if you are seeking optimum health at this time in your life, there are also certain foods that you must avoid. Rather than sound like a broken record (most of you are aware that these foods are potential troublemakers), I'll just list them with a firm reminder that they ultimately are not worth the trouble they cause: alcohol, sugar, caffeine, white flour, refined, processed foods, and salt.

Exercise

Why there is a tendency to slow down as we get older, I don't know. But it is so important to our physical and emotional health to keep active. We exercise when we're younger without much effort; it is part of the active life-style of the young. When we are older, it seems we must plan it into our lives, and it takes more effort. Yet the benefits are tremendous.

Exercise ensures strong, healthy bones and aids in preventing osteoporosis; it is one of the surest ways to keep calcium in the bones. The connective tissue of the cartilage, ligaments, and tendons becomes more resilient and the bones become more dense. Many of the aches and pains of the joints begin to disappear.

Exercise can also directly benefit women during menopause by positively influencing the hormonal system. Both the production and use of hormones are maximized by sufficient activity. A well-functioning endocrine system nourished by good eating habits and exercise improves the entire physical and emotional experience of menopause.

Other benefits include a stronger heart, capable of pumping more blood with less effort. Capillaries are added to the blood vessel system, enabling more oxygen and nutrients to be carried to cells throughout the body. This increased circulation renews vitality and energy. An added benefit is seen in the skin; it takes on a vibrant new look.

Whatever form it takes, exercise should be a vital part of your life. Though gyms and health clubs offer a great deal, they cannot substitute for the great outdoors. Don't neglect "life exercise," the physical workouts that get you outside while playing, working, and enjoying nature.

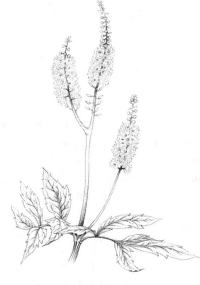

black cohosh

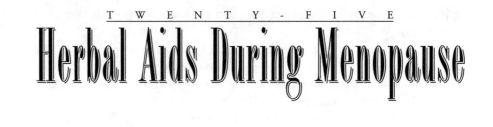

Strengthening and Toning Remedies

The following formulas strengthen and tone the endocrine system. The adrenals, which take on the role of producing estrogen after the ovaries cease to, often need a boost during this transitional time. Each of these blends contains herbs that help revitalize the adrenal glands.

In order for herbs to be effective, they must be used consistently. Unlike some forms of medicine, herbs do not promise instant cures or relief, but used regularly over an extended period of time, they gradually ensure steady, long-lasting results.

ENDOCRINE TONIC FOR MENOPAUSE

1 part licorice
1 part wild yam
3 parts sassafras
3 parts sarsaparilla
1 part vitex (chaste berry)

1 part ginger
1 part cinnamon
1 part dandelion root
½ part orange peel
¼ part dong quai

To Make:

Mix the herbs together. Adjust taste. For each quart of tea use four to six tablespoons of herb mixture. Simmer over a very low heat for twenty minutes. Strain. Drink three to four cups daily for three months or as long as needed. The herbs may be simmered several times before being thrown out. Make a quart of tea each day and drink it throughout the day. It may be refrigerated and drunk cold.

ENDOCRINE TONIC CAPSULES FOR MENOPAUSE

1 part black cohosh
2 parts kelp
1 part spirulina
1 part ginger
1 part motherwort

1 part wild yam root
1 part licorice
2 parts yellow dock root
½ part dong quai

To Make:

All herbs must be in powdered form. If possible, buy them already powdered. If not, you can powder them in coffee grinders and/or nut grinders. (But if using your coffee grinder, be forewarned; it will *never* be good for grinding coffee again. You coffee will taste like herbs and vice versa). Mix together thoroughly. Put in size "00" empty gelatin capsules (available at natural food stores and pharmacies) or rice paper. Take two capsules three times daily for three months or as long as needed.

ENDOCRINE TONIC TINCTURE FOR MENOPAUSE

2 parts wild yam

1 part sarsaparilla

1 part blue cohosh

2 parts false unicorn root

1 part dong quai

3 parts sage

3 parts licorice

3 parts dandelion root

To Make:

Mix herbs together. Put two ounces of the mixture in a wide-mouthed bottle and cover with one pint of good-quality brandy or vodka. Cover with a tight-fitting lid and place in a shaded, warm area. Let your tincture sit for four to six weeks. Shake once a day to mix herbs and alcohol together. Strain through a strainer lined with cheesecloth. Rebottle the herbal liquid. It is now ready for use. Recommended dose: one-fourth teaspoon diluted in tea or juice three times daily for three months or longer.

Another herbal mixture that many women have used before and during menopause with excellent results is Dr. Christopher's Change-Ease formula. Dr. Christopher was a famous herb doctor of this century. This formula is available at many natural food stores. The formula contains the following herbs: black cohash, sarsaparilla, ginseng, licorice, false unicorn root, holy thistle, and squaw vine.

Herbs are very concentrated in vitamins and minerals available in a form that is readily assimilated by the human body. The following tea formula will help ensure that you are getting adequate calcium and other essential minerals and vitamins in your diet. It is pleasant-tasting and can be enjoyed throughout the day. I usually make a couple of quarts of this daily and serve it to the whole family.

MENOPAUSE HIGH-CALCIUM FORMULA

1 part comfrey

1 part oat straw

1 part horsetail

1 part borage

2 parts nettle

3 parts peppermint

1 part chamomile

To Make:

Mix herbs together and adjust flavors to suit your taste. Use four to six tablespoons per quart of water. Pour boiling water over the herbs and let steep for thirty minutes. Drink two to four cups daily.

The following tea blend contains no caffeine but will, if used over a period of time, restore vitality and energy. Unlike caffeine-rich foods, it does not deplete the system, but contributes to a slow, steady increase of energy.

4 parts sassafras

1 part dong quai

1 part ginseng

1 part ginger

2 parts licorice

2 parts ginkgo leaf

2 parts gota kola leaf

1 part cinnamon chips

⅛ part orange peel

To Make:

Mix herbs together, reserving the ginkgo and gota kola leaves. Use four tablespoons of the root mixture per quart of water. Simmer over very low heat (with lid on pot) for thirty minutes. Remove from heat and add one teaspoon each of ginkgo and gota kola. Cover pot and let steep for thirty minutes. Strain and drink as desired. The suggested amount is one cup twice daily. You can reuse the herbs for two to three pots of tea before they are depleted.

The Crone represents the wise old woman in each of us and symbolizes that time of life when wisdom is sought. Biologically, she corresponds to the menopause cycle of a woman's life. She holds the key to wisdom and maturity gained from life experience. She is the keeper of dreams, the shaman within, and a spirit friend who can guide us on our spiritual quest. She is little understood in our society and, rather than being respected and honored, she is feared and ridiculed. The sum of our collected experiences as women, the Crone is a formidable force if not reconciled with. She makes herself known in one form or another. It is best to listen to her guidance and respond. This special candy is in her honor.

CRONE CANDY

1 cup sesame butter

½ cup (or more) honey

2 vials royal jelly (available in
   natural food stores)

Coconut, carob chips and/or powder,
   ground nuts, chopped fruit, etc.,
   to taste.

1 tablespoon spirulina

3 tablespoons bee pollen

3 tablespoons dong quai powder

2 tablespoons ginseng powder

To Make:

Mix honey and sesame butter into a paste. Stir in the remaining ingredients and mix well. Adjust flavors to taste. Roll into balls. Eat and enjoy!

Hot flashes, also called flushing, flushes, or sweats, are not fully understood, although they occur in about 75 percent of women during menopause. Every woman's experience of hot flashes is different. They can be absolutely unpredictable, or occur like clockwork. For some women they last but a second or two, while for others the hot, flushing sensation lasts for minutes. In some parts of the world, hot flashes are considered a sign of well-being, and women welcome them. For most women in our country, the sensation is regarded as unpleasant, though I have met women who welcome the warm, tingling feeling.

There are several hypotheses as to what causes hot flashes. One theory is that they result from vasomotor instability. This affects the nerve centers and the flow of blood, which in turn produces a prickly, hot sensation. Another theory is that the pituitary gland increases its production of the ovary-stimulating hormone FSH (follicle-stimulating hormone) in response to the decreased production of estrogen and progesterone. The large amounts of FSH in the blood cause an upset in the intricate glandular balance in the body. Hot flashes may occur as a result of the body attempting to achieve a new hormone balance. Yet another explanation is that the hormone changes taking place irritate the blood vessels and nerves, causing the blood vessels to overdilate and produce a hot feeling. Whatever the cause, "hot flashes" create an uncomfortable sensation in part because they are unfamiliar and unpredictable.

With the use of herbs and diet it is possible to exert some control over the length and time of hot flashes and even, in some cases, to eliminate them completely. The following suggestions have significantly diminished hot flashes for many women.

❦ Switch to a grains-based diet and eliminate all sugars and sugar-rich foods (including fruit and fruit juice).

❦ Take Dr. Christopher's Change-Ease formula (available in natural food and herb stores). Take two tablets three times daily at the onset of hot flashes and continue for three months.

❦ Concentrate on foods rich in calcium and vitamin E. (See pages 210 and 213) Take 400–600 I.U. of vitamin E daily. (Take only 50–150 I.U. of vitamin E daily if you have diabetes, high blood pressure, or a rheumatic heart.)

❦ Take ginseng daily to normalize the body's response to hot and cold and to relieve hot flashes.

❦ Drink several cups of sage tea daily. (Use regular garden sage.) Use one tablespoon sage per cup of water. Infuse it for twenty minutes. Sage is a "yang," grounding herb and many women have found it helps relieve hot flashes.

The following herbal formulas have also been used successfully to normalize hot flashes.

TEA FOR HOT FLASHES

2 parts sage
1 part blue vervain
2 parts motherwort

2 parts blessed thistle
½ part rosemary
¼ part ginseng

To Make:

Mix herbs together. Add one teaspoon per cup of water that has been boiled. Let steep, covered, for thirty minutes. Strain and drink in small amounts as needed throughout the day—one-fourth cup every hour, for example.

TINCTURE FOR HOT FLASHES

2 parts wild yam
1 part licorice
1 part black cohash

1 part ginseng
1 part false unicorn root

To Make:

Follow directions for making tinctures on page 66. Take one-fourth teaspoon diluted in warm water or tea three times daily or as often as needed.

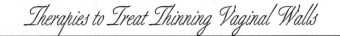

Therapies to Treat Thinning Vaginal Walls

The thinning of the mucous membranes, along with a loss of elasticity in the walls of the vagina, causes an uncomfortable sensation of dryness in many women during the menopause cycle. The thinning of the vaginal lining results from the ovaries' decreased production of estrogen. This thinning does not always cause problems, but it can be painful if the lining of the vagina becomes inflamed, dry, and rough. Estrogen creams and pills are the common allopathic solution for this problem, but these products have serious risks and should be used with caution and awareness.

Though the medical name, *atrophic vaginitis,* makes this situation seem as if it is a disease, it is not. It can be remedied with simple loving care and understanding. Above all, follow a good solid nutritional program during your menopausal years. This, more than anything, will help prevent the vagina from becoming overly dry and thin.

The following are suggestions for preventing and/or remedying the problem:

❧ Take 400–600 I.U. vitamin E daily. (Take only 50–150 I.U. daily if you have diabetes, high blood pressure, or a rheumatic heart.)
❧ Drink at least two quarts of water and/or tea a day.
❧ Take two tablets of Dr. Christopher's Change-Ease formula three times a day.
❧ Apply the following herbal ointment whenever the vagina feels dry and irritated.

1 part comfrey leaf and root   1 part calendula
1 part St. John's wort
Follow instructions for making an herbal salve on page 55.

❦ Aloe vera/slippery elm paste is often used to soothe and lubricate an inflamed, dry vagina. Mix enough slippery elm powder into the aloe vera gel to form a thickish paste. Apply inside the lips and up into the vagina. It will feel very cool and soothing.

❦ Always lubricate a dry vagina before having sex so as not to further irritate the tissue. Use the Herbal Ointment above for its soothing, healing herbal properties, or the oil from a vitamin E capsule. (Use a capsule that has 400 or more I.U.'s of vitamin E.) Cocoa butter, coconut oil, and other fruit or vegetable oils such as almond oil and apricot oil also make nice natural lubricants.

❦ Exercise the PC muscle (the pubococcygeus). This marvelous muscle, stretching from the tail bone to the pelvic bone, supports all the internal pelvic organs and is directly related to the health of the vagina. If not exercised on a regular basis, the PC will, like any muscle, weaken and eventually atrophy. Lack of PC muscle tone can contribute to urinary incontinence, prolapsed uterus, lack of sensitivity in the vagina, dryness, and less pleasurable sex. With regular PC exercise, the entire pelvic region will become stronger and healthier. Fresh blood is drawn to the vaginal tissue, creating thicker walls and more moisture. The supporting muscles will become stronger, and there will be an overall improvement in the health of the vagina.

The Kegel Exercises

Exercising the PC muscle is easy. It is naturally stimulated by any activity where you must squeeze and release the pubococcygeus such as in sexual intercourse and in urinating. There is also a set of exercises developed specifically for the PC. The Kegel exercises, developed by Dr. Kegel in 1940 as a nonsurgical remedy for urinary incontinence, can be done anywhere, anytime. Do them when you're driving, standing in line at the grocery store, or watching TV. No one will ever suspect what you're up to.

First, identify the PC muscle. It is the muscle used to stop urination and tighten the anus. Kegel exercises are a concentrated tightening and releasing of that muscle. For best results, it is suggested that you work up to doing 200 Kegels a day (this only takes about ten minutes a day). Alternate between fast and slow contractions. Spread the exercises out during the day, starting with 50 in the morning, 100 in the afternoon, and 50 again in the evening. Like any exercise, it is important to begin gradually, work up, and be consistent. Find a time of day or activity that works for you and go for it! The results are certainly worth the time it takes.

Dealing with Water Retention

Women in menopause often experience water retention and the many symptoms related to it: bloating, swelling, depression, mood swings, and emotional outbursts. During menopause the hormones are changing considerably. These hormones, especially estrogen, help to regulate the fluid balance. Unusual fluctuations of estrogen cause the body's sodium level to rise, which in turn causes the cells to retain more water. These slight variations in body chemistry make a profound difference in the ecology of our systems. Even a few ounces of excess water can cause breast tenderness, swelling, depression, and anxiety.

The element of water relates to our emotions and feelings. When we are deficient in body fluid, we experience a dryness of feelings; sometimes we may feel hot, eruptive feelings such as anger. When we have excess water in our systems, we often become overly emotional, weepy, and depressed.

The solution is *not* to limit your fluid intake. Quite the contrary. Water is a natural diuretic, essential to cellular health, and necessary in correcting the problem of water retention. Many women make the mistake of resorting to diuretic pills, which actually upset the sodium/potassium balance and further aggravate the problem. But water retention can be easily corrected.

❦ Throw the salt shaker out the back door. At least take it off the table and leave it out of your food when cooking. Avoid salty foods. It may take a couple of weeks to appreciate the marvelous wholesome flavor of unsalted food, but once your taste buds get used to it they'll be shocked at the amount of salt found in most food.

❦ Drink two quarts of water and/or tea daily. Unsweetened cranberry juice is a refreshing tonic for the kidneys and urinary system. Dilute and sweeten it with a little honey if necessary. If unsweetened cranberry juice is unavailable, Ocean Spray will do.

❦ Drink three cups of the following natural diuretic tea daily.

MILD DIURETIC TEA FOR MENOPAUSE

1 part chickweed	1 part pipsissewa and/or uva ursi
2 parts nettle	2 parts cornsilk
1 part oat straw	

To Make:

Use four to six tablespoons of herb mixture per quart of water. Add herbs to cold water and slowly bring to a simmer over low heat. Remove immediately from the stove. Keep pot tightly covered. Let infuse for twenty minutes. Strain. Drink three to four cups daily.

❦ Take a good-quality calcium/magnesium supplement each day and/or drink Menopause High-Calcium Formula (see page 217).

❦ Exercise enough to work up a sweat and get your circulatory system moving. Hot and cold baths are excellent to improve circulation. Saunas and jacuzzis, followed by a cold or cool shower, work as well.

Several of the symptoms experienced during difficult menstruation are present for some women during menopause. Those delicate imbalances of hormones have a definite way of letting us know when something is awry. Lower backache can often be caused by water retention and/or stress. If chronic backache is a problem for you during menopause, follow the general suggestions given on pages 216–18 and those under "Dealing with Water Retention" on pages 221–22.

❦ When experiencing back pain, take two tablets of valerian root every two hours. For faster relief, use valerian tincture. Use one-fourth teaspoon of the tincture, diluted in one-half cup warm water or chamomile tea, every hour or as needed.

❦ Gently massage the lower back. Ideally this is done by a friend, but it can be done, if need be, on yourself. Use the Backache Oil formula given below. It's a rather unusual formula and has an earthy odor. I first made it for a friend who had severe back problems. It was so helpful in relieving her pain that I continued to make it, with good results. Though it will not smell very pleasant (valerian either smells like the rich warm earth or like dirty socks, depending on your sense of smell), it is very effective.

BACKACHE OIL

½ part chamomile flowers
1 part valerian root
¼ part ginger
½ part sassafras

Olive oil or peanut oil (any good vegetable oil will do)
Eucalyptus or sage essential oil to improve the scent

To Make:
Follow directions on page 50 for making oils.

❦ Drink a mixture of equal parts of pennyroyal tea and chamomile tea. Infuse the tea following the instructions on page 47.

❦ Take hot herbal baths, using pennyroyal, lavender, and/or chamomile herbs. They are wonderfully relaxing. Place the herbs in a large cloth bag or handkerchief and tie to the nozzle of the tub. Let hot water course through it for a few minutes, then adjust the temperature. Jacuzzis and saunas are also very relaxing and will generally soothe away a backache. Do not attempt to carry the world on your shoulders; it is very hard on the back muscles and generally causes a lot of stress and tension.

HERBAL
HEALING
FOR
WOMEN

•

224

Osteoporosis

A crippling, degenerative disease, osteoporosis is marked by a gradual loss of bone mass, which can lead to skeletal deformities and fractures, especially of the hips. A rising concern for women, it is estimated that upward of 25 percent of American women have varying degrees of osteoporosis. It is more prominent in women than men, due to the hormonal changes of menopause, dietary differences, and general lack of exercise. Though osteoporosis and the effects of it are most noticeable in older women, bone loss begins in our early to midthirties and becomes more prevalent after menopause due to changes in estrogen levels.

I believe the rapid rise in osteoporosis is due in part to our high-protein, high-fat diet. It has been known by biochemists for years that a high-protein diet causes bones to lose calcium.

This information is largely ignored by the medical community. The rapid bone development that occurs in many American children due to high-protein diets contributes to a weak skeletal structure. The remainder of the diet can't support this rapid bone growth, resulting in a porous and unsubstantial skeletal structure that rapidly loses density in later years.

Calcium, long regarded as essential for a healthy skeletal structure, is largely obtained from dairy foods. To ensure the best calcium absorption, foods with a calcium/phosphorus ration of 2:1 are ideal. Dark-green leafy vegetables, some nuts and seeds, and seaweeds generally contain a 2:1 ratio. The calcium/phosphorus ratio in milk is less than ideal: a 1:1 ratio. The American Dairy Council advises drinking four glasses of milk a day to ensure we're getting our proper calcium intake and to guard against osteoporosis. We are the only country in the world that drinks that much milk, and also the country with the highest rate of osteoporosis.

Though calcium is essential for building strong bones, the best sources of calcium are not from milk products, but from nuts, seeds, grains, and vegetables. Seaweeds, those humble vegetables from the sea, are the number-one source of digestible assimilated calcium for the body. Though calcium is essential for healthy bones, lack of calcium alone does not cause osteoporosis. There are countries in the Orient where calcium intake was always relatively low and osteoporosis was not a problem until the introduction of a Western high-fat, high-protein diet.

An overemphasis on the Twiggy look could also be a contributor to the high rise of osteoporosis. In our teenage years and in the active years of midlife, lack of proper nutrition is often sacrificed for the popular thin look. Osteoporosis is most prevalent in small-boned, thin women. Perhaps if we placed as much emphasis on eating well and exercising adequately as we do on fitting into the latest fashion, we would begin to see a decrease in osteoporosis.

Lack of proper exercise is probably the number-one contributor to osteoporosis. We've become a sedentary society. Our bodies, which long to run and jump and dance in graceful movement, have become the victims of the restrictive clothes we wear, the sedentary jobs we work at, and the television shows that turn us into couch potatoes. Without the exercise our bodies yearn for, our bones get stiff and brittle. Exercise has not only been shown to prevent osteoporosis, but also to alleviate the symptoms of it. A recent study in the United States showed that menopausal women who exercised vigorously for one hour each day for a year increased bone calcium levels by one-third. Exercise insures proper bone density and helps alleviate demineralization of the bones. It is also an excellent antidote to the hormonal and metabolic changes of menopause.

Though it is generally felt by the medical profession that osteoporosis is not reversible, Dr. John Lee, a doctor from my hometown of Sebastopol, California, feels otherwise. He conducted a study of 100 women in his family practice who all had varying degrees of osteoporosis. Using a combination of a low-protein, low-fat diet, exercise, vitamin and mineral supplements, and low doses of estrogen and transdermal progesterone, he reversed osteoporosis in all these women.

The following steps should be taken to prevent and/or reverse osteoporosis:

❦ Eat a low-protein, low-fat diet.
❦ Reduce the amount of dairy you consume. Do not rely heavily on dairy products as a source of calcium.
❦ Reduce your intake of substances known to contribute to calcium loss. Among these are coffee (each cup robs the body of 5 milligrams of calcium), carbonated beverages, alcohol, salt, and sugar.
❦ Eat a diet rich in dark-green leafy vegetables, nuts, seeds (sesame seeds are remarkably high in digestible calcium), tofu, molasses, and seaweeds.
❦ Find an exercise routine that works for you and that you enjoy, then stick to it. Resistence-type exercises, such as weight lifting and free weights are the best kind of exercises for building bone density. However, any type of exercise is beneficial, including such nonstressful exercise as yoga and walking. Remember, exercise is the surest way to slow down the advances of osteoporosis.
❦ Take calcium supplements. Though they will neither prevent nor correct osteoporosis, they do provide extra insurance against the disease. A natural biochelated calcium supplement in the amount of 1000–1500 milligrams is recommended daily for women susceptible to osteoporosis.
❦ Nourish and support the endocrine system to prevent the hormone imbalance that contributes to osteoporosis. See pages 216–8 for herbal formulas that tone and strengthen the endocrine system.

Estrogen Replacement Therapy

ERT drugs are today's "pie in the sky" for menopausal women. They effectively mask many of the symptoms of menopause. They make wrinkles less apparent by pumping up the cells with water, they lubricate the vaginal lining, and they alleviate hot flashes. There is also evidence that ERT therapy helps prevent the bone loss that causes osteoporosis, and protects postmenopausal women from heart disease.

Sounds pretty good? Yes, but estrogen replacement therapy can have serious side effects, too. There are several known risks involved in its use, and the possible long-term effects of taking it are still unknown. The most serious side effect of ERT is cancer of the endometrial lining of the uterus. The average incidence of endometrial cancer in women of postmenopausal age is one in 1000. For women who have been on estrogen therapy for two to four years, this percentage increases four to eight times; and for women on estrogen therapy for over seven years, the percentage increases fourteen times.

There are other side effects. All the symptoms of water retention, such as weight gain, breast tenderness, depression, and excessive mood swings, are possible with ERT. Breakthrough bleeding is another of the most common side effects. Another possible consequence is an increase in the size of existing benign tumors of the uterus.

But perhaps the worst side effect of all is the masking or postponing of this natural and important cycle of a women's life. We developed a pill to regulate our menstrual cycles and our birthing rhythms. We've now made a pill to control the processes of aging. Choosing to ignore the few remaining rites of passage we have as women, we become alienated from our sources of power. Though for some women ERT is a necessary and important guarantee of well-being, others are put on it for simple or minor complaints. We're told that these synthetic hormones will postpone the aging processes associated with menopause and alleviate the symptoms. It's time to ask ourselves why we would want to postpone menopause. Is there something wrong with aging naturally? With her wrinkles and strong hands, her rounded body, and her gray hair, my grandmother was a gorgeous woman. What is wrong with that image as a model to grow old by? Have you seen pictures of the older women of the native tribes? There is something very earthy and strong about them. They are still the pillars of their tribes. I hang their pictures around my room so I can withstand the bombardment of images that embody our culture's obsession with youth. I want reminders that it is possible to age naturally and gracefully.

I've had the honor of being close friends with many elderly women. I've made sure my daughters, too, share time with my older friends. What examples these strong older women are to us! There was no one more lively than my neighbor and herbal ally, Adele Dawson. At eighty-six, Adele could run circles around any of her younger cronies. When she died just a few weeks ago, I think we were all as surprised as we were saddened by her sudden death. How could anyone so alive die? Juliette De Baircli Levy in her late seventies still travels the world living the life of a gypsy and communing with the peasant people she loves so much. The years have slowed her down some, but her spirit is still wild and free. My daughters recently had the opportunity to spend a day with Tasha Tudor, well-known artist, herbalist, and master gardener. Well into her seventies, this marvelous women is a powerful inspiration to them. And to me.

Though there are certainly situations where it is medically necessary to take estrogen replacement therapy, continue to work with your natural cycles by implementing the dietary and life-style changes you feel are appropriate. Allow yourself to experience the gift of aging. Awaken to the spirit of the Crone, the wisdom of the elders. Do not think that the drug is the magic pill of youth that will cure everything. *You* are still in control and are ultimately responsible for the health of your body as it journeys through this rite of passage.

If you decide not to take ERT or wish to discontinue its use, the following suggestions may be helpful:

❦ Take 400–800 I.U. of vitamin E daily (50–150 I.U. if you have diabetes, high blood pressure, or a rheumatic heart).

❦ Take six tablets of Dr. Christopher's Chang-Ease Formula (available in natural food stores).

❦ Take two tablets of dong quai twice a day and/or two tablets of ginseng twice a day.

❦ Enjoy one to two one-inch round balls of Crone Candy daily (see page 218 for recipe).

❦ Make the following formula into both a tea and tincture. Mix one-fourth teaspoon of the tincture into each cup of tea and drink two to four cups daily.

ROOT TEA FOR MENOPAUSE

2 parts wild yam	1 part false unicorn root
2 parts licorice	2 parts sage
3 parts sarsaparilla	1 part cinnamon
1 part vitex (chaste berry)	½ part black cohosh
1 part ginger	

To Make:

Use four to six tablespoons of herb mixture per quart of water. Add herbs to cold water and bring to a slow simmer over low heat. Simmer for twenty minutes, then strain. Drink two to three cups daily. To make as a tincture, see directions on page 66. Take one-fourth teaspoon three times daily.

Avoid or decrease your consumption of refined, processed foods, sugar, and caffeine-rich foods such as coffee and black or green tea.

If you are already on ERT therapy but wish to discontinue it or cut back on its use, do so *slowly* and *gently*. Each day shave off a tiny bit of your standard ERT dose with a sharp knife or razor. Do this over a long period of time while *increasing* those items that stimulate your body's inherent health and balance. If you reach a point where you feel you are decreasing ERT too quickly, stay at that dosage until your body stabilizes again. Then continue with the program. This process of balancing and reawakening the body's natural ability to create its own hormones may take several months, but it has proven effective for many women.

For most women the best suggestions for a congenial menopause cycle are to stay active, healthy, and happy. Continue to pursue life, to love and be loved. Find new interests and/or continue to develop your old ones. Do not fall prey to the myth that this is not a productive time. The only production we are no longer capable of is reproduction.

Though both confusing and exciting, menopause is a time of quiet power and inner strength. We have tasted and drunk from life's deep well. We have made love. Had babies. Climbed mountains. Danced. And cried deeply. Having experienced much that life has to offer, called on by the Great Mystery, we continue to explore life from a new vista.

Our biggest ally at this time is the Crone, the Old One, the Wise Woman of every culture. Where does she exist in our culture? You may have to seek hard to find her, but she is there, buried deep within your heart, waiting to be heard and understood. She carries the gifts of herbs, wisdom, and acceptance. She invites the child within you to wake up and play. She is the mother of youth and the gateway to wisdom gained from experience. And we, each of us who are women of menopause, stand at her threshold awaiting her gifts if we only dare seek.

Part Seven

Materia Medica for
WOMEN

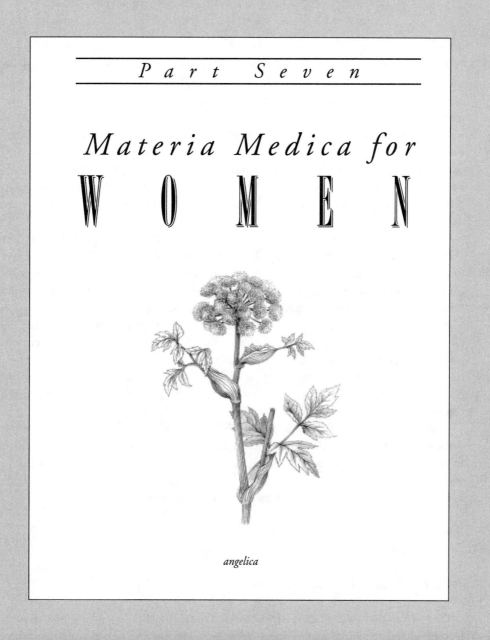

angelica

The physician treats, but nature heals.

—Hippocrates

The following is a listing of herbs that have been mentioned frequently throughout this book. Though it is always difficult to decide which herbs to include in a listing such as this, I have tried to keep the selection limited to those herbs that are particularly useful for women.

I've always felt it a requisite when studying herbs to reference *each* herb you're planning to use in at least three different herb books. Because herbs are such multifaceted characters, no one book will give you a complete picture of who it is or what it can do. But reading about it in several books will paint a more complete picture for you and give you a broader understanding of the depths and possibilities of each herb you are working with.

Reading will fill your head with the wonderful facts and stories about each plant, but herbalism is more than book learning. The best possible way to learn about each herb is to experience it. If, after you've read about it, the herb seems like one that is appropriate for your situation, try it. The taste, the smell, the effect of the herb on your being is the best laboratory you have for determining its effectiveness.

Every herb is replete with legends that take us back to ancient times. Though they often seem quaint and antiquated, these stories provide valuable insights into the current uses of the plants. Without getting too carried away, I've included some of these historical references. When the information is available, I've also included information on chemical constituents and clinical studies. Taken together, this information provides a colorful, multidimensional picture of the plant.

Throughout my years of working as an herbalist, each of the following herbs has become a familiar plant ally, close to my heart. Though a few are rather exotic and difficult to come by, most are common and familiar, the everyday plants of the simpler. Look in your own backyard or neighborhood for these treasures. You'll find half of the plants mentioned in this Materia Medica growing abundantly there.

Angelica
Angelica archangelica, A. sylvestris, and related species
Umbelliferae
Parts used: roots, stems, seeds, and leaves

One of the most widely used of European plants, Angelica has a long and colorful history. Called the "herb of the Angel," Angelica was revealed to a Benedictine monk when he was pleading to God for a cure for the plague. Angelica does have strong antimicrobial and antiseptic properties that may have been helpful in aiding patients with bubonic plague (though judging by the number of deaths, I'm not sure I would say it had much success with that disease). It was also commonly called "the root of the Holy Ghost" and was associated with St. Michael, to whom it appeared in a dream. Under the ward of Michael the Archangel for whom it was named, it was considered a panacea and was especially valued for warding off evil spirits. For centuries, angelica has been brewed in "Carmelite water," a special long-life elixir. It is also the main ingredient in Swedish bitters, a famed tonic that is still readily available and hailed for indigestion, headaches, and general maladies.

Angelica is composed of a variety of essential oils, bitter principles, and coumarin compounds, among other things, giving it a complex range of actions. A warming, decongesting herb, angelica promotes circulation, and energy throughout the body. Its concentration of bitters makes it an excellent digestive aid, one that is used both for sluggish liver and for poor digestion. It warms the bronchials and is used for congestion, flus, and colds.

Angelica has a special affinity for the female reproductive system and has been used as a birth tonic, to relieve congestion of the pelvis, and for menstrual irregularities. Its warming, decongesting properties are often helpful in easing painful and cramping menstruation. It is also used to aid in the expulsion of the placenta after childbirth.

There are several varieties of angelica. The Chinese variety, dong quai, is one of the most widely used herbs in the Orient. It is called the "female ginseng" and is used as a tonic for the reproductive system. Many herb books suggest using dong quai and angelica interchangeably. Though dong quai and angelica are botanically similar, I'm convinced, after observing the actions of both of these herbs for many years, that they have different though compatible properties. Dong quai, taken over a long period of time, is more useful for toning and building the reproductive system. Angelica has a stronger, more medicinal action. It stimulates circulation to the pelvic region and serves to break up long-standing stagnation in the reproductive system, stimulating suppressed menstruation. Both herbs are valuable for women. I suggest using angelica more for specific medicinal purposes and dong quai as a long-term tonic and building herb.

Angelica is still found growing wild throughout North America. In Europe, however, where it has been used for hundreds of years, it has been overharvested and is seldom found in the wild any more. A very beautiful plant, it stands out in any landscape, its very stateliness commanding attention. *One must be very careful when harvesting angelica, as it can easily be confused with poison hemlock* which is DEADLY poisonous. As when harvesting any herb, be sure it is the herb you want. (See Appendix I for a list of books to help in herb identification.)

Because of its emmenagogic properties, angelica it is not recommended during pregnancy. It is a safe, nontoxic plant but should only be used sparingly. Do not use it over an extended period of time.

Black Cohosh
  Cimifuga racemosa
  Ranunculaceae
  Parts used: rhizomes and roots

Though black and blue cohosh are unrelated, they are often used together and have a synergistic, not interchangeable, relationship with one another. Termed "cohosh" by the Algonquian Indians in reference to "rough" roots, both plants grow in similar habitats. They have long been valued for their positive effects, both in menstruating women and in women undergoing labor and childbirth. However, these two plants have distinct differences as well. While blue cohosh is primarily associated with blood flow to the pelvic area, black cohosh maintains its effects through its estrogenlike action. It has a regulating and normalizing effect on hormone production and is often used in formulas to balance and regulate female hormones.

Though primarily known for its effects on the female reproductive system, black cohosh is also highly regarded as a nervine and muscle relaxant and has been successfully used for headaches, pain, and muscle spasms. Its anti-inflammatory action makes it useful for arthritis, and for muscular and neurological pain.

Many of its uses come to us from Native Americans, but it was adopted and used frequently by the early settlers and herbal doctors. Eclectic physicians believed black cohosh to be one of the most useful and powerful of uterine tonics, and some of the early patent medicines contained high concentrations of the herb. It was the main ingredient in Lydia Pinkham's famous "Vegetable Compound" and was drunk by women throughout the early nineteenth century to relieve menstrual stress and nervous tension. Though largely ignored by the orthodox medical community in America, black cohosh is included in formulas to promote menstruation in several European countries, and similar varieties are used in the Chinese pharmacopeias.

In women's formulas black cohosh is used in combination with blue cohosh to stimulate uterine contractions and is often given during the last week of pregnancy to prepare the uterus for childbirth. It has proven helpful when the birth date is long overdue and there is a possibility that either mother or infant is in stress. Because of its estrogenic qualities, black cohosh has a special affinity with menopausal women and is used in formulas to balance and regulate hormone production during menopause. Black cohosh is used to bring on delayed menstruation and is also helpful to relieve the stress and nervous tension accompanying the menstrual cycle.

A wonderful woman's herb, black cohosh thrives in rich woodland soil. It is a beautiful, stately plant with long spikes of white fairylike flowers that bloom in the late summer and fall.

Though nontoxic, it should not be used during the early trimesters of pregnancy because it is a uterine stimulant and can cause premature contractions. It is often used at the end of pregnancy, however, to stimulate labor.

Black Haw
  Viburnum prunifolium
  Caprifoliaceae
  Parts used: bark of root, trunk, and branches

Black haw is used similarly to its cousin, cramp bark. Both viburnums are excellent for "quieting" the uterus and are used for threatened miscarriage, uterine cramps, and dysmenorrhea. Black haw has powerful relaxant and sedative effects on the female reproductive system and is useful when there is tension and stress in those organs. It has a strong reputation for preventing miscarriage, and was used by the Native Americans and pioneer women for this purpose.

To their shame, slave holders in their perversion used it also. It was common practice for landowners to rape their women slaves to increase their slave holdings. Slave women, familiar with the use of herbs, would drink the readily available cotton root bark, a potent abortifacient herb. Knowing of this practice, the slaveowners often forced women slaves to drink a concoction of black haw every day to prevent abortion. This custom is recorded in *King's American Dispensatory*: "It was customary for planters to compel female slaves to drink an infusion of black haw daily whilst pregnant to prevent abortion from taking the cotton root."

Scopoletin, a chemical constituent of black haw, is a powerful uterine relaxant. The plant also contains valerianic acid, a sedative factor found also in valerian. The salicin in black haw, a main ingredient in aspirin, may contribute to its anti-inflammatory and pain-reducing effects. Rich in steroidal saponins that serve as precursors for hormone production by the liver, black haw is an excellent herb during menopause.

There have been no reported cases of toxicity and no known side effects from using black haw.

Blessed Thistle
Cnicus benedictus
Compositae

Parts used: leaves, roots, flowers, and seeds
This lowly plant has evoked quite an impressive list of names, including our lady's thistle and holy thistle. Though regarded by farmers and gardeners as an invasive weed, blessed thistle has long been valued by herbalists and healers around the world. It is rich in the bitter glycoside cnicin, which stimulates digestive enzymes and bile secretions. It is also high in mucilage, tannin, and contains small amounts of essential oil.

Blessed thistle and its close cousin, milk thistle *(Cardus marianus),* are both excellent tonics for the liver and digestion. Both are known to repair damaged liver cells. A distinctive bitter, blessed thistle can be used as a digestive aid before meals. It also has a specific stimulating and toning effect on the liver, which makes it beneficial for most hormonal imbalances. Blessed thistle is often used in combination with other hormonal regulators for women who have menstrual difficulties. But Blessed Thistle is most widely known for its ability to stimulate blood flow to the mammary glands and thus increase and enrich the flow of mother's milk. It is often combined with fennel, raspberry leaf, and other, less bitter herbs to make an effective and tasty tea.

I find thistles a remarkable group of herbs and honor them for their tenacity and hardiness. They are found growing throughout the world and endure the harshest of environments. There are no poisonous members of this large family. Most are edible and most are valued for their medicinal actions. Finding a way to use them is often more difficult than finding them. Most have thorns, thistles, and little prickles that tend to keep the timid away. Blessed thistle is remarkably easy to grow and is a lovely, mysterious, low-growing plant. My husband doesn't allow me to grow my thistle patches anywhere near our house and gardens. I plant little patches of them in our most distant acres and they seem quite happy there, neglected and left alone in dry sunny fields.

Blue Cohosh
 Caulophyllum thalictroides
 Berberidaceae
 Parts used: roots and rhizomes (berries poisonous)

When I first moved to New England I was delighted to find blue cohosh, an herb I had used for years but had never seen, growing in abundance. A beautiful, tall plant with blue-green stems, an unusual leaf structure, and lovely (but poisonous) deep blue berries, blue cohosh is easy to recognize in the eastern hardwood forests.

Formerly known as papoose root and squaw root, blue cohosh was commonly used by Native American women during the latter stages of pregnancy to ensure an easier labor and childbirth. Dr. Shook, an early physiomedical herb doctor, stated, "This exceedingly valuable herb is well called 'women's best friend' for the reason that it is much more reliable and far less dangerous in expediting delivery in those cases where labor is slow and very painful. This is a very old Indian remedy. They believed it to be the best parturient in nature, and it was the habit of their women to drink the tea several weeks before labor."

Early eclectic medical doctors and physiomedical herbalists used blue cohosh in the manner of the Native American women. They prescribed it for easing childbirth and labor. It was listed in the U.S. *Pharmacopoeia* from 1882 until 1905 as a labor inducer and was generally given during the last few weeks of pregnancy. It was also used before pregnancy to prepare the uterus for childbirth.

It is still widely used among herbalists today for the same purposes and is considered one of the best uterine stimulants and menstrual stimulants available. Caulosaponin, a chemical found in blue cohosh, actively stimulates uterine contractions and promotes blood flow to the pelvic region. A strong medicinal herb with very active properties, blue cohosh should be used in a responsible way. I've found it very helpful in cases where labor is long and drawn-out and the mother's energy is waning. I've also used it when labor is delayed for such a length of time as to be threatening to the mother and infant. Blue cohosh tincture often helps facilitate labor, contractions, and childbirth.

A very powerful emmenagogue, blue cohosh will help bring on a suppressed or delayed menstruation. The herb also has powerful antispasmodic properties and is helpful for relieving menstrual cramps and general pain.

Caulosaponin, one of the active constituents of blue cohosh, has been under clinical observation by the scientific community. Isolated from the mother plant and injected into animals in laboratory situations, caulosaponin has produced a narrowing of the arteries. Scientific studies then go on to suggest from these very limited (and, I might add, inhumane) studies that blue cohosh may be responsible for human heart damage. Caulosaponin is only one chemical contained within the chemical blueprint of blue cohosh. To isolate it, test it on clinically doomed animals, then pronounce it damaging, as in this case, seems ludicrous, especially when the plant has been used for so many hundreds of years and continues to be used safely and effectively.

There are precautions, however, that need to be taken when using blue cohosh. The herb should *not* be used during the early trimesters of pregnancy. It can, and has been known to, cause premature uterine contractions, leading to miscarriage and/or abortion. Use it only as a medicine in specific dosages, not as a tonic or food herb. Use it specifically for stimulating uterine muscle contractions to bring on suppressed menstruation, and for easing the pains and cramps of the menstrual cycle. Blue cohosh is generally used in combination with other herbs and is often used with black cohosh. Though unrelated, black and blue cohosh have a synergistic relationship with one another. They work best in combination for menstrual disorders and for inducing labor.

Chamomile
Matricaria chamomilla, Anthemis nobile, and related species
Compositae
Parts used: flowers, leaves

There are few medicinal plants as well loved as chamomile. It is generally regarded as one of the finest and safest of medicinals and is used for all manner of disorders. In European sanitariums, chamomile is still served to patients, a welcome alternative to the caffeine-rich drinks that are available in hospitals in the United States. It can be drunk daily as a pleasant relaxing beverage tea or used effectively for extreme nerve stress and nervous system disorders. Chamomile is one of the plants that I describe as having "soft power": though a gentle plant, it is also a powerfully effective medicine.

The seemingly endless list of problems chamomile is said to help can all be traced to its effects on the nervous system and digestive system, as well as to its anti-inflammatory action. Azulene, a major active chemical in chamomile, is a beautiful blue volatile oil. This oil has anti-inflammatory, antibacterial, and anodyne properties. Azulene is easily destroyed by heat, so chamomile should always be prepared by infusing rather than decocting.

Chamomile is characterized by a bittersweet flavor. The bitter principles in it stimulate the gastric juices, making it excellent for the liver and digestive system. The longer the flowers are infused, the more its bitter principles are released. For a strong, bitter tea, steep chamomile for at least twenty minutes or longer. For a more gentle, relaxing tea, infuse the flowers for five to ten minutes.

Chamomile is commonly used for stomach stress, digestive complaints, nervous system disorders, inflammation in the joints, and for wounds. It is an excellent remedy for all manner of women's disorders and is especially valuable for problems arising from stress, anxiety, and tension. Chamomile is an excellent healing agent in douche formulas and sitz baths and is used frequently for this purpose in commercial preparations.

My favorite evening nightcap is a simple mixture of equal parts of chamomile and rose hips, with just a pinch of stevia. I find it delicious, calming, and gently soothing to the spirit after a long day. Try sipping this tea while enjoying the calm of a warm chamomile bath. And when you tuck yourself into bed, have a little pillow of Chamomile to put beside your head. (To make a sleep pillow, see page 250.)

Chamomile is also a wonderful herb for infants and children and is a favorite remedy for colic and digestive disorders. Baby's first bath is a special delight when it is made with chamomile flowers. Not only fragrant, a chamomile bath is calming to a small child and, I think, reassures its little spirit that the world is a good place to be born into. Beatrix Potter's famous children's story about Peter Rabbit demonstrates chamomile's special appropriateness for children and its calming effects on them. When little Peter Rabbit is chased by Farmer John with a pitchfork, Peter hops back to his mother who quickly fixes him a cup of chamomile tea and puts him to bed.

Chamomile is a favorite cosmetic herb the world over and is wonderful for the hair and skin. I've recently seen a whole slew of new cosmetics on the market featuring this little flower. I enjoy it best in simple preparations, such as facial steams, herb baths, flower waters, and homemade creams and lotions. (For some of these recipes, see pages 96–104.)

There are many varieties of chamomile on the market and every herbalist has her personal favorite. For medicinal purposes, I prefer the bitter Hungarian chamomile *(C. recuitita)*. I also love the beautiful *A. nobile* and *M. chamomilla* for flavor and tea. Experiment with the different kinds to find your favorite. They all have similar properties and flavors. Do beware of picking "wild chamomile," however. Many plants that look like chamomile are not. When I lived in the mountains of the Pacific Northwest, I was excited to find myself surrounded by a sea of "wild chamomile." You can imagine my delight as I brewed up a cup of this abundant wild herb. But after one sip of that extremely bitter tea, I knew I had the wrong herb. I was lucky: dog weed is only mildly toxic. Many plants of the composite family look alike and are easily confused.

Though chamomile is generally considered safe and nontoxic and can be used with no residual buildup or side effects, there are a few people who experience allergic reactions to it. Chamomile belongs to the large composite family of plants, which cause allergies in some people. If you suffer from allergies brought on by pollen-bearing plants, it would be wise to exercise caution the first time you try a cup of chamomile tea. In my many years as a practicing herbalist, I have seen only two cases of chamomile-caused allergies. The symptoms are wheezing, itchy eyes, and a swollen, inflamed throat.

Comfrey
Symphytum officinale and related species
Boraginaceae
Part used: entire plant

Twenty years ago, while walking down a back country road with a group of friends, I was struck by a young aspiring Hell's Angel on a Harley-Davidson. Thrown into a ditch next to a little plant called self heal, I sat up only long enough to see bones sticking out of my right leg, laid back down, and decided to let the universe take care of it. Two surgeries and several months later, I was informed that my leg was not healing and would require additional surgery and the insertion of a permanent metal plate that would extend from my knee to my ankle. I wasn't eager to have this surgery and decided to take matters into my own hands.

For the next several months I drank and ate copious amounts of comfrey, learned to maneuver quite gracefully in my full-leg cast, and continued to visit my doctor on a regular basis. It was his monthly task to inform me that I was being foolish and that, given the condition of the bones, my leg would not heal. I always assured him that it might, and I just wanted time to try. I discovered 110 ways to cook comfrey, juice comfrey, and drink comfrey. I believe I turned a bit green around the gills. It took eighteen grueling months, but it was a joyous day when my cast came off. I had a healed bone and didn't need a metal rod in my leg.

Comfrey is a marvelous herb and is one of the best-known healing herbs of all times. Its very name, symphytum, means "to heal." Comfrey has been touted for centuries for its bone-mending qualities, for its healing effect on ulcers, and for its general soothing effect on the mucous membranes. It contains tannin as well as mucilage in its chemical composition, making it not only soothing but constrictive and healing for wounds, cuts, and tears. It also contains steroidal saponins, making it particularly beneficial for reproductive and hormonal imbalances. Rich concentrations of allantoin, a cell-proliferant that stimulates the growth of connective tissue and cartilage, make comfrey a specific for broken bones, torn cartilage, swellings, and bruises. Along with all its specific healing properties, comfrey is also a delicious and nourishing food herb. It contains high amounts of digestible plant calcium, iron, protein (up to seven times more protein than soybeans contain!), B vitamins, and vitamin A, among other things.

It was a favorite herb of most early herbalists and was written about for centuries in the old herbals. Hildegard of Bingen, famous visionary, saint, and herbalist of the Benedictines, recommended it for wounds in the eleventh century. Paracelsus, Pliny, Gerard, Dioscorides, and Culpepper were all fans of the herb and recommended it highly. Down through the ages in most parts of the world comfrey was recognized as one of the great healing herbs. Indeed, comfrey maintained a scrupulous reputation—right up to the present day.

In 1968 an independent Japanese scientist first reported finding pyrrolizidine alkaloids, substances that are regarded as potentially hepatoxic and carcinogenic, in comfrey. What a furor that report caused! Once considered one of the all-time great healing herbs, comfrey now sits on trial as a possible carcinogen. Austrian studies confirmed the Japanese reports. Pyrrolizidine alkaloids are found in concentration in the young leaves and roots of comfrey. From the scientific community the news filtered into the herbal community and spread like wildfire. A recent headline in one newspaper stated: "Warning! Comfrey Tea Can Kill You."

Though it is important to be open to the possible dangers of comfrey, it is just as important to sift through the information and misinformation and form an opinion based on fact, rather than on hysteria. The truth of the matter is that most plants contain chemicals that are potentially harmful. These chemicals form a synergistic relationship, often nullifying and/or strengthening certain aspects of one another. As Michael Tierra states in *The Way of the Herbs,* "Plants have a dynamically complex biochemistry. In many instances this allows for small amounts of substances, which when isolated and concentrated might otherwise be poisonous, to be quite safe and harmless." The sum total of these hundreds of chemicals determines the personality, or action, of the plant. Judging a plant's action on the basis of a single chemical component is like judging a person's character on the basis of a single personality trait.

Comfrey is rich in allantoin, calcium salts, and mucopolysacharrides, all of which are cell builders and serve to neutralize the cell-inhibiting action of the pyrrolizidine alkaloids. It is also important to note that the pyrrolizidine alkaloids found in comfrey are in a "N-oxide," or organic state, unlike those used in laboratory studies. These organic compounds are more likely to be degraded when digested in the human body.

Another important issue to consider is the nature of the tests conducted. Once identified, the alkaloids were isolated and injected into laboratory animals in proportions far greater than would normally be ingested in medicinal use. The animals developed liver damage and cancerous tumors. Another experiment was done on six-week-old laboratory rats, doomed to death from their first day of life. They were fed comfrey root as fifty percent of their total diet. After a time, the rats did develop tumors, which merely proves one of the standing laws of science: that every substance or chemical is a poison if we consume enough of it. Or as Paracelsus said several hundred years ago, "All things are poison and nothing is without poison. It is the dosage that makes a thing poisonous." (It is interesting to note that comfrey is used extensively as a fodder for dairy and beef cattle throughout the Pacific Northwest with no ill effects. In fact, farmers there grow fields of comfrey because of its beneficial role in increasing milk production and the overall health of the herds.)

Studies conducted in Washington found very minute amounts of pyrrolizidine alkaloids in comfrey. Some plants tested had none at all. An independent researcher in the United States found that of three samples tested for pyrrolizidine alkaloids, one was negative, the second contained only trace amounts, and the third contained one part per million.

Because of these laboratory findings, an attempt was made to collect case histories of individuals who used comfrey and later developed liver toxicity. However, of the thousands of people who use comfrey worldwide, only three somewhat questionable cases have been identified, none of which points conclusively to comfrey as the culprit. In 1984 there was a case of veno-occlusive liver disease in a forty-nine-year-old woman who had been taking comfrey-pepsin tablets for four months. The *American Journal of Medicine* reported a case of a woman who reportedly drank as many as ten cups of comfrey tea a day and handfuls of the tablets, and developed veno-occlusive liver disease. The third reported case of veno-occlusive liver disease was that of a twenty-three-year-old New Zealand man who died of liver failure. He was said to have eaten four or five steamed comfrey leaves every day for one to two weeks before he died.

Not having access to the complete case histories on these patients, I can make no statement of whether, in fact, comfrey is the only possible cause of the liver pathology. Even if it is, three cases out of tens of thousands, perhaps millions, of people who use comfrey is not statistically significant enough to ban its use. If our pharmaceutical industry were subject to such standards, we would have no drugs on the market at all.

Mark Blumenthal, editor of the highly respected magazine *HerbalGram,* states, "The comfrey incident might have looked different if it had been put into context of a toxicity scale. One such scale is the HERP index, which classifies the cancer-causing potentials of various substances. Extrapolating from the HERP index, former U.S. Department of Agriculture botanist James Duke, Ph.D., calculates that less than one-fifth an ounce of brown mustard is twice as cancer-causing as comfrey tea, which has roughly the same cancer-causing potential as a peanut butter sandwich. Wine is 144 times more cancer causing than an equal amount of comfrey tea."

But the comfrey controversy continues to rage. Banned in Canada, it is awaiting its fate in the United States. Some herbalists continue to use comfrey, basing their faith "on the empirical evidence of the conservative ages" and ignoring current data. Most herbalists are taking a discerning stand, recommending small amounts of comfrey for internal purposes (awaiting pending information) and continuing to use it externally. Some herbalists, caught up in the fervor of the tests, have discontinued its use altogether and urge others to do so. As for me, until the evidence and the hard facts are much more compelling, I will continue to use comfrey for myself and recommend it judiciously for my clients. Meanwhile, the Austrian company that conducted the original tests verified that the tests were inconclusive. In Japan, where the alkaloids were first discovered, the doctors still continue to recommend comfrey for cirrhosis of the liver.

Through it all, comfrey continues to grow unabashedly. A large luxurious plant, its carefree attitude seems to say, "If you doubt my safety, don't use me! I've been around a long time. I'll outlast the controversy."

Please note: Because of the controversy surrounding the safety of comfrey, I have left it out of many recipes throughout this book that I would otherwise have included it in. It is still included in several formulas for external use as there is absolutely *no* evidence or indication that it is harmful when used externally. It is best to avoid comfrey during pregnancy.

Cramp Bark
Viburnum opulus
Caprifoliaceae
Parts used: bark, young stems, and root bark

Possibly one of the best uterine nervines, cramp bark is remarkably effective for relaxing the uterine muscles. It is among my favorite remedies for menstrual cramps. I've also found it invaluable in cases of threatened miscarriage due to nerve stress and uterine tension. As Dr. John Christopher, one of the famous herb doctors of this century, writes in *The School of Natural Healing,* cramp bark is "possibly the best female regulator-relaxant that we have for the uterus and ovaries, and is especially useful for painful and difficult menstruation and for nervous afflictions during pregnancy that threaten abortion."

Rich in valerianic acid, the same constituent found in valerian, cramp bark's sedating and relaxing actions are specific to the reproductive system. A high tannin content makes it beneficial in cases of excessive menstrual bleeding. It is often recommended as a tonic and remedial herb for women who bleed excessively during their menstrual cycle. It is an invaluable herb for use during menopause by women who find themselves bleeding excessively due to changes in hormones. I've also found it helpful for women who have double menstrual cycles each month.

Though a strong medicinal herb, cramp bark can be safely used over an extended period of time. There are no known side effects or reported toxicities.

Dandelion
  Taraxacum officinale
  Compositae
  Parts used: root, leaf, and flowers

Though not generally considered an herb specifically for women's problems, dandelion is high in plant estrogens and is utilized in many formulas for women. It is one of the outstanding healing herbs, and like comfrey, has been lauded throughout the centuries by every great herbalist.

The root is considered the herb par excellence for the liver and is used for all liver disorders, digestive upsets, and gall bladder problems. As a specific herb for the liver, it also benefits the female reproductive system by helping to regulate and normalize hormone production.

The leaf, too, is of great value as a remedial herb. A specific for kidney and urinary problems, dandelion leaf is one of the safest and most effective diuretics available. But while its diuretic properties are as pronounced as those of most synthetic drugs it does not, as is so often the case with synthetic diuretics, deplete the system of potassium. In fact, dandelion leaf is rich in natural potassium, which feeds the body's own reserves.

Dandelion leaf is highly effective for menstrual bloating, PMS, and the breast tenderness associated with water retention. Its gentle but effective diuretic qualities aid the kidneys in eliminating excess water held in the body during hormonal changes. Dandelion leaf is also invaluable to women going through menopause. The root supplies essential nutrients needed by the liver to help produce and regulate the production of hormones. The leaf aids the kidneys in eliminating excess water and toxins from the system.

Both the root and leaf of dandelion provide essential nutrients to the system. Considered a food herb, dandelion is a rich source of vitamins A and C, iron, calcium, and potassium, as well as many other trace minerals. It has long been valued as an early spring vegetable and is eaten in many cultures in the world today. In the United States, with our unsophisticated taste buds, appreciation for the feisty bitter greens is low. But in France and many other European countries, its bitter flavor is prized and the greens are frequently included in salads.

Each cup of dandelion greens provides 7000–13,000 I.U. of vitamin A. You don't need to eat much to get your weekly quota. I generally recommend including a few dandelion greens in your evening salad. Marinating the steamed dandelion greens in an olive oil, honey, and vinegar dressing overnight almost completely rids them of bitterness. And it is a delicious way to enjoy this marvelous plant.

No known toxicity has ever been reported.

Dong Quai
  Angelica sinensis
  Umbelliferae
  Part used: root

This is one of the most useful of female tonic herbs. It has often been called "the female ginseng," though both men and women can use the herb successfully. Gentler in action than its Western cousin, angelica, dong quai (also called dong qui and tang kwei) is excellent when used over an extended period of time for strengthening and balancing the uterus. Though dong quai has no specific hormonal action, it exerts a regulating and normalizing influence on hormonal production through its positive action on the liver and endocrine system.

It can be used to treat almost every gynecological imbalance because of its strengthening and building qualities. It is nourishing to the blood and has a mild stimulating and cleansing action on the liver. It also has mild nervine properties which calm and relax the system.

Dong quai is a specific for menstrual irregularities, for dysmenorrhea, and for delayed or absent menstrual cycles. It is an excellent herb to help ease women into menopause and is highly recommended for use during menopause if difficulty arises. It is also a good toning herb to use for young women just entering their menstrual cycles. Its highly specific mode of action seems to benefit every woman's problem. It is nonestrogenic in action, yet balances and regulates hormonal production.

Dong quai may stimulate bleeding and is not recommended for use during menstruation or for the duration of pregnancy. If you are taking dong quai over an extended period of time, it is suggested that you use it until one week before the menstrual cycle, discontinue its use during the bleeding time, and resume it at the end of the cycle.

Dong quai is readily available in most herb stores, but better quality dong quai is often found in Chinese herb stores. It comes in many shapes and forms. The whole root is small and whitish and looks like carved ivory. It is definitely feminine in nature. The whole root may be grated or chopped and made into tea or tinctured. But the root in its whole form is a little difficult to work with. My favorite way to purchase the root is sliced and pressed. The root is shaved into whole slices, then pressed and cured. It is aromatic, exotic-looking (the pieces often look like the vagina), and easy to use. Dong quai is also available as powder, extract, and tincture.

A potent herb, dong quai is totally safe and nontoxic and can be used over an extended period of time. However, sometimes the strong flavor and action of the herb causes gastric upset. If so, take it in combination with other herbs. It is not recommended for use during menstruation or pregnancy.

False Unicorn Root
  Chamaelirium luteum
  Liliaceae
  Part used: root

Doug Elliott, famed woodsman, herbalist, and well-known storyteller from North Carolina, tells a story about false unicorn root in his book, *Roots: An Underground Botany and Forager's Guide.* "The long trailing roots of this plant, so the legend goes, possessed not only extremely beneficial healing properties, but extraordinary magic. So beneficial was it for the people that used it that the Devil himself became angered and tried to change the qualities of the root from good to bad. The power and goodness of this plant was so strong, however, that his attempts were always thwarted. Finally, the Devil flew into a rage and personally bit off every one of the roots. His rage was so searing that to this day the roots have not been able to grow back. But the remaining stub is still imbued with good medicine, and every spring it is able to put forth the tall spike of beautiful blazing-star blossoms as a reminder that the power of goodness can always avert the forces of evil."

This marvelous and very beautiful plant has long been honored for its beneficial effects on the female reproductive system. False unicorn root contains steroidal saponins which are precursors of estrogen. It is considered amphoteric in action, normalizing and balancing hormonal production. It is generally considered a uterine tonic and has been used in formulas to prevent miscarriage, to curb morning sickness, and to help reestablish muscle tone in prolapse of the uterus. Eclectic doctors in the early 1900s used false unicorn root for infertility in both men and women. Dr. King, a well-known eclectic physician and author of *the* authoritative eclectic textbook, *King's American Dispensatory,* stated, "I have found this plant to possess a decidedly beneficial influence in cases of sexual lassitude in both sexes. In diseases of the reproductive organs of females, and especially of the uterus, it is one of our most valuable agents, acting as a uterine tonic, and gradually removing abnormal conditions, while at the same time it imparts tone and vigor to the reproductive organs."

Because the plant is known by many common names and often confused with other plants, be certain you are purchasing *Chamaelireum luteum* for medicinal purposes. Do not confuse it with *Helonias bullata,* a federally recognized endangered species. False unicorn's gently curved root, which resembles a unicorn's horn, gives the plant its most common name. Its also called blazing star because of the spike of starlike blossoms that form on it each spring. The rather bitten-off appearance of the root gives rise to the legend of Devil's Bite, another common name for *Chamaelireum.* In several of the old textbooks, *Chamaelireum luteum* is often referred to as true unicorn root (known today as *Aletris farinosa*). Though they have been used interchangeably, probably more due to name than to action, *Chamaelireum* is used specifically for the reproductive system, while *Aletris,* or true unicorn root, has a direct action on the gastrointestinal tract and is used for digestive disturbances. I have not found them to be interchangeable in action.

Though this plant is considered a tonic herb and is often recommended for use over a long period of time, dosages should be regulated. *Large* amounts can cause vomiting and nausea. What constitutes a "large amount" I can only guess, because neither I nor my peers have had experience of this effect of *Chamaelirium* use. However, old textbooks suggest this as a possible side effect. I have always used false unicorn root in combination with other herbs and generally suggest three to four cups of tea daily.

Ginger
  Zingiber officinale
  Zingiberacea
  Part used: root

Both because of its delicious flavor and its remarkable healing qualities, ginger root has long been honored the world over. One of the most widely used medicinal herbs in modern China, it was first mentioned in the *Pen Tsao Ching (The Classic Book of Herbs)*, written by emperor Shen Nung around 3000 B.C. He valued ginger for much the same reasons we do today. An excellent warming herb, ginger promotes circulation throughout the entire system. It is especially indicated for women's reproductive problems, digestive disturbances, and for respiratory and bronchial problems. As an ancient Indian proverb puts it, "Every good quality is contained in ginger."

Ginger is a specific remedy where there are problems associated with congestion in the reproductive system. It directs blood to the pelvic area and helps relieve pelvic blockages. Its antispasmodic properties relax the smooth muscles and thus help alleviate menstrual cramps.

Ginger is also an excellent digestive aid and is as useful as any allopathic drug for both morning and motion sickness—without the side effects. A particularly pleasant way to enjoy this "medicine" is to suck on candied ginger. And hot ginger tea served with honey and lemon offers a delicious way to treat colds, menstrual and digestive cramps, morning sickness, and poor circulation. Placed directly over the pelvic area, ginger is also an effective poultice for cramps.

Ginger may be used either fresh or dried. Keep some of both on hand. Fresh ginger is sold in most supermarkets and natural food stores. The fresh root is more effective and tastes better than the dried root. It stores well in the refrigerator or a cool dry place. To use, just grate the root with a hand grater and use in teas, cooking, baths, and poultices. The dried ginger is good for blending into premixed herb formulas.

Because Ginger is traditionally used to promote menstruation, there is some concern in the scientific community that it may stimulate uterine contractions and thereby trigger miscarriage. In the long recorded history of ginger's use, there is no record of this ever occurring or any indication that it was ever used for this purpose. In fact, it is highly recommended and often used for morning sickness throughout pregnancy.

Ginger is a nontoxic culinary herb that can be safely used over an extended period of time. There are no known side effects from using ginger root.

Hops
  Humulus lupulus
  Cannabinaceae
  Parts used: female flower bracts and golden pollen (for medicine); young shoots and leaves (for food)

My two young hops vines come from hundred-year-old Vermont stock. Though only a couple of years old, they are already climbing the roof of the house. A vigorous grower, hops has been cultivated for hundreds of years. Pliny, the ancient Greek naturalist, grew hops in his garden and enjoyed the fresh young shots and leaves of the plant as an early spring vegetable. He also gave the plant its current name, lupus, or "willow wolf," in reference to the way the plant intertwines around willows and other plants. For centuries hops has been employed as a medicine and has been valued as a nerve tonic and sedative herb. It contains properties similar to those of valerian and may be used in much the same way, though valerian is stronger than hops as a pain reliever and muscle relaxant. Hops is rich in bitter principles and is considered a primary digestive sedative and nervine herb. It is also one of the best herbs for inducing sleep, and is used successfully for insomnia.

Now considered the primary herb in the brewing of beer, hops was originally added not for flavor, but for its natural preservative properties. Because of its extremely bitter flavor, it was not widely accepted at first and created quite a stir among the drinking crowd. But its digestive qualities and relaxing effect, along with the fact that it was so easy to cultivate, soon made it a favorite among brewers. Today it's the most widely used plant in the brewing industry. Many of the early herbalists considered beer brewed from hops to be a medicinal tonic and recommended it in moderation as a medical treatment for nervous stress.

Though it is most widely used today as a sedative for insomnia, stress, and tension, hops also has strong estrogenic properties. It is excellent for regulating and balancing hormonal production, and especially for treating those imbalances due to stress and nervousness. Hops is also useful for stimulating milk production.

Hops' estrogenic effect is a rather recent *rediscovery.* When hops was first cultivated in large amounts for the brewing industry, female hops pickers who worked in the fields for several weeks noted that their menstrual cycles arrived prematurely and that the young girls who picked hops got their menstrual cycles earlier. At the same time, men who picked hops were known to have a lessening of sexual desire. Hops began to develop a reputation as a sexual depressant for men and a sexual stimulant for women. This observation led to the discovery that hops contains high concentrations of plant hormones that have estrogenlike effects on the female system. The amount of these plant hormones found in fresh hops is considerable and the effects of using it for regulating and balancing the hormonal action is quite remarkable. The hormonal effects lessen as the plant dries. The suppressing factor for men also seems to be fairly pronounced and seems to be related to hormone-type chemicals found in hops, although the actual factors have not been determined. For its hormone-regulating action, the plant is more effective when used fresh. It is also effective if tinctured fresh.

For its nervine and sedative properties, the plant is most effective dried. In the late summer and early fall, the female plant produces hundreds of strobiles, or leaf bracts. They look like green pine cones and are often mistaken for the flower part. Tucked inside the leaf bract is the tiny fruit and a wonderful golden pollenlike substance (actually shiny glands) rich in lupulin, the active constituent of hops. This pollenlike substance is valued by herbalists for its sleep-inducing qualities and its gentle but powerful nervine properties.

Because hops is so rich in volatile oils, it is one of the traditional herbs used in sleep or dream pillows. The volatile oils are released by the pressure of sleeping on the pillow and affect the brain directly through the olfactory center. Hops may be used by itself in the pillow, but is often combined with roses, chamomile, and lavender. To stimulate dreams, mugwort may be added. (For directions on making dream pillows, see the entry for mugwort.)

The only known side effect of hops is rare cases of direct-contact dermatitis caused by harvesting the pollen (unless one were to consider its anaphrodisiac effects on men detrimental).

Lady's Mantle
Alchemilla vulgaris, A. xanthochlora
Rosaceae
Parts used: primarily the leaf, but often whole plant

For many centuries, lady's mantle was believed to possess magical healing qualities. Its botanical name, *Alchemilla,* reflects its alliance with the ancient alchemists, who used it as a base for many of their alchemical formulas. Dew seems naturally drawn to *Alchemilla,* and on any spring morning hundreds of sparkling jewels line the edges of the plant's rounded green leaves. This special moisture was traditionally considered a holy water that could purify and cleanse all illness.

My neighbor and herbalist friend, Adele Dawson, told me of the time she was leading a garden group through her semiwild gardens. The rain had just ceased that morning and the lady's mantle was gloriously bedecked with silvery dew. Adele was telling the group how the alchemists had once used this dew to treat most illnesses when a woman interrupted. She had a painful open sore on her lip that simply wasn't healing in spite of several medications. Did Adele think lady's mantle might help? Adele reiterated that what she was sharing was simply hearsay and that it wasn't known for sure what effects, if any, the plant might have. But the woman was eager to try, and she and Adele collected several dew-laden leaves. A few days later she called Adele to report that the herb had worked wonders and that she was busy planting a lady's mantle garden.

I knew little about this magical plant until I traveled to a women's healing festival in the high Alps of Switzerland. There the plant has a rich living tradition and is still honored as an herb for women. Found both in the wild and in cultivated gardens, it grows close to the earth, reflecting the earth's heartbeat. It collects the morning dew and wears it like fine jewels. Its flowers are small, greenish, and lacy like the green hair of the fairy queen, Tatiana.

It has been used the world over. Arabs claimed that regular use of lady's mantle would ensure fertility, and it's still sold in Middle Eastern markets for this purpose today. Culpepper, sometimes ridiculed for his bizarre remedies, used the herb for "flagging breasts," but interestingly, the women of Switzerland still use poultices of lady's mantle to firm and tone breast tissue.

The plant has been used throughout history to treat menstrual irregularities and difficulties. Rich concentrations of tannin make it especially valuable in curbing heavy or excessive menstrual flow. It also contains salicylic acid and has sedative properties, as evidenced by its ability to alleviate cramps and painful menstruation. Lady's mantle is commonly used in douche formulas for minor vaginal irritations. During the menopause years, the magic and gentle power of lady's mantle can be quite helpful.

Though difficult to find in herb stores, lady's mantle grows easily and should be cultivated in every woman's garden for its beauty and usefulness. It has no known toxic or side effects and is recommended both as a remedial and a tonic herb.

Lavender
Lavendula officinalis and related species
Labitatae
Parts used: flowers and leaves

Lavender is one of my favorite herbs for nerve stress and tension. It has a special affinity with women's spirit. Often thought of as a delicate ornamental, lavender is not only beautiful and aromatic, but pungent and powerful. Native to the Mediterranean, where it grows wild on the sun-drenched hills, it has traveled far and wide and has taken up residence in gardens everywhere. With its lovely, lavender blue flowers and fragrant pungent odor, it has entwined itself into the hearts of women everywhere and is a very useful herb if we but open to its strengthening and empowering qualities.

Lavender has long been valued for its ability to bring courage and strength to the user. Traditionally, sprigs of lavender were tied in bundles and placed in the hands of women in labor. Squeezing the fragrant bundles was believed to give them added strength and courage during childbirth. Lavender has long been used to calm nervous stress and is especially useful during menopause and menstrual difficulties. During the Middle Ages it was a valued remedy for hysteria. I've found it can be very healing to women undergoing periods of intense stress to place sprigs of lavender and lavender oil in the rooms of their home. Its essence brings calmness and inner strength to the user.

Though beautiful and fragrant, lavender is a potent herb and is best used in combination with other herbs when taken internally. For headaches, lavender should be combined with melissa (lemon balm) and skullcap. For muscle spasms and cramps, it works wonders when combined with valerian. For depression, lavender should be mixed with borage flowers. Because of its exceptionally high concentration of volatile oils, lavender is also very effective when used externally, and it is often found in herbal baths, steams, and massage oils. Hot water opens the pores, and the volatile oils are rapidly absorbed and diffused throughout the body. It's like immersing oneself in a giant cup of calming tea. Lavender baths are excellent for pregnant women and are highly recommended during the entire pregnancy. For people who are bedridden, lavender sponge baths are invigorating, refreshing, and revitalizing.

Today most women are introduced to lavender as a potpourri and sachet herb. Though certainly these are two of its many uses, lavender is far more than just a lovely aromatic flower. A potent healing plant, it is a crone among herbs—wise, ancient, and powerful.

There are no reported side effects or toxic reactions from the use of lavender.

Licorice
Glycyrrhiza globra
Leguminosae
Part used: roots

Long ago it was discovered that the root of Glycyrrhiza, when extracted and boiled down into a thick syrup, made not only a delicious candy but an effective herbal medicine. Some 50 percent sweeter than sugar, it effectively masks the taste of bitter medicinals and serves to harmonize or blend the other herbs in a formula.

Licorice has long been used as a remedy for stomach and heart problems, for indigestion, and for coughs and other bronchial and respiratory problems. It holds an honorary place in the *Pen Tsao Ching,* the classic book of herbs written by Shen Nung over 5000 years ago, and is still one of the most widely prescribed herbs in China, where it is termed the "peacemaker." As popular elsewhere in the world, licorice was a favorite remedy of the Greek, Roman, German, and English herbalists. Hippocrates, considered the father of modern medicine, used this herb frequently and called it *glukos riza (glycyrrhiza),* or sweet root. And the great herbalist/abbess Hildegard of Bingen included it in her materia medica.

Licorice is of special importance to women and has been used in women's formulas for centuries. It has estrogenic and other steroidal properties and is used to normalize and regulate hormone production. Glycyrrhizin, a major component of licorice root, is structurally similar to adrenal cortical hormones. It has proven especially helpful in treating adrenal exhaustion, infertility due to hormonal imbalance, menopausal dysfunction, and Addison's disease. Singers love to chew on the whole roots of licorice to soothe their throats and strengthen their voices. I particularly appreciate this herb because it weaves the flavors and effects of other herbs into a smooth mellow brew—very useful when you're mixing up some of those bitter herbs! However, not everyone appreciates the sweetness or enjoys the flavor of licorice. If too much is used in a formula, the tea becomes overly sweet and unpleasant-tasting. Some women have an aversion to its flavor.

Licorice has been used for centuries by large numbers of people and has, until recently, been considered completely safe and nontoxic. Quite by accident, a Dutch pharmacist discovered that a cough syrup made from licorice extract was very popular with people suffering from ulcers. Patients claimed their stomach ulcers responded far better to their licorice-based cough syrup than to their regular ulcer medication. Further studies confirmed these claims and extracts of licorice were commonly prescribed for stomach ulcers. But as the ulcers cleared up, patients began to experience water retention and elevated blood pressure. Upon further investigation, it was found that the high concentrations of glycyrheticinic acid in licorice achieved effects similar to those of the adrenal hormone ACTH; they caused retention of sodium and potassium and, consequently, a rise in blood pressure. Licorice quickly went from being a favorite medicinal herb to being an entry on the herbal "blacklist."

Though it is important to use licorice with caution if you're a possible candidate for high blood pressure and/or water retention, it should be noted that there have only been twenty-five reported cases of high blood pressure and or water retention caused by licorice root in the world. All of these were caused by very concentrated extracts of licorice and licorice products, not by the whole herb in its natural form. In fact, most of the cases of licorice overdose have resulted from eating too much licorice candy. Being a licorice lover myself, I can appreciate the dilemma. It is interesting to note that licorice in its natural form is high in asparagine, which counteracts the water-retentive activities of glycyrheticinic acid. However, since there have been several cases of licorice-related water retention leading to high blood pressure, pregnant women or women with a tendency toward high blood pressure, kidney, or urinary-tract problems should avoid extended use of licorice root.

Motherwort
  Leonurus cardiaca
  Labiatae
  Parts used: primarily the leaf, but often the whole plant

Motherwort has long been noted as an herb to treat both the heart and the female reproductive system. Its botanical name, *cardiaca,* stems from the Latin word for heart. Its common name, motherwort, means herb (wort) for the mother. In ancient days, motherwort's traits were described in such quaint language as "dispelling melancholy vapors from the heart," and for "calming the trembling of the heart." Seventeenth-century herbalist Nicholas Culpepper wrote of motherwort, "It took the name Motherwort because it settles mothers' wombs and is a wonderful help to women in their sore travail [delivery] . . . it also provoketh women's courses [menstruation]." In ancient China it was used to promote longevity due to its heart-strengthening abilities, and in Greece and Rome it was honored as a remedy for both physical and emotional problems associated with the heart.

Scientific studies conducted in China, Europe, and the United States confirm the traditional uses of motherwort. Concentrations of leonurine and stachydrine, chemical constituents that promote uterine contractions, have been found in motherwort, substantiating its traditional use for promoting delayed menstruation and hastening childbirth. Glycosides, also found in motherwort, have the effect of lowering blood pressure, which directly reduces stress on the heart muscle. (A Chinese legend has it that a sage who drank motherwort tea every day lived to be 300 years old.) Motherwort has amphoteric qualities that allow it to change and adapt to the situation. As well as being a stimulant to the system, it also has sedative qualities, making it both a uterine stimulant and a sedative.

Motherwort's strong emmenagogic properties stimulate menstrual bleeding, making it an herb of choice for delayed menstruation. It is also an excellent remedy for menstrual cramps, specifically those accompanied by scanty menses; because of its emmenagogic properties, it is not generally recommended for menstrual cramps associated with heavy bleeding. The amphoteric qualities of motherwort make it both a sedative and stimulant herb for menstrual stress, tension, delayed menstruation, water retention, and PMS. For insomnia and pain associated with menstruation and/or childbirth, motherwort is an excellent herb. I generally combine it with skullcap and/or valerian as a pain inhibitor.

Motherwort is a member of the mint family and, like most mints, it grows easily and willingly. Give it a little place in the garden with rich soil and plenty of moisture and it will thrive happily, providing years of bountiful harvest.

Because of its ability to stimulate uterine contractions, it is not recommended during pregnancy, except during the last few days, when it is used to stimulate labor. It is, however, used effectively and safely during the actual labor to facilitate childbirth.

Mugwort
  Artemisia vulgaris
  Compositae
  Part used: leaves

Mugwort is a member of a powerful family of herbs. Ruled by the goddess Artemis, this family has an illustrious past. Artemis, goddess of the moon, childbirth, and war, has been immortalized as a voluptuous blond. In fact, she was a woodland nymph who ran wild and free with the creatures of the woods, and was a protector of wild things, not the huntress she was later made out to be. Her plants were the fragrant herbs that grew freely on the hillsides. She used these aromatic plants for healing the wounded animals, aiding women at childbirth, and caring for the injured warriors who fled to the woodlands. Though the Artemisia family is somewhat ignored by current herbalists, it remains a favorite of many wise women practitioners and is cherished by elder herbalists. It is certainly a favorite of that wise old gypsy herbalist, Juliette de Bairacli Levy. She mentions it often in her talks about animals, child rearing, and women's problems.

Mugwort is one of the most common and widely used herbs of the Artemisia family. A vigorous, lanky plant, it is found growing wild throughout the world. It has a distinctive, refreshing fragrance that is reminiscent of the dry Mediterranean hillsides and the Aegean sea. The smell alone is invigorating and uplifting. Mugwort is often one of the herbs used in smudging, a ceremonial burning of herbs to uplift the spirit.

Mugwort is, without doubt, a bitter and has a valued place as a liver stimulant and digestive aid. (All bitter herbs stimulate gastric juices and aid in digestion.) Mugwort, in combination with other bitters, can be taken before and after meals to alleviate sluggish digestion, constipation, and gas. Mugwort also has mild nervine properties that are useful in treating stress and nervous tension. Because of its bitter principles and nervine qualities, Mugwort was one of the original herbs used in the brewing of herbal beers. Thus its name: the herb (wort, the original word for herb) of the cup (mug).

In China, mugwort is used extensively and, in the form of moxa, is a very familiar remedy. Moxa is a system of treatment, often combined with acupuncture, in which an herb is dried, rolled into cones (like incense cones) and placed on certain meridian points of the body. The moxa is then lit and allowed to burn down close to the skin. The heat and pungency of mugwort stimulate the point, and energy moves through. This treatment works wonderfully. Michael Tierra, author of *The Way of Herbs* and a licensed acupuncturist, states that, in some cases, it is more effective than acupuncture needles.

Mugwort is most widely known and respected for its beneficial effects on the female reproductive system. It is a uterine stimulant and aids in bringing on delayed or suppressed menstruation. When the menstrual cycle has been absent for a long time, mugwort is one of the best herbs to use. Ruled by Artemis, goddess of the moon, mugwort stimulates the natural rhythms in women. Drink mugwort tea for several days around the full moon—and wear red.

Mugwort is also excellent for young women just entering their moon time. It helps regulate their cycles and has been used for this purpose for centuries. Because of its extremely bitter taste, it should mixed with other herbs, such as melissa and lavender, or used in tincture form. Mugwort can also be used in the bath and is very pleasant when mixed with lavender flowers.

Because of its connection with Artemis and moon energy, mugwort is affiliated with the dream world. A favorite "dream time" herb, it is used in dream pillows, as a dream tea, and in dream balms to rub on the temples at night. It does activate and stimulate the dreams of many women and seems to help one to journey into the moon-time world.

To make a dream pillow, fold a piece of 8" x 8" fabric in half, and then sew two of its sides together, leaving one side open for stuffing. The fabric should be beautiful and soft. (Cotton and velvet are lovely to use.) Often women choose to embroider these pillows with moons and stars. Stuff the pillow with a dried mixture of:

4 parts mugwort
1 part lavender
1 part hops
1 part chamomile
1 part roses

Sew the pillow closed and place it next to your head at night. Fluff it before sleep to release the odors.

Mugwort is a nontoxic herb. Because of its emmenagogic properties, it is not recommended for use during pregnancy. It should be mentioned, however, that there have been no reported cases of miscarriage or abortion due to the use of mugwort, and in China it is actually used to prevent miscarriage.

Nettle
Urtica dioica
Urticaceae
Parts used: primarily the leaf, but often the whole plant, including the seed

Nettle may be one of the herbal wonders of the plant "queendom." Its usefulness can be traced to antiquity and its popularity as a medicine and a food has hardly waned. True, if you've never been introduced to the virtues of herbs, you've probably never even heard of the positive side of nettle. As a matter of fact, the very word probably conjures up visions of painful welts and dermatitis. But nettle is beloved in the herbal community and is one of my personal favorites.

Long valued as both a food and a medicine, nettle has an ardent following in many parts of the world. In ancient Greece and Rome it was cultivated as a tasty food and used medicinally in remedies for gout, rheumatism, and poisonous snake and insect bites. The tough fibers of the stalk were used in fabric making. Remnants of nettle fabric have been found in burial shrouds that date back to the Bronze Age, and it is still used today by survivalists to make cordage and fabric.

Nettle is a gourmet green. Lightly steamed tender young nettle tops, served with olive oil, lemon juice, and a bit of feta cheese, make a delicious dish. Another tasty way to prepare nettle is to gather the tender tops in the early spring and layer them, fresh and raw, in a large pot or glass jar. (Do not cook them.) Cover them with a mixture of one part cider vinegar and one part olive oil, then let the herbs marinate in the dressing for several weeks or months. The vinegar and oil will preserve and "pickle" them, and you can enjoy them all through the winter months. My favorite way to serve nettle is to use it in place of spinach in the Greek dish, spinach pie. Mixed with rice, ricotta, and feta cheese, steamed nettle is sandwiched between layers of butter and phyllo. Nettle is enjoyed a hundred different ways by wild food enthusiasts and has a zealous gourmet following.

Its reputation as a specific remedy for general female problems and as a tonic during pregnancy stems from Native American tradition. Native American women used it as a tonic throughout pregnancy and as a remedy for hemorrhaging during childbirth. Nettle is still used to enrich and increase the flow of milk and to aid in restoring and rebuilding the mother's energy following childbirth. As a general female tonic there are few substances that surpass it. It is excellent for young women entering their moon cycles and for women in menopause. Nettle helps reduce water retention, is excellent for correcting symptoms of PMS, and is a specific remedy for excessive menstruation. Because of its high vitamin K content, it helps control and prevent hemorrhaging. The high concentrations of vitamins and minerals found in nettle are easily assimilated and provide a wealth of nutrients to the system. It is one of the best sources of digestible plant iron and is rich in calcium, vitamin A, and chlorophyll.

Even the sting that gives nettle its nasty reputation has been used for centuries as a remedy—and a successful one at that—for arthritis and rheumatism. In a rather unusual treatment, the fresh stalks of nettle were used to flog the arthritic patient in the areas of inflammation. The formic acid (the same acid found in the sting of bees and ants) contained in the stinging hairs of the nettle agitates the skin instantly upon contact, causing irritation and raising welts. The counter irritation produced by nettle, as well as the fresh supply of blood carried to the area, alleviates the deeper pain and blockages of arthritic inflammation. This treatment is still used by some courageous and adventuresome souls today. One of the great characters in the herbal community, Dr. James Duke, Ph.D., a respected authority on medicinal plants for the U.S. Department of Agriculture, reported using the fresh juice of stinging nettles on his gout and experiencing instant relief.

A rather recent discovery regarding nettle is its use in the treatment of hay fever and other allergies. Quite by accident, a lab technician at the Eclectic Institute in Portland, Oregon, an institute that specializes in plant research and product development, found that taking freeze-dried nettle capsules almost instantaneously relieved his hay fever symptoms. Surprised and delighted, he shared this information with his colleagues. Several others in the lab tried it and reported the same excellent results. In response, the National College of Naturopathic Medicine in Portland, Oregon, conducted several clinical studies and confirmed the findings. Freeze-dried nettle capsules relieved symptoms of allergies and hay fever significantly in 70 percent of the test group. Research on whether fresh or dried nettle can also help allergy sufferers is underway.

If there is one plant that quickly teaches people how to talk to it, it is nettle. If you approach it wisely, quietly, and with respect, you can pick the plant with your bare hands. If you are uncertain, the plant will sting you rather rudely. I have always enjoyed showing people how to pick nettle greens in this way. At first, they can hardly believe that they are picking the greens with their bare hands. It is like a delicate dance between the plant and the harvester. But, watch out! If you get out of rhythm, or move too quickly, you'll probably be stung!

Altogether, nettle is a fine food, medicine, and powerful plant. It is recommended for use over an extended period of time. Contact with the fresh plant can produce a painful dermatitis, however. (The best remedy for nettle rash is nettle juice and/or fresh yellow dock leaf poultices.) There have been a few reported cases of swollen membranes and allergiclike reactions when the plant has been ingested raw! I always recommended that the plant be cooked, dried, or pickled before use, though I myself enjoy the taste of nettles eaten fresh in the field.

Pennyroyal
   Hedeoma pulegioides (American pennyroyal) and *Mentha pulegium*
   Labiatae
   Parts used: leaves and flowers

Lovely, fragrant, and unassuming, pennyroyal has acquired one of the worst, and in some ways the most undeserved, reputations among herbs. Historically noteworthy, it was used by the legendary herbalists Gerard, Culpepper, Dioscorides, and Pliny, and enjoyed an honored spot in the repertoire of healing herbs for several centuries. At one time considered a safe, nontoxic plant, it was included in the *U.S. Pharmacopoeia* from 1831 until 1931. It was indicated for colds, flus, digestive disturbances, suppressed menstruation, and other women's complaints.

In the early 1900s, chemists began distilling the oil from the plant. It was assumed, since the herb was such an innocuous substance, that the oil would be safe as well. And it is, *so long as it is used properly and for its intended purpose. The essential oil of pennyroyal is extremely potent. (Most essential oils are.) Taken internally, even in small doses, pennyroyal oil can be extremely toxic.* As a menstrual aid, pennyroyal herb carries blood flow to the pelvis and stimulates uterine contractions. It has also been used as an abortifacient. Sometimes women have assumed that, because the herb was effective, the oil would work even better as an abortifacient. It has been a fatal assumption. In 1970 two young women died from drinking pennyroyal oil. Though bottles of the essential oil are clearly labeled "toxic" and herb books state the precautions, these women ignored the warnings. Doses as small as two teaspoons of essential oil can send a woman into convulsions.

It is important, however, not to confuse pennyroyal herb and pennyroyal oil. Pennyroyal herb is nontoxic and safe to use. It is an excellent herb for colds, stomach upsets, and suppressed menstruation. It is simply one of the best herbs known to stimulate blood flow to the pelvis and to stimulate suppressed menstruation. It is an excellent herb for alleviating menstrual cramps and tension. It is also recommended during labor to facilitate contractions and to stimulate delayed or prolonged labor. *But the herb has been used to stimulate abortions and is not recommended to use during the early trimesters of pregnancy.*

Though the oil has such a deadly reputation, it, too, has many time-honored uses. Pennyroyal's name is derived from the Latin word *pulex,* which means flea. And pennyroyal oil is an excellent flea and insect repellent. It is used in many commercial brands of insect repellents. When backpacking, I look for a campsite near a fresh patch of pennyroyal. It helps keep the bugs away, makes a delicious, refreshing tea, and is fragrant and is lovely to lie beside, a true friend in the wild.

Pennyroyal oil should only be used externally! Rubbed over the pelvic region (being careful to keep it away from the sensitive vaginal lips), pennyroyal oil will successfully ease cramps and promote the menstrual cycle. But use the oil sparingly. It is very potent and will have a dramatic effect if overused.

Pennyroyal herb, as well as pennyroyal oil, has a reputation as an abortifacient. For this purpose, however, the herb must be drunk in enormous quantities and be combined with other uterine stimulants, so there is little danger of accidentally drinking too much pennyroyal tea. It works by stimulating uterine contractions and causing blood to flow to the pelvic region. The herb is nontoxic and doesn't poison the system as is often purported. It would take an estimated seventy-five gallons of tea to equal the potentially toxic dose of pennyroyal oil. Women who have drunk large amounts of the herb tea in hopes of aborting, but who have failed to do so, have had healthy children. Pennyroyal herb does not poison the fetus.

Though I would like to see the pennyroyal controversy placed in proper perspective, there are strong precautions that should be heeded when using the herb. Both the leaf and the oil should be avoided when pregnant. *The* oil *of pennyroyal should always be used with respect, knowledge, and caution. Never take pennyroyal oil internally.*

Raspberry Leaf
Rubus idaeus, R. strigosus
Rosaceae
Parts Used: primarily the leaf, but often the whole plant for medicinal purposes.

For centuries raspberry leaf was recognized as a powerful uterine tonic by indigenous people throughout the world, but the herb's uses as an aid in childbirth were largely ignored in the West until the 1940s. At that time, several reports were published in prestigious medical journals extolling raspberry leaf's extraordinary effects on the uterus and pelvic region, and the herb quickly became famous in the United States and Europe. Such scientific studies and the traditional uses of the raspberry leaf both confirm its role as an exceptional aid in pregnancy and childbirth.

The presence of fragarine, an alkaloid found in rich concentrations in the leaf, contributes to the plant's potency as a pregnancy tonic. Fragarine, in combination with several other of the plant's constituents, serves to tone and relax the pelvic and uterine muscles. It is a rich source of many vitamins and minerals and is particularly high in calcium, iron, phosphorus, potassium, and vitamins B, C, and E.

In the early days of my herb shop, if anyone walked in to purchase raspberry leaf, they were either pregnant or buying the herb for someone who was. This wonderful tonic herb was largely ignored by everyone else. Fortunately, things have changed. Raspberry leaf is now recognized not only for its value during pregnancy, but also as a woman's herb in general. (It's also a great herb for men.) Its astringent properties make it a good remedy for excessive menstruation. The high concentration of vitamins and minerals, especially calcium and iron, make raspberry a wonderful nutritive tonic for use during all of the cycles of womanhood.

Raspberry leaf serves as an excellent all-purpose herb, with many other applications in herbal medicine. Because of its high concentrations of tannin, it is a valued remedy for diarrhea and dysentery. Recent studies demonstrate its usefulness in lowering blood-sugar levels. It is also used for reducing fevers and stopping excessive bleeding. It can be an effective treatment for many childhood illnesses, including fevers and diarrhea, and it is a fine general tonic for building healthy bones and teeth.

Considered by many the "herb supreme" for pregnant women, raspberry leaf is a safe, nutritive, uterine tonic. It is generally recommended for use during the entire nine months of pregnancy. As a pregnancy tonic, it provides a rich supply of vitamins and minerals. It supplies the extra calcium and iron needed during this period and, because of its fragarine content, actually tones and firms the pelvic muscles. It has amphoteric, or adaptive, qualities. Raspberry leaf serves as both a uterine relaxant and stimulant, thus causing a regulating action in the uterus. Raspberry leaf also aids in cleansing the afterbirth from the system and is used to enrich and increase the flow of milk.

Both cultivated and wild raspberry leaves are used. *Rubus idaeus,* the cultivated variety, is generally available in most herb stores. But the wild variety, *R. strigosus,* is considered more potent and carries with it the indescribable, yet discernable, strength and vitality of things that belong to the wilderness. If you have raspberry growing near you, pick the leaves (be sure they are unsprayed), dry them, or use them fresh. Raspberry leaf tea is a refreshing beverage and can be drunk warm or at room temperature.

The herb has no contraindications, does not produce any residual side effects, and is generally considered a safe and effective herb in all of the above situations. Raspberry leaf tea is one of those herbs that has been used for centuries by many different people around the world. Though it has received good press by the scientific community, its real value has been established by the actual experience of thousands of women over hundreds of years.

Shepherd's Purse
  Capsella bursa pastoris
  Cruciferae
  Parts used: leaves, stems, and seeds

Also called mother's heart, this humble little weed is often neglected as a healing herb. Yet it is one of the best herbs to stop hemorrhaging and has a prominent place in the first-aid kits of most midwives. Its high concentrations of tannin, tyramine, and other amines are what make it such an excellent remedy for excessive bleeding after childbirth. Though the scientific community has largely ignored it, tests have confirmed that shepherd's purse is high in oxytocin, a uterine contractor.

I've found the herb most beneficial as a specific remedy for hemorrhaging and excessive menstrual flow. Either by itself or combined with yarrow and taken frequently throughout the day, it will arrest heavy bleeding. Taken several days before the onset of menorrhagia, it will lessen the flow considerably. Its antibleeding properties also make shepherd's purse a useful first-aid item for nosebleeds, deep wounds, and cuts. Because of its high concentrations of tannin, it can be used to treat diarrhea and dysentery, though there are other herbs more specific for these problems.

Shepherd's purse grows wild throughout the United States and is especially found in gardens, orchards, and fields. It is a rather inconspicuous little plant, named after its heart-shaped seed packets. Shepherd's purse does not have a long shelf life and is most effective when used fresh. It also tinctures easily and can be tinctured fresh from the field or garden. If you're lucky enough to have a good supply of shepherd's purse growing wild near you, encourage its growth. It is a wonderful little first-aid herb. The young leaves have a peppery, mustardlike flavor and may be added to salads and other vegetable dishes.

There are no known toxic side effects or reported cases of toxicity from using shepherd's purse, even over an extended period of time.

Squaw Vine
Mitchella repens
Rubiaceae
Part used: leaves; berries edible

A low-growing forest creeper, Mitchella is a delight to come upon in densely carpeted forests. Also known as partridge berry, Mitchella produces bright-red fruit in the late fall. Though somewhat inconspicuous in its native habitat, this little herb has a well-earned reputation as a woman's tonic. Indigenous to the North American continent, squaw vine was first used by Native American women to aid in pregnancy and childbirth. Considered one of the finest herbs for toning and nourishing the uterus, squaw vine is often mixed with raspberry leaf for the perfect pregnancy tonic. The combination is highly valued by women who have previously had difficult childbirths. Used throughout pregnancy, it helps ensure a smooth, safe birth.

Squaw vine is recommended for infertility resulting from hormone imbalance. Its high concentrations of saponins provide the necessary building blocks for balanced hormone production. It is rather humbling to realize how many plant allies provide steroidal substances needed for human reproduction!

It is also a favorite herb for painful, irregular menstruation. Taken for several weeks or months, it will often correct even the most persistent menstrual problems. Squaw vine is equally good for men. It is used in formulas for infertility due to low sperm count and is also an excellent tonic for the prostate gland.

A true tonic herb, squaw vine is nontoxic and produces no residual buildup or toxicity, even when used over an extended period of time.

Valerian
Valeriana officinalis and related species
Valerianaceae
Part used: root

One of the most potent herbs known for the nervous system, valerian is powerful, safe, and very effective. Its name is derived from the Latin word *valere,* "to be well," "be strong." It has a long and colorful history and has been highly regarded as an herbal medicine for centuries. Hildegard of Bingin, famous abbess/herbalist of Germany, used it as a sedative in the twelfth century. In the 1500s Gerard claimed it to be one of the most popular remedies of his time. Today, in spite of its distinct and somewhat offensive odor, valerian continues to be one of the most popular medicinal herbs in the world. In Europe, where it has been known for centuries, it is used in hundreds of over-the-counter drugs and is relied on as a medicine for tension.

There is no finer herb for stress and nervous-system disorders. Though potent, it is perfectly safe to use and is neither habit-forming nor addictive. Valerian is effective both as a long-term nerve tonic and as a remedy for acute problems such as headaches and pain. It is one of the best herbs known for insomnia and/or restless sleep. Having once gone through a bout of insomnia, I know how well valerian works. I kept a bottle of the tincture by my bed, and when I would wake in the night, haunted by the troubles of the day, I'd take a few sips of the tincture and read a paragraph or two from a boring book, and I'd be back to sleep in no time.

Valerian has powerful tonic effects on the heart and is often recommended in combination with hawthorne berries for high blood pressure and irregular heartbeat. I've also used it effectively in combination with hawthorn berries for altitude sickness. On a trip in the high Andes, I and a group of women friends relied heavily on our valerian-hawthorn tincture to curb altitude sickness.

A favorite antispasmodic herb, valerian relieves the symptoms of spastic coughing and muscle twitching and is specific whenever there is muscle and joint tension. The herb can be mixed with licorice root, coltsfoot, and mullein leaf for a soothing cough remedy.

Sometimes called moon root and Undine's herb, valerian has a special affinity with women. Because of its muscle-relaxant properties, it is an excellent treatment for alleviating menstrual tension and stress. Combined with cramp bark, it effectively relieves menstrual cramps. During menopause, valerian provides stability and grounding in what is sometimes a traumatic time for women. Though the smell of valerian is a bit ripe at times, I frequently combine it with ginger and lavender in a massage oil for menstrual cramps. This oil has also been used successfully during labor.

Often compared to the smell of dirty socks, the odor of valerian is offensive to many users. But, oddly enough, others love it. I find it earthy, rich, and pungent. The odor is actually an indicator of the strength of the root: the riper the better. The flavor is not like the odor; it definitely doesn't *taste* like dirty socks! When fresh, the odor is faint and somewhat sweet. As the plant dries, the active ingredients are released and the odor becomes more pronounced.

Valerian is dose-dependent; in other words, in order to be effective, sufficient quantities must be used. For some women, a sufficient amount may be one-fourth teaspoon of the tincture (or one-fourth cup of the tea) taken three times daily. For others, it may be necessary to take upwards of one to two teaspoons of tincture (or a couple of cups of tea) every few hours. Don't be afraid to take adequate amounts of this herb. Begin with low doses and increase until you feel the relaxing effects of valerian. The herb is non-habit forming and will not make the user groggy. You can tell that you have taken too much valerian if you experience either a "rubbery" feeling in your muscles—as if they are *too* relaxed—or a feeling of heaviness. Cut back the dosage so that you feel relaxed but alert.

Though generally considered an altogether safe, nontoxic herb, valerian does have one rather unusual characteristic that is interesting to know about. High concentrations of essential oils, including isovalerianic acid and valerianic acid, contribute to the relaxing effects of valerian. A conversion is necessary in the digestive process for these acids to be effectively used by the system as nervines and sedatives. If this conversion doesn't take place, valerian may act as a stimulant and further agitate an already stressed person. The first time you use valerian, be aware of this possibility. Some 95 percent of the people who use valerian find it a relaxing sedative herb. In about 5 percent of the population, valerian acts as a stimulant. If you're one of the 5 percent, discontinue use.

Vitex
   Vitex agnus casus
   Verbenaceae
   Parts used: fruit and berries

Named agnus casus (chaste) by the Greeks, vitex, or chaste tree, early gained a reputation for calming sexual passions. The Arabs used it to cure insanity and it is still available in Egyptian bazaars today as a "calming agent in hysteria." Gerard, a famous herbalist of the 1500s, wrote that "the seeds and leaves are good against pain and inflammations of the uterus." Vitex was fed to temple priestesses to suppress libido and used by monks and priests to subdue desire, which is the source of its folk names "monk's pepper" and "chaste berry." In some Mediterranean countries, the lovely flowers are still strewn before the feet of novices as they enter the temples. A chaste berry syrup was available in France in the 1800s and used for "repressing the desires of Venus." Vitex is not a true anaphrodisiac, however. Nor is it sexually stimulating, as a French herbalist, Cazin, believed it to be. The truth is that vitex neither suppresses nor increases libido. It is a normalizing herb for the reproductive system. In the words of David Hoffman, "Vitex will always enable what is appropriate to occur."

Long acknowledged in the ancient world as a valuable medicinal herb, this lovely shrub has only recently been introduced into the herbal materia medica of the United States. Because of the interest surrounding the herb, extensive research and clinical studies have been conducted on it and much is known about the effects of the plant on the human body. Vitex has a stimulating effect on the pituitary gland, which, among other functions, regulates and normalizes hormone production. Studies verify that vitex increases the production of luteinizing hormones, enhancing the progesterone cycle. At the same time it inhibits the release of the follicle-stimulating hormone, FSH, and normalizes the estrogen cycle. It is an excellent herb for restoring and regulating the estrogen/progesterone balance.

Vitex's normalizing and balancing action is particularly beneficial in treating painful and irregular menstruation, infertility, PMS, menopausal problems, and other hormonal imbalances. It has been found helpful in the treatment of endometriosis and is also useful in normalizing the system after discontinuing birth control pills. Because it stimulates the production of prolactin, vitex is often given to nursing mothers to help ensure a healthy supply of milk. As a birthing aid and to stimulate the milk flow, take vitex one week before the birthing date and for ten days thereafter.

Vitex may be used for acute situations but it is most effective if taken over a prolonged period of time. For chronic problems, such as menstrual irregularities, endometriosis, infertility, and delayed menstruation, vitex should be taken for up to one year or longer. No side effects have ever been reported from extensive and extended use of this plant. It is one of the most useful herbs for women and should definitely be included in your herbal pantry.

Wild Yam
Dioscorea villosa, D. paniculata, D. mexicana, and related species
Dioscoreaceae
Part used: root

Wild yam is valued both in the herbal and scientific communities for its powerful effect on regulating hormone production. Steroidal saponins that yield diosgenin are found in high concentrations in many species of wild yam. These plant steroids provide essential building blocks needed in the production of both progesterone and cortisone. Until recently, wild yam was the sole source of the diosgenin used in the production of contraceptive pills. It also provides the base of many different steroidal drugs manufactured today. Amazingly, 50 percent of the raw material needed for steroid synthesis is still provided by wild yam. Considered the most widely used herb in the world today, it is estimated that over two hundred million prescriptions a year are sold containing its derivatives.

Long before wild yam was used in the synthesis of sex hormones and contraceptives, it was highly regarded by the herbal community and used in its entirety for normalizing hormone production. Though primarily regarded as a progesterone-producing herb, it acts to regulate the ratio of progesterone to estrogen in the system.

Unlike contraceptives synthesized from the plant, wild yam in its natural state has no known side effects and is nontoxic. It is one of the most widely used herbs for problems caused by hormone imbalance and is used effectively for menstrual distress, miscarriage, infertility, menopause and endometriosis.

But it also has many other properties and has been used in folk medicine over the centuries for many different ailments. It is commonly recommended for liver complaints, digestive disturbances, morning sickness, and lung inflammation. Greatly valued by Chinese herbalists, wild yam was first mentioned in the *Pen Tsao Ching* in 25 B.C. It is still used in China for problems associated with the spleen, kidneys, liver, and lungs.

As a primary liver tonic herb, wild yam activates and stimulates liver activity. High concentrations of steroidal saponins provide the building blocks required by the liver to synthesize sex hormones. Whenever both the liver and reproductive system are implicated as the cause of hormone imbalance, wild yam is the herb of choice to use in the formula.

Wild yam has no known side effects and is nontoxic. It can be used over an extended period of time with no harmful effects.

Yarrow
Achillea millefolium
Compositae
Part used: leaves and flowers

When Achilles was born, his mother, holding him firmly by the heel, dipped him head first in a bath of yarrow tea. Wise Woman that she was, she knew that this would protect him from all harm. And it did—until he was wounded in the very heel his mother had held him by. Nonetheless, the yarrow bath had protected him in other respects, and during the Trojan wars Achilles used yarrow to stanch the bleeding of his soldiers. To this day, yarrow is considered a prime remedy for wounds and hemorrhaging. When regular medicine was in short supply during World War I, yarrow was used on the wounds of injured soldiers.

The legends surrounding yarrow are many. When the Chinese first created the oracle for consulting the I Ching, an ancient book of wisdom, the area around the oracle was cleared. The first plant to grow back was yarrow. The long, strong stalks of the yarrow were perfect for "casting" or consulting the oracle. In many cases, coins have replaced the yarrow stalks today, but the traditional consultant still uses this time-honored method.

Yarrow has a long association with witchcraft, which essentially means it was used by the wise women healers of Europe. Since much of what comes to us from Europe about women during the Middle Ages is still shrouded in the darkness and the terror of the witch-hunts, many of the healing herbs they used still bear the scars of those horrid times. Yarrow, an herb much used by the wise women for female disorders, carries tales of being used as a "flying herb" (would that it was!), used in "dark brews," and for "calling in the spirits."

Both beautiful and powerful, yarrow has figured as a prominent healing herb in both the physical and spiritual realms. Though not generally considered a specific herb for women, I include it in this list of women's herbs because it is highly effective as a treatment for easing menstrual cramps and aiding in labor and childbirth. Though it serves many other purposes, it deserves a prime place on this woman's materia medica.

Either used alone or in combination with shepherd's purse, yarrow will decrease heavy menstrual bleeding. Taken several days before the menstrual cycle begins, it serves to lessen the flow and prevent the problem of cyclic hemorrhaging. Its antibleeding properties are due to concentrations of tannin and astringent actions. It is often combined with shepherd's purse and used by midwives to prevent excessive bleeding following childbirth.

Amphoretic in action, yarrow has both stimulating and sedative actions which excite the uterine muscles while at the same time relaxing them. Yarrow is useful for stimulating delayed or absent menstrual cycles. Either by itself or combined with uterine relaxants, yarrow helps ease menstrual cramps and uterine tension.

High concentrations of volatile oils in yarrow stimulate blood flow to the surface of the skin and aid in elimination via the pores. It is one of the best diaphoretics known and is an excellent aid during fevers and pelvic congestion.

I have generally recommended the white yarrow commonly found growing wild throughout the United States as the most medicinal of the yarrows. However, when I was recently in Switzerland teaching at a large women's conference, the audience quickly informed me that the pink yarrow was the strongest of the medicinal yarrows. In the alpine meadows throughout Switzerland, it was the *pink* yarrow that was found growing in wild profusion.

Through centuries of recorded use and scores of clinical studies, yarrow has proved a safe, nontoxic herb. However, because of its stimulating action on the uterine muscles, it is one of the herbs generally not recommended for use during the early stages of pregnancy. I might add, however, that yarrow has never been known to precipitate an abortion and, as far as I know, has never been used for this purpose.

Books on Healing, Health, and Herbs

FOUR BASIC HERBALS FOR THE BEGINNER/INTERMEDIATE

There are many excellent herbals available. The following are the medicinal herb books I recommend most often for beginner/intermediate herbalists. Each of these books gives a clear overview of herbalism and provides accurate, sincere information. And each has been written by an herbal practitioner.

❦ *The Family Herbal* by Barbara and Peter Theiss. Rochester, VT. Healing Arts Press, 1989.

Applying their experience as parents, pharmacists, and herbalists, the Theisses have written an excellent beginner's guide to the practical application of medicinal plants in family health care. The book has wonderful photographs.

❦ *The Holistic Herbal* by David Hoffman. Scotland: Findhorn Press, 1983.

David Hoffman's book explores herbology in the context of Gaia, the living earth. It's a beautiful weaving together of both the scientific and the spiritual aspects of herbs and comes recommended for the beginner.

❦ *A Modern Herbal* by Mrs. Maude Grieve. New York: Dover Publications, 1971.

Originally published in the 1930s, this is hardly a "modern herbal" anymore, but nevertheless, it is a wonderful and informative two-volume set. *A Modern Herbal* is still many herbalists' favorite book. It contains information on the growing, cooking, medicinal uses, and chemical constituents of herbs.

❦ *The Way of Herbs* by Michael Tierra. New York: Simon & Schuster, 1990.

Drawing from his extensive studies of East Indian, Native American, Ayurvedic, and Chinese herbal systems, Tierra combines their various practices into a harmonious blend he terms "Planetary Herbology."

HERB BOOKS ESPECIALLY FOR WOMEN

As more and more women become interested in herbs, there is a growing number of herbals being written by and for women. These are some of my favorite *medicinal herb books for women*.

❦ *Artemis Speaks: V.B.A.C. Stories and Natural Childbirth Information* by Nan Koehler. Occidental, CA: Jerald R. Brown, 1985. Available from Jerald R. Brown, Inc., 17440 Taylor Lane, Occidental, CA 95465.

Primarily an herbal about natural childbirth and pregnancy, this book offers valuable information for pregnant women. It contains a special section on vaginal birth after caesarean (V.B.A.C.), which includes information from women who have had V.B.A.C. It is a wonderful, earthy guidebook written by an experienced herbalist and midwife.

❦ *Healing Yourself During Pregnancy* by Joy Gardner. Freedom, CA: Crossing Press, 1990.

This is a practical, sensitive book for the pregnant woman. A potpourri of information, comfort, and experience from a very talented herbalist.

❦ *Hygieia: A Woman's Herbal* by Jeannine Parvati. Monroe, UT: Freestone Press, 1978.

A woman's classic, this book is full of wonderful lore, formulas, and herbal information written by an inspiring herbalist and midwife.

❦ *Natural Child Care* by Maribeth Riggs.

Though not a book on women's health, this herbal will prove invaluable to many women who are seeking natural and herbal remedies for children. It provides sound practical holistic health strategies for infants and children.

❦ *Natural Healing in Gynecology* by Rina Nissim. New York, NY: Pandora Press, 1986.

This is a very comprehensive approach to alternative healing methods for women's health problems. Rina's book is of special interest because she is able to compare the relative success rates of Western and Eastern therapies using herbal and natural methods.

❦ *Nature's Children* by Juliette de Baircli Levy.

This is one of my favorite little herbal tomes. Juliette writes poetically and spiritedly about the uses of herbs for children. A classic, this book is recommended for women to read regardless of whether they have children or not.

❦ *Women's Herbs: Remembering Our Roots* by Deb Soule. ME: Blackberry Books, forthcoming.

This is a sensitive and wise approach to herbalism and women. Deb Soule is a practicing herbalist who writes from personal experience.

❦ *The Wise Woman Herbal for the Childbearing Years* by Susun Weed. Woodstock, NY: Ash Tree Publishing, 1986.

A favorite herbal about pregnancy, childbirth, and the newborn, written in simple, easy-to-understand language.

❦ *The Wise Woman Herbal for the Menopausal Years* by Susun Weed. Woodstock, NY: Ash Tree Publishing, 1992.

An excellent wise woman book full of practical wisdom for the menopausal woman.

A SELECTION OF OTHER GOOD HERBALS

These are some of my other favorite books about herbs. All are excellent, fascinating, and worth reading.

❦ *American Materia Medica Therapeutics and Pharmacognosy,* edited by Finely Ellingwood. Portland, OR: Eclectic Medical Publications, 1983. Available from Eclectic Medical Publications, 11231 S.E. Market St., Portland, OR.

Another of the outstanding textbooks published by the Eclectic Medical Society in the early 1900s. It is still an excellent reference and is used by serious students of herbalism.

❦ *Ayurveda, the Science of Self-Healing* by Dr. Vasant Lad. Santa Fe, NM: Lotus Press, 1984.

This fine introduction to the basic principles of Ayurvedic herbal medicine is written by one of the outstanding Ayurvedic practitioners in this country.

❦ *Back to Eden* by Jethro Kloss. Loma Linda, CA: Back to Eden Books, 1988.

This classic is often termed the herbal "bible." It is full of excellent information, formulas, and recipes.

❦ *Between Heaven and Earth* by Efrem and Harriet Korngold. New York: Ballantine Books, 1991.

This is a lucid and penetrating introduction to Chinese medicine.

❦ *Discovering Wild Plants* by Janice Schofield. Anchorage, AK: Northwest Books. 1989.

This is one of my favorite wild herb identification books. The pictures are excellent and the information about each plant is interesting and thorough. The book covers the edible and medicinal uses of herbs and provides recipes for each plant. Though the book focuses on the herbs of the Pacific Northwest, I have found it applicable to plants on the East Coast as well.

❦ *The Healing Herbs* by Michael Castleman. Emmaus, PA: Rodale Press, 1991.

This is one of my favorite sources of information on both the scientific and folkloric aspects of herbs. Michael has done an outstanding job of researching the historical uses of plants.

❦ *Herbal Medicine* by Rudolf Fritz Weiss, M.D. U.S. distributor: Medicina Biologica, Portland, OR.

An outstanding medical botanical reference, this book is particulary recommended for the more advanced student of herbalism.

❦ *The Herbs of Life* by Lesley Tierra. Freedom, CA. Crossing Press, 1992.

An excellent and simple explanation of Chinese and Western herbology. This book was written for the beginner/intermediate student and is an excellent introduction to medicinal herbology.

❦ *Herbs: Partners in Life* by Adele Dawson. Rochester, VT: Inner Traditions, 1992.

Written by one of my favorite elder herbalists, this book is alive with the spirit, essence, and wisdom of herbalism.

❦ *Herbs and Things* by Jeanne Rose. New York: Grosset and Dunlap, 1969.

Another of the herbal classics, Jeanne's book is a wealth of information, historical references, recipes, and formulas.

❦ *The Illustrated Herbal Encyclopedia* by Kathi Keville. New York: Bantam Doubleday, 1992.

This comprehensive encyclopedia is written by a well-known herbalist. It is beautifully illustrated with color photographs.

❦ *The Illustrated Herbal Handbook* by Juliette de Bairacli Levy. London: Faber and Faber, 1982.

Juliette has been my mentor and friend for many years, and all her herbals are favorites of mine. Each captures the spirit and essence of herbs, and brings the art of herbalism alive. *The Illustrated Herbal Handbook* is her general herbal. *Nature's Children* is an excellent book on raising children herbally. Juliette also has several herbal books on animals: *The Complete Herbal Handbook for Farm and Stable, The Complete Herbal Book for the Dog,* and *Cats Naturally.*

❦ *King's American Dispensatory,* edited by Harvey W. Felter. Portland, OR: Eclectic Medical Publications, 1983. Available from Eclectic Medical Publications, 11231 S.E. Market Street, Portland, OR.

First published during the latter part of the nineteenth century, this outstanding two-volume materia medica is a landmark work on eclectic medicine and the clinical uses of North American herbs.

❦ *Medicinal Plants of the Mountain Southwest* by Michael Moore. Santa Fe, NM: Museum of New Mexico Press, 1979

One of the great herbalists of our day, Michael Moore writes in a highly informative and entertaining manner. I love all his books. This one is a jewel.

❦ *The New Age Herbalist* by Richard Mabey. New York: Collier Books/Macmillan, 1988.

A visual treat, this well-organized herbal is full of photos and drawings. It covers the body systems and the corresponding herbs in a clear, succinct manner and provides very up-to-date material. This is the "coffee table" medicinal herbal.

❦ *Roots: An Underground Botany and Forager's Guide* by Douglas B. Elliott. Old Greenwich, CT: Chatman Press, 1976.

Doug is a fascinating storyteller, a woodsman, and an herbalist. His book offers all herb lovers a rare opportunity: the chance to look and learn about the mysterious "other half" of plant life that lies just beneath our feet.

❧ *School of Natural Healing* by Dr. John Christopher. Provo, UT: Biworld, 1976.

This is an herbal classic written by one of the great herb doctors of the century. *The School of Natural Healing* was originally published as Dr. Christopher's home study course and makes an excellent reference textbook.

❧ *The Web That Has No Weaver* by Ted Kaptchuk. New York: Congdon and Weed, 1983.

An excellent introduction to Chinese medicine, this is another of my favorite books on this ancient system of healing.

GENERAL BOOKS ON WOMEN'S HEALTH

Although several of the following books on women's health do not offer herbal or natural therapies, they provide conventional and allopathic remedies and are excellent general references. Use them in conjunction with books offering natural therapies to arrive at more educated and informed decisions. Some have excellent pictures of the female anatomy and are wonderful just to look at.

❧ *The Complete Guide to Women's Health,* by Carroll and Bruce Shephard. New York: Penguin Books, 1985.

A well-organized and thorough guide to women's health problems from a conventional point of view. Though it provides little in the way of information about alternative or natural healing, it offers information on the various medical tests available and the symptoms of women's diseases. It has great pictures and charts. I must say, however, that I object to the section on cosmetic surgery.

❧ *Everywoman's Medical Handbook* by Dr. Miriam Stoppard. New York: Ballantine Books, 1988.

This is a rather simplistic A-to-Z guide to women's health from a conventional allopathic point of view. The charts and pictures are good, but again, I object to the section on cosmetic surgery.

❧ *Menopause Naturally: Preparing for the Second Half of Life* by Sadja Greenwood, M.D. Volcano, CA: Volcano Press, 1989. Available from Volcano Press, P.O. Box 270, Volcano, CA 95689.

A friendly, supportive book for menopausal women. The chapter on nutrition is especially helpful.

❧ *Natural Medicine for Women* by Julian and Susan Scott. New York: Avon Books, 1991.

This is a good reference that provides information on a number of natural healing modalities, including yoga, homeopathic remedies, herbal medicine, and meditation for various women's health problems.

❧ *The New Our Bodies, Ourselves: Updated and Expanded for the '90s* by the Boston Women's Health Book Collective. New York: Simon & Schuster. 1992.

This is quite possibly the most complete sourcebook available on women's health issues. It is an excellent reference written by and about women. Though it addresses the major issues of women's health primarily from an allopathic point of view, herbs and natural therapies are also included.

❧ *A New View of a Woman's Body* by the Federation of Feminist Women's Health Centers. New York: Simon & Schuster, 1981.

This book is worth having just for the pictures. There are great illustrations of the reproductive anatomy of women's bodies and photographs of clitorises and vulvas that are very instructive. This book contains good information on self-examinations, birth-control methods, and the various health problems of women.

❦ *WomanCare: A Gynecological Guide to Your Body* by Lynda Madaras and Jane Patterson. New York: Avon Books, 1984.

This book is well organized, complete, and easy to understand. While it includes no alternative choices or natural therapies, it does contain much medical data. It identifies the symptoms of various women's health problems and carefully explains the different medical treatments available.

BOOKS ON GENERAL HEALTH

There are many excellent books available these days on natural health. The following are my favorites.

❦ *The Art of Good Living* by Svevo Brooks. Boston: Houghton Mifflin Co., 1986.

This beautiful, simple classic is a practical and poetic guide to good living. Providing "simple steps to regaining health and the joy of life," this book inspires the reader.

❦ *Food and Healing* by Annemarie Colbin. New York: Ballantine Books, 1986.

This is one of my favorite books on the relationship between food and healing. It enables one to make intelligent, conscious choices about the way we eat and how it will affect our well-being.

❦ *Natural Health, Natural Medicine* by Andrew Weil, M.D. New York: Houghton Mifflin, 1990.

Andrew's book is a wonderful source of information on various health problems. His advice, drawn from his personal experience as a doctor, is sound, intelligent, and sometimes refreshingly controversial. Considered by some to be the "finest book on natural medicine."

❦ *Staying Healthy with the Seasons* by Elson Haas, M.D. Millbrae, CA: Celestial Arts, 1981.

This lovely book presents healing and health in relationship to the four seasons. It addresses food, herbs, and preventive and curative therapies in a very simple and holistic manner.

Herb Resource Guide

Herb stores are springing up around the country and many natural food stores now offer a large selection of herbs. Whenever possible, buy your herbs locally. If, however, you are unable to get good-quality herbs close to home, the following sources offer excellent quality herbs and/or herbal products. They are all small mail-order companies owned by herbalists.

❦ **Avena Botanicals, Box 365, West Rockport, ME 04865**
This is a source of exceptional quality products. Avena herbalist, Deb Soule, grows the herbs used in her products in her lovely herb gardens and/or wildcrafts them herself. She has a special line of products for animals as well as one for women.

❦ **Dry Creek Herb Farm, 13935 Dry Creek Road, Auburn, CA 95603**
Shatoiya Jones, herbalist and organic gardener, has developed a line of excellent natural cosmetics using herbs from her garden. She supplies these and other fine home-made herbal products through the mail.

❦ **Gaia Herbs, 62 Old Littleton Road, Harvard, MA 01451**
This company provides high-quality fresh plant herb extracts and tinctures to many stores throughout the country. You can also mail-order directly from Gaia Herbs.

❦ **Green Terrestrial, P.O. Box 41, Route 9W, Milton, NY 12547**
Wise Woman herbalist Pam Montgomery wildcrafts and/or grows her own plants and makes a wonderful line of medicinal herbal products.

❦ **Herbalist and Alchemist, P.O. Box 458, Bloomsbury, NJ 08804**
As well as an excellent selection of organic and wildcrafted herbal tinctures, Herbalist & Alchemist also offers exceptional-quality Chinese herbs and herbal products.

❦ **The Herb Closet, 104 Main Street, Montpelier, VT 05602**
This small, collectively owned and operated herb business offers over 400 bulk botanicals as well as an extensive line of tinctures, salves, capsules, and herb books.

❦ **The Herb Wyfe, 17 West Main Street, Wickford, RI 02852**
This small shop offers a fine selection of herbs, oils, containers, and other materials needed for making your own herb products.

❦ **Island Herbs, c/o Ryan Drum, Waldron Island, WA 98297**
Ryan wildcrafts all his own herbs and is highly respected for the exceptional quality of the plants he supplies. The seaweeds he harvests are superb.

❦ **Jean's Greens, RR 1, Box 57, Medusa, NY 12120**
This small company has a wonderful selection of fresh dried organic and wildcrafted herbs, as well as oils, containers, beeswax, and other materials needed for making herbal products. The owner, Jean Argus, also has a line of her own teas: "Ease Dis-Ease Teas."

❦ **Jeanne Rose's Herbal Products, 219 Carl Street, San Francisco, CA 94117**
Well-known herbalist and author Jeanne Rose makes a wonderful line of natural cosmetics and herbal products.

❦ **Mountain Rose, P.O. Box 2000, Redway, CA 95560**

A small herb company nestled in the coastal mountains of northern California, Mountain Rose supplies bulk herbs, beeswax, books, oils, containers, and, also, a complete line of my formulas.

❦ **New England Botanicals, P.O. Box 6, Shelburne Falls, MA 01370**

Wise Woman herbalist Gail Ulrich offers an excellent line of herbal tinctures and medicinal products that she makes herself.

❦ **Sage Mountain Herb Products, P.O. Box 420, East Barre, VT 05649**

This is a small, family-run business that provides exceptional quality tinctures and other herbal products. All products are formulated by me, Rosemary Gladstar, and are made of organically grown and/or wildcrafted herbs.

❦ **Simpler's Botanicals, P.O. Box 39, Forestville, CA 95436**

This small business located on the grounds of the California School of Herbal Studies offers a line of exceptional handcrafted herbal and aromatherapy products made by experienced herbalists.

❦ **Traditional Medicinal Herb Tea Company, Sebastopol, CA 95472**

Though certainly no longer a small company, Traditional Medicinals continues to offer an excellent line of formulas (the original blends having been formulated by me, Rosemary Gladstar). These teas are excellent for the woman who does not care to mix or blend her own formulas. Traditional Medicinal products are available in most natural food and herb stores across the country. Several pharmacies and supermarkets nationwide also carry them. The formulas especially created for women include: Female Toner, Mother's Milk, PMS Formula, Pregnancy Tea, and Women's Liberty.

❦ **Trinity Herbs, P.O. Box 199, Bodega, CA 94992**

Trinity is a small wholesale herb company that sells quality bulk herbs in quantities of one pound or more.

❦ **Wild Weeds, P.O. Box 88, Redway, CA 95560**

A small herbal emporium, this mail-order business was initially started to supply correspondence-course students with the herbs and herbal materials they needed. It's a wonderful resource for bulk herbs, herbal products, containers, and many of the items needed to make your own herbal products.

APPENDIX III

Herbal Newsletters and Educational Resources

Newsletters

❦ *The American Herb Association Newsletter,* P.O. Box 1673, Nevada City, CA 95959
❦ *The Business of Herbs,* North Winds Farm, Route 2, Box 246, Shevlin, MN 56676
❦ *Foster's Botanical and Herb Reviews,* P.O. Box 106, Eureka Springs, AR 72632
❦ *HerbalGram,* P.O. Box 201660, Austin, TX 78720
❦ *The Herb Companion,* 201 East Fourth Street, Loveland, CO 80537
❦ *The Herb Quarterly,* P.O. Box 548, Boiling Springs, PA 17007
❦ *Medical Herbalism,* P.O. Box 33080, Portland, OR 97233
❦ *The Northeast Herb Association,* P.O. Box 146, Marshfield, VT 05658
❦ *Planetary Formula Newsletter,* c/o Roy Upton, P.O. Box 533, Soquel, CA 95073
❦ *The Wild Foods Forum,* 4 Carlisle Way, N.E., Atlanta, GA 30308

Educational Resources

❦ American Herb Association (AHA), P.O. Box 1673, Nevada City, CA 95959
❦ American Herbalist Guild (AHG), P.O. Box 1127, Forestville, CA 95436
  These two organizations both publish directories of the classes, seminars, and correspondence courses offered in the United States. There is a small fee for their directories.
❦ *Edible and Medicinal Herbs* by Dr. Sharol Tilgner, Wise Woman Herbals, P.O. Box 328, Gladstone, OR 97027
  A very informative video on identifying wild and edible plants. It's a good beginners' guide.
❦ *Edible Wild Plants* by Jim Meuninck and Dr. Jim Duke, Media Methods, 24097 North Shore Drive, Edwardsburg, MI 49112
  A lively, entertaining field guide to wild plants by two well-known experts. Jim also produces a variety of other herbal videos.
❦ *The Garden Speaks* by Raylene Veltri, Earth Alive Videos, P.O. Box 336, San Geronimo, CA 94963

This is a lovely journey into the heart of the plants. Raylene leads us gently and poetically through her garden, introducing us to the plants and their healing and edible uses. I wouldn't classify this as an identification video so much as an experience with the plants.

❧ *Herbal Preparations and Natural Therapies* by Debra Nuzzi, Morningstar Publications, 997 Dixon Road, Boulder, CO 80302

This professionally produced video is the next best thing to attending classes. In four comprehensive hours Debra skillfully teaches the art of making herbal preparations.

❧ *Northeast Herbal Association,* P.O. Box 146, Marshfield, VT 05658-0146

This organization publishes a newsletter and directory of herbalists and herbal activities in the eastern part of the United States.

❧ *The Science and Art of Herbalism: A Home Study Course* by Rosemary Gladstar, P.O. Box 420, East Barre, VT 05649

Written in an inspiring and joyful manner, *The Science and Art of Herbalism* is designed for students wishing a systematic, in-depth study of herbs. It contains a degree of knowledge and a lively student-teacher interaction not found in most home study courses. The course emphasizes the foundations of herbalism: wildcrafting, earth awareness, and herbal preparation and formulation. Though it instills in the student the skills necessary to practice herbal home health care, it doesn't ignore the rich spirit and essence of herbs. The heart of the course is the development of a deep personal relationship with the plant world.

❧ *The Seeker Press,* P.O. Box 299, Battle Ground, IN 57920

This small company specializes in herbal videos. Some of the topics are unusual and wonderful.

❧ *Women to Women,* One Pleasant Street, Yarmouth, ME 04096

Dr. Christiane Northrup of *Women to Women,* a women's health center, has produced some excellent audio cassettes for women. Included in the series are such cassettes as *Endometriosis, Menopause,* and *PMS and Co-dependency.* Dr. Northrup is an excellent lecturer and presents a very holistic medical approach to women's problems.

Abortion References

Because it is so difficult to get information on alternative methods of abortion, I wish to include the titles of three very sensitive and sensible booklets on the subject.

❧ *Abortion: A Personal Approach* by Joy Gardner. 1985. Healing Yourself Press, R.R. 1, Winlaw, BC V0G 2J0, Canada.

This sensitive, compassionate book is written by a woman who has assisted many women and couples through such difficult times, using her skills as a counselor and healer.

❧ *Self-Ritual for Invoking Release of Spirit Life in the Womb* by Deborah Maia. 1989. Mother Spirit Publishing, P.O. Box 893, Great Barrington, MA 01230.

A very inspiring and deeply moving account of one woman's experience in using her inner wisdom and power as guidance through this difficult process.

❧ *A Woman's Book of Choices: Abortion, Menstrual Extraction, Ru-486* by Rebecca Chalker and Carol Downer. 1992. New York: Four Walls Eight Windows.

Available by writing to Four Walls Eight Windows, P.O. Box 548, Village Station, New York 10014.

Your Personal Health Profile

If you are not ready to alter your way of life, you cannot be healed.
—Hippocrates

One of the main purposes of this book is to help you gain control of your own health. There are times when the guidance of a professional health practitioner (preferably one who is holistically minded) is definitely needed and should be sought. This is especially true whenever there is a question as to the severity of the situation. But for many health problems, we can, with simple remedies and dietary changes, develop health programs that will correct the imbalances. Working with the guidance of a professional health practitioner, we can also design our own programs and be in control of our health even while receiving more mainstream medical treatment. I have included the following information to serve as a guideline for planning health strategies.

Allow yourself plenty of time to fill this health form out. Answer each question as honestly and completely as possible. When you have finished, put it down for a couple of days before you begin designing a personal program for yourself.

NAME

DATE OF BIRTH

ADDRESS

OCCUPATION

PRESENT HEALTH STATUS

Check each column where symptoms apply and elaborate in the space provided below if necessary. Please indicate with a (✓) any symptoms that you sometimes experience; use two checks (✓✓) to indicate those that occur often; use three checks (✓✓✓) for those that are a major concern.

Cardiovascular

_____ High blood pressure

_____ Low blood pressure

_____ Pain in heart

_____ Poor circulation

_____ Swelling in ankles

_____ Previous stroke or heart murmur

Muscles/Joints

_____ Backache/upper or lower

_____ Broken bones

_____ Mobility restriction

_____ Arthritis/bursitis

Eyes, Ears, Nose, and Throat

_____ Asthma

_____ Earaches

_____ Eye pains, dry/wet

_____ Failing vision

_____ Hay fever

_____ Sinus infection

_____ Sinus congestion

_____ Sore throat

_____ Tonsils

_____ Hearing loss

Urinary/Kidney

_____ Excessive urination

_____ Water retention

_____ Burning urine

_____ Kidney stones

_____ Lower back pain

_____ Dark circles under eyes

_____ Itchy ears/eyes

_____ Emotional insecurity

Skin

_____ Boils

_____ Bruises

_____ Dryness

_____ Itching

_____ Varicose veins

_____ Skin eruptions

Respiratory

_____ Chest pain

_____ Difficulty breathing

_____ Cough

_____ Tuberculosis

_____ Congestion

Gastrointestinal

_____ Belching

_____ Colitis

_____ Constipation

_____ Abdominal pain

_____ Liver problems

_____ Gallstones

_____ Ulcers

_____ Indigestion

Please add any comments on any of the symptoms checked above that you feel will give a more complete overview of your present state of health. _____ _____

Specific Health Facts

___ Do you have allergies? To what? _____

___ Are you allergic to any medications? Which ones? _____

___ Are you allergic to any foods? Which ones? _____

___ Do you take any regular medications, either prescribed or over-the-counter? Please list. _____

___ Do you take regular vitamin, mineral, or herbal supplements? Please list.
_____

___ Have you had any operations? What and when? _____
_____

___ Have you had any major injuries/accidents? What and when? _____
_____

___ Have you had any major illness or hospitalizations? What and when? _____
_____

Specific Women's Problems
Please check any of the following problems that you are currently experiencing.

General

___ Fibroid

___ Uterine cysts

___ Endometriosis

___ Cervical dysplasia

___ Pelvic pain (When and for

how long?)

___ Painful intercourse

___ Swelling of hands, feet, ankles

___ Vaginal infection (What type and

for how long?)

___ Breast pain (When in cycle?)

___ Breast lump (Does it change with

cycle?)

___ Vaginal itching, discharge

(For how long?)

___ Difficulty in conceiving

___ General fatigue, exhaustion

___ Anemia

___ Headaches (Migraines?)

___ Pelvic inflammatory disease

___ Infertility

___ Genital herpes

___ Shortness of breath

___ Anemia

Menstruating Women

___ Irregular menstrual cycles

___ Heavy menstrual bleeding

___ Bleeding between menstrual cycles

___ Painful menstrual cramps

(What degree of severity?)

___ Absence of menstrual cycle

(For how long?)

___ Dramatic mood swings around

menstrual cycle

Menopause

___ Hot flashes

___ Dramatic mood swings

___ Dry vaginal lining

___ Osteoporosis

___ Break-through bleeding

___ ERT therapy

Common Physical Activities

YOUR
PERSONAL
HEALTH
PROFILE
•
275

___ Sitting at a desk (How long each day?)

___ Sitting in a car (How long each day?)

___ Jogging/running

___ Calisthenics

___ Aerobics

___ Swimming

___ Weight lifting

___ Walking

___ Other _____

___ Standing (How long each day?)

___ Yoga

___ Tai chi

___ Hiking

___ Bike riding

___ Horseback riding

___ Tennis

___ Bending/lifting

___ Do any of the conditions above aggravate a current health condition? _____

_____

___ Please describe your program of physical fitness. _____

_____

Please check each item listed below if it is included in your daily or usual diet.

____ Red meat

____ Fish

____ Poultry

____ Fruits

____ Vegetables

____ Raw foods

____ Grains

____ Nuts

____ Seeds

____ Fermented foods

____ Butter

____ Milk

____ Cheese

____ Yogurt

____ Sugar

____ Honey

____ Baked goods

____ Desserts

____ Coffee

____ Black tea

____ Herbal tea

____ Alcohol

____ Vitamins

____ Protein supplements

____ Food supplements

____ Cigarettes

Elaborate on your dietary habits.

What do you like about them and what

would you like to change?   _____

_____

_____

Do you now follow or have you ever

followed a restricted diet? Please describe

and indicate when.   _____

_____

_____

_____

_____

Past Health Problems

List all major health problems you've had in the past five years.

Problem   Year

_____

Contraceptive History

List the kind(s) of contraceptives you have used, if any, and for how long.

Birth control pills _____

IUD _____

Diaphragm _____

Condoms_____

Rhythm _____

Mucous method _____

Astrological _____

Chemical spermicides _____

Pregnancy History

List each pregnancy you have had, including miscarriages and abortions.

Pregnancy/Date   Miscarriage/Date   Abortion/Date

_____

_____

_____

Family History

Circle any significant family health history: diabetes, cancer, disease, mental illness, asthma, tuberculosis, gout, epilepsy, thyroid problems, obesity.

Other _____

Current State of Emotions and Feelings

Please take a moment to answer the following questions:

Are you able to express your feelings and emotions? _____

Is there an excess of stress in your life? _____

What is causing the stress? _____

Are you satisfied with your job? _____

If you are in a relationship, are you satisfied with it? _____

Are you lonely? _____

If there is one thing in your life you would like to change right now, what is it? Can you change it? _____

Are you a "nervous type" person? What are the things that make you most nervous?

_____

Have you a "Super Woman" complex? _____

Do you sleep well? _____

Do you dream? Do you remember your dreams? _____

Are you satisfied with your general energy level? _____

Do you often feel exhausted and fatigued? _____

Is it easy to wake up in the morning? _____

Which of these feelings predominate in your life: joy, happiness, anger, sadness, fear, sympathy, worry, depression? _____

If you were to choose one or two emotions that seem dominant in your life they would be _____ and _____ .

Please indicate the approximate dates and describe the nature of any traumatic experiences you have had in the past seven years (divorce, loss of lover, loss of job, change of residence, injury, death, etc.) _____

Year   Event

_____

_____

_____

_____

Designing a Personalized Health Program

There are several factors to take into account before designing your program:

❧ Look over the above form and get an overview of the major areas of concern. Note the *number one* area of physical concern. Note your current emotional status. Sum these up for yourself. Note any outstanding features that stand out on this form. When filling out this kind of health form and focusing on our personal health problems, it can often seem as if everything is falling apart. The secret is to look for the *key* problems. If I am having problems with my liver, I can develop digestive disturbances, menstrual imbalances, extreme feelings of anger, PMS, heavy bloated feelings, etc. If, rather than treating all the symptoms individually, I treat my liver with a well-planned health program, the other symptoms will gradually disappear.

❧ It is often helpful to write a personal health summary after filling out a health form. (See the letter written by Marie Ann below. It's a very good example of a personal health summary.)

❧ Do not design a program that will be impossible for you to follow. Keep your life-style in mind and be realistic about your level of commitment. It is far better to design a moderate health plan that you can realistically follow than to design a lavish one that is doomed to failure.

❧ Prepare your medicines so that you can readily take them. You have many choices, as you've seen throughout this book. If it is easier for you to take capsules rather than tea, then plan accordingly.

❧ It is always best to have the guidance of a holistically minded practitioner to work with and/or to review your health program with.

❧ Be consistent with your program. Six to eight weeks is a reasonable time to test out a program designed to treat a mild chronic health problem. If, after that time, you don't notice a significant change, it may be necessary to make adjustments to it. Adjust your diet, formulas, exercise program, etc., as necessary. Even the best-designed program needs to be altered periodically to respond to the progress you are making. In addition to adjusting it to reflect your progress, you may want to adjust it for the seasons, the climate, and the weather.

❧ A well-designed holistic health program takes the emotional and spiritual aspects of a person, as well as their physical condition, into account. In fact, these factors may be the most important considerations in healing. There are many forms of therapy to help women through emotional and physical crises. Don't neglect counseling, guidance, dream work, massage therapy, relaxation techniques, gardening, and other forms of therapy that may help to heal your inner being.

❧ When planning your herbal strategy, it is important to include one or two tea formulas. These teas should be formulated to taste good, since you will be taking them for several weeks, but they should also be specific to the problem. A general dosage of tea for a chronic health problem is three to four cups daily. Also, include one or two tinctures. The tinctures can be formulated to be specific and strong, since the flavor of the formula is not so important. A general tincture dosage for a chronic problem is one-half teaspoon three times daily. Capsules may also be included. A general capsule dosage for a chronic problem is two capsules three times daily.

Your Own Health Program

Your Key Physical Areas of Concern

_____

_____

_____

Your Key Emotional Areas of Concern

_____

_____

_____

Your Dietary Program
What foods to include: _____
_____
_____

What foods to eliminate: _____
_____
_____

Your Exercise Program
Daily_____ How much time _____
_____

Weekly_____ How much time _____
_____

Your Herbal Supplements

Formula	What form	How much	How often
1. Tea Formula			
2. Tincture Formula			
3. Capsule Formula			

Your Vitamin/Mineral Supplements

Formula	What form	How much	How often

Your Additional Supportive Therapies
(Sitz baths, massage, counseling, etc.)

1. _____
2. _____
3. _____
4. _____

Your Goals:

_____
_____

Weekly reports

Week 1. _____
Week 2. _____
Week 3. _____
Week 4. _____
Week 5. _____
Week 6. _____

At the Completion of Your Program

Did you follow the program? _____
What was the easiest part for you to follow? _____
What was the most difficult part for you to follow? _____
Did you meet your expectations? _____
Were you satisfied with the results? _____

A Sample Health Program

The Earth is a patient healer. One of her most important teachings is to be patient.

—Wabun Wind

A woman wrote to me who had been suffering from menstrual problems for several years. We met briefly and I felt that herbs would definitely complement the program she was already pursuing. After we exchanged the following letters, we met again to individualize and customize her program further. I'm including these letters because I feel they represent a good overview of a woman accepting responsibility for her own health and her willingness to utilize several different health modalities in her healing process.

Dear Rosemary,

About seven years ago I started having extremely difficult periods. They weren't especially heavy, but I had intense pain, chills, sweats, and nausea for several hours, usually on the first day. I finally was given a prescription for anaprox which worked wonders. I took one or two pills a month for several years. Around that same time, my gynecologist discovered a polyp on my cervix and I had it surgically removed, along with a D&C (under anaesthesia). The doctor thought this might alleviate the cramps, but it didn't. So I relied on the anaprox until about three years ago, when I started having very heavy bleeding. I went to a person for shiatsu and dietary treatment, resumed a more or less macrobiotic diet (which I had followed strictly for a year some time before, around 1980) and took Chinese herbs in the form of teas that I brewed. The combination seemed to be good, because I stopped having the intense pain and sweats, etc. and have gotten by ever since with just aspirin (ibuprofin) and no anaprox in several years. However, the bleeding remained heavy.

So I went to a gynecologist last spring. She thought my uterus seemed large and suggested ultrasound, as she suspected fibroids. The ultrasound showed one large (tennis-ball-size) fibroid at the top of the uterus, protruding upwards from the uterine wall. She and I both agreed it was not dangerous; the bleeding was heavy but manageable and I should just keep watch to make sure it didn't grow much more. I went back after three to four months, and things seemed about the same.

That was in June. In August and October I had clotting again (like I haven't had in a year or so) that brought on really heavy bleeding. I was glad I was at home both times, as it would have been a real mess to be out somewhere. This got me a little alarmed and feeling as though I had to stay close to home on my menstrual days. I must say, though, that all three times I've had the heavy clotting and bleeding things have been unusually stressful—a grueling project at work, my father being close to death, and distressed, middle-of-the-night phone calls from an exboyfriend. I mention this because I feel there's a definite emotional component to the condition.

I have a new and very wonderful relationship now (since September) and feel that this will be beneficial. However, my new manfriend is a real meat-and-potatoes type and makes me apple pie and French toast and venison stew to show his devotion! I realize all this can be worked on, but I hate to have serious dietary restrictions. I'm quite thin (105 pounds, 5'3") as it is, and I never feel very nourished on macrobiotic fare (although I like it). I'm also not an enthusiastic cook and think of eating out as a primary source of fun and an opportunity to be social with friends, etc. Philosophically, I don't agree with too much dietary emphasis, although I always go for whole foods, low sugar or no sugar, and natural ingredients whenever I have a choice.

Herbs make great sense to me and I feel that this is a health care route that my system will respond to. I do welcome additional dietary recommendations and am conscious of following them as much as possible. I guess the rigidity of a full year of strict macrobiotics was a bit too much, I react a little against food taboos!

I went to a nutritionist in Los Angeles whom other people in our company see when we're there on business. I liked her very much, and she recommended a vitamin regimen based on a long consultation and the results of blood tests I'd had taken earlier. As a consequence, I've been taking a couple of multivitamins, C, bioflavonoids, black current seed oil, Mega-Co-Q enzyme, Iron, A, E, zinc, and wheat germ oil. She's just recently suggested adding B_6 and betacarotene. She also recommended pau d'arco tea which I've only recently begun drinking—2 times a day.

As you can see, it's a bit much! But I manage to take them all without too much trouble. I keep it up because I seem to have more energy and a stronger immune system. I feel better, even though the menstrual symptoms have not improved noticeably.

A Few Days Later

Went to the gynecologist who found the fibroid to be about the same size. She did an endometria biopsy, the results of which I'll have sometime next week. However, neither she nor I expect to find any abnormalities. She doesn't seem keen on doing anything invasive yet, but gave me literature on D&Cs and a procedure that injects dye into the uterus to look for cysts, polyps, etc. (in case it's something other than the fibroid causing the bleeding).

I also have some midcycle spotting (not unusual in women my age, I'm told) and a clear, waterlike discharge about a week or a few days before menstruation (which no one seems to have any clue about). It's strange, because it happens every month, several times over the course of a couple days, with no apparent explanation.

Another annoying symptom I've had for about a year is itching around the outside of the anus. Again, the doctor can find no apparent cause. I'm constipated—or I should say, have some difficulty with bowel movements—a good bit of the time, so this may be the sole reason for the itching, but I'm not sure. I've tried a couple of different oils and creams externally a *few times, but without much effect. Fortunately, it's not too bad—I just wonder what it's about.*

Regarding exercise, I walk two to three miles several days a week and play tennis once or twice a week—so I feel in good physical condition. I'm active with the community, especially theater and singing, and perhaps have pushed too hard in recent years. I mange the editorial department of a publishing company and the job can be rather stressful.

I've followed a meditation practice for years—nothing fancy, but very nourishing. I find I'm in an "off" phase with this practice in recent months, preferring to rest or get my home organized—feeling much more domestic than spiritual! I'm sure it would be good for me to use the visualization and meditation tools that are available to me, but it's not coming as naturally as I might have expected. I've also been in love for three months and rather distracted (but very happy!). I'd really like to be healthy in every way and hope that some herbal assistance might be of real benefit.

Thank you for reading this long epistle. I very much appreciate any thought or suggestions you have.

With all good wishes,

Marie Ann

Dear Marie Ann,

What a joy to get to know you via the mail, though I might add, I'm sorry about the circumstances that compel you to write. Your letter fairly bubbles with enthusiasm, energy, and inner resources—all excellent assets for personal healing. Perhaps being in love has something to do with it! In any case, you are off to a good start. Your vitamin program, physical level of activity, and awareness levels will all be helpful in trying to correct the imbalances that harbor in your reproductive area.

It sounds like the problem is a fairly long-standing one and could quite possibly, as you suggest, stem from old pain or blockages in the reproductive area. You might, as you hinted, use some of your meditation skills to focus in on your pelvic area and bring warmth to that area. Get the energy flowing and moving through there. It's always a nice exercise to take your hands and warm them by rubbing them vigorously together, then placing them over your pelvic in a gentle, firm, healing manner. Imagine that your womb is the center of the universe and wholesome. A nice time to do this is right before bedtime and upon rising.

The herbal suggestions I am making for you are all quite common and have been recommended to many other women in similar situations. If you have a need to feel closer, more connected to the herbs, then I suggest reading about them in David Hoffman's book, *The Holistic Herbal;* Michael Tierra's book, *The Way of Herbs;* and/or Barbara and Peter Theiss's book, *The Family Herbal.* I would suggest that you make a fairly strong commitment to the herbal program for three months. The program I suggest may seem time-consuming and something of a bother at first. But after you're followed it for a week or two, you'll find it becomes quite easy, and the general improvement (in energy and overall good feeling) you'll notice will make it even easier to keep on track. Once you begin the program, it's important to continue. If you feel that you may lack the commitment to follow it closely for three months, I'd suggest thinking hard about whether to begin at all. Herbs work, but they work best in a slow, natural way. They need us to work with them.

What I would suggest is a fairly rigorous program for three months: taking herbs and vitamins, keeping a watchful eye on your diet (not necessarily being restrictive, but eating soundly and wisely), and doing castor oil packs over your pelvic region several times a week. You will know within three months' time if this program is benefiting you. Your menstrual cycles should show a marked improvement, with bleeding becoming less severe. Generally, there is a feeling of overall vitality and zest, as the first chakra area regulates physical "juice" and vitality. [Chakras are energy centers in the body. They correspond to the endocrine system in western physiology.] If you have questions along the way, don't hesitate to call.

❦ Continue following the vitamin suggestions recommended to you. I'm glad to see you are taking black current seed oil. It is higher in GLA and less expensive than evening primrose oil. Though the initial investment seems high, I recommend buying all your herbs and vitamins in large quantities. This will not only save you money, but reduce the risk of your running out of something and discontinuing part of your program.

❦ Diet is important. But diet need not be restrictive in your case. Rather than looking at excluding lots of things, I would look at including certain items and setting simple dietary guidelines that you are willing to adhere to, such as cutting back on sugars (both natural and otherwise); cutting back on coffee and other high-caffeine substances, including chocolate; and cutting back on dairy foods and red meat. (These are all estrogenic foods and you want to cut back on foods that are estrogenic in nature.) Emphasize such foods as dark green leafy vegetables, miso, protein-rich legumes, grains, chicken, fish, and fruits. Basically, eat for wellness, health, and vitality. Right now you are wishing to heal yourself. Without creating a sense of denial, create a diet that you know makes you feel good. Need anything more be said?

Here are some other suggestions for your wellness program:

❦ Castor oil packs over the pelvic region three times weekly. These are messy, but they come highly recommended and have been very effective for many women. They were made famous through the works of Edgar Cayce. [See page 156 for instructions.]

❦ Sitz baths. This is another old fashioned but highly effective treatment. Once you get past the initial shock of it, it starts to feel great. The pelvic area begins to fairly glow. A sitz bath will take about one half hour but is neither messy nor complicated. [See page 113 for instructions.] This treatment gets the blood flushing into the pelvis and helps heal any blockages. It will not create a heavier menstrual cycle.

❦ To help regulate and control heavy bleeding, eat seaweed throughout the month. Really, try it! Get dulse, hizike, kelp, arame, etc., and eat some every day in soups and salads. Heavy bleeding is often due to thyroid imbalance, and seaweed helps regulate, nourish, and feed the thyroid better than anything else. Are you one of those people who can't stand seaweeds? Then take kelp tablets, though it is a rather expensive way to eat this food (rather like eating broccoli in capsules). But in any event, please do try to eat lots of seaweed during the week. What I do each day is make a cup of miso soup and add lots of seaweed to it. I also toast kelp in a heavy cast-iron skillet. Both kelp and dusle are excellent when prepared this way.

❦ One week before your menstrual cycle is to begin, take a tincture of shepherd's purse and yarrow in combination. Take one-half teaspoon three times daily. When your cycle begins, take the tincture as often as needed; this can be up to one-fourth teaspoon every half hour if needed. Continue until bleeding decreases.

❦ Dong quai is suggested as a daily tonic for women's health and health problems. It can be taken in capsule form, tincture, or by nibbling on the root. Do not take it during menstruation; it may stimulate bleeding. Take it throughout the month and discontinue it as soon as you start bleeding, then start again when the bleeding stops.

❦ I also like to recommend a good-tasting medicinal tea to drink with your herbal program. It is warming, healing to make, and reminds one of the traditions we are following—how rooted they are in our psyches and beings. Medicinal teas also help us to cut back on consumption of less healthy drinks. The following tea is what I would suggest for you. Remember, it should taste good to you! So if you need to adjust the flavors a bit, please do so.

3 parts wild yam	2 parts sassafras
1 part licorice	1 part sarsaparilla
2 parts vitex	2 parts cinnamon
3 parts dandelion root	1 part pau d'arco
1 part ginger	

These suggestions, along with your vitamin program, will make for a fairly intensive program. You may find it more sensible to cut back on a few things, selecting those that seem the most sensible, the most feasible, and the most resonant with you. I definitely recommend the tinctures, seaweed, sitz baths, and tea. I would also suggest that you continue to take the black current seed oil. I am not a big fan of vitamins, though I recognize their value, and I think that at this time they may be helpful to you. At a later date, you may choose instead to take Floradix, an excellent natural vitamin/mineral formula in liquid form made by Bioforce. I definitely recommend it during menstruation if you feel tired and listless from heavy bleeding. I've used it myself with excellent results. It even tastes good!!

In good medicine,

Rosemary

APPENDIX VI

Quick Reference to Formulas

QUICK
REFERENCE
TO
FORMULAS
•
287

Index